"The hallmark of our evolutionary flourishing is coll book is a stunning example of its power. Editors K taken two of the most influential therapies of our t mitment therapy and positive psychology—and ha both clarifies and deepens the discoveries that have each. By establishing seven foundations of well-being that are both scientifically based and practically oriented, they enable a coherent and fascinating look at the role of mindfulness and an array of potent, cutting-edge therapeutic strategies. This fresh synthesis is destined to be a landmark in the literature of emotional healing and spiritual transformation."

—Tara Brach, PhD, author of *Radical Acceptance* and *True Refuge*

"This is a 'greatest hits' collection of essays in practical, positive psychology. Organized by the editors' groundbreaking framework of the seven foundations of well-being, this book is a superb combination of solid theory, research, and evidence-based practice. Immediately useful to any psychotherapist, mindfulness teacher, or business coach."

—Rick Hanson, PhD, author of *Buddha's Brain*

"Unifying two important fields—positive psychology and acceptance and commitment therapy—Kashdan and Ciarrochi's volume contains multiple gems of contributions from the preeminent figures in psychology. Whether you are an expert or a novice, a student or a mental health professional, you will learn a great deal from this book."

—Sonja Lyubomirsky, professor of psychology at the University of California, Riverside, and author of *The How of Happiness* and *The Myths of Happiness.*

"To every innovator working to create new tools and technologies for increased well-being: *Mindfulness, Acceptance, and Positive Psychology* should immediately go to the top of your must-read list. The new research and provocative ideas in this collection will undoubtedly spark countless fresh ideas and help shape, for the better, the next wave of life-changing, positive interventions. This book will give an invaluable edge to designers and developers who want to ground their creative work in leading-edge scientific research."

—Jane McGonigal, PhD, author of the *New York Times* bestseller *Reality Is Broken*

THE
MINDFULNESS & ACCEPTANCE
PRACTICA SERIES

As mindfulness and acceptance-based therapies gain momentum in the field of mental health, it is increasingly important for professionals to understand the full range of their applications. To keep up with the growing demand for authoritative resources on these treatments, *The Mindfulness and Acceptance Practica Series* was created. These edited books cover a range of evidence-based treatments, such as acceptance and commitment therapy (ACT), cognitive behavioral therapy (CBT), compassion-focused therapy (CFT), dialectical behavioral therapy (DBT), and mindfulness-based stress reduction (MBSR) therapy. Incorporating new research in the field of psychology, these books are powerful tools for mental health clinicians, researchers, advanced students, and anyone interested in the growth of mindfulness and acceptance strategies.

Visit www.newharbinger.com for
more books in this series.

mindfulness, acceptance, AND positive psychology

the seven foundations of well-being

EDITED BY
TODD B. KASHDAN, PhD
AND
JOSEPH CIARROCHI, PhD

CONTEXT PRESS
An Imprint of New Harbinger Publications, Inc.

Publisher's Note

Distributed in Canada by Raincoast Books

Copyright © 2013 by Todd B. Kashdan & Joseph V. Ciarrochi
        Context Press
        An Imprint of New Harbinger Publications, Inc.
        5674 Shattuck Avenue
        Oakland, CA 94609
        www.newharbinger.com

Cover design by Amy Shoup; Text design by Tracy Marie Carlson; Acquired by Catharine Meyers

Library of Congress Cataloging in Publication Data

Mindfulness, acceptance, and positive psychology : the seven foundations of well-being / edited by Todd B. Kashdan, Joseph Ciarrochi.
    p. cm. -- (The context press mindfulness and acceptance practica series)
    Summary: "Edited by two leading mental health professionals, Mindfulness, Acceptance, and Positive Psychology is the first book to successfully integrate key elements of acceptance and commitment therapy (ACT) and positive psychology to promote healthy functioning in clients. By gaining an understanding of "the seven foundations of well-being," professionals will walk away with concrete, modernized strategies to use in clinical or private practice. A must-have read for any mental health professional interested in synthesizing ACT and positive psychology to help clients realize their full human potential"-- Provided by publisher.
  Includes bibliographical references and index.
  ISBN 978-1-60882-337-6 (pbk.) -- ISBN 978-1-60882-338-3 (pdf e-book) -- ISBN 978-1-60882-339-0 (epub) 1. Positive psychology. 2. Acceptance and commitment therapy. 3. Well-being. I. Kashdan, Todd. II. Ciarrochi, Joseph.
  BF204.6.M56 2013
  150.19'88--dc23
                     2012040516

Printed in the United States of America

15   14   13
10 9 8 7 6 5 4 3 2 1   First printing

For the six ladies that created, guided, or nourished my lust for life: Roxanne, Selma, Sarah, Raven, Chloe, and Violet

—T.B.K.

To Ann Bailey, for her unwavering love and support

—J.C.

Contents

Alphabetical List of Contributors

Dermot Barnes-Holmes, *National University of Ireland, Maynooth*

Yvonne Barnes-Holmes, *National University of Ireland, Maynooth*

Robert Biswas-Diener, *Portland State University, Positive Acorn*

Sarah Cassidy, *Smithsfield Clinic, Co. Meath, Ireland*

Joseph Ciarrochi, *University of Wollongong, Australia*

Mairéad Foody, *National University of Ireland, Maynooth*

Barbara L. Fredrickson, *University of North Carolina at Chapel Hill*

Eric L. Garland, *Florida State University*

Russ Harris, *Private Practice, Melbourne, Australia*

Laura Harty, *George Mason University*

Steven C. Hayes, *University of Nevada*

Todd B. Kashdan, *George Mason University*

Nadezhda Lyubchik, *Portland State University*

Elizabeth Malouf, *George Mason University*

Lance M. McCracken, PhD, *Health Psychology Section, Psychology Department, Institute of Psychiatry, King's College London*

Mindfulness & Acceptance for Positive Psychology

Louise McHugh, *University College Dublin*

Leslie Merriman, *Colorado State University*

Kristin Neff, *University of Texas at Austin*

Acacia C. Parks, *Hiram College*

Bryan Roche, *National University of Ireland, Maynooth*

Karen Schaefer, *George Mason University*

Kelly Sheline, *Colorado State University*

Michael F. Steger, *Colorado State University, North-West University, South Africa*

Ian Stewart, *National University of Ireland, Galway*

June P. Tangney, *George Mason University*

Dennis Tirch, *Weill-Cornell Medical College, American Institute for Cognitive Therapy*

Robyn D. Walser, *National Center for PTSD and TL Consultation Services; California*

Kerstin Youman, *George Mason University*

CHAPTER 1

The Foundations of Flourishing

Joseph Ciarrochi

University of Wollongong, Australia

Todd B. Kashdan

George Mason University, USA

Russ Harris

Private Practice, Melbourne, Australia

Are humans innately good and compassionate (Rousseau, 1783/1979) or are they nasty and brutish (Hobbes, 1651/2009). This question has troubled philosophers for centuries, and when we look at the history of humankind, there is no simple answer. You can find great acts of love and kindness in our past, but also intense hatred and cruelty. We had the renaissance, but we also had the dark ages. We invented penicillin but we also invented nerve gas. We built churches, cathedrals, and hospitals, but we also built atom bombs and concentration camps. For every historical figure who has struggled for equality and compassion (Martin Luther King), we can find one who has fought equally hard for discrimination and cruelty (Adolf Hitler). Humans are capable of anything.

So the question should not be about the basic nature of humanity. Rather, the key question is, "Can we create a world where the best side of humanity finds expression?" Positive psychology and Acceptance and Commitment Therapy (ACT) share a common answer: Yes.

Both perspectives focus on human strengths and aim to promote human flourishing. They often have overlapping technologies, particularly in the area of goal setting, psychological strengths, mindfulness, and the clarification of what matters most (values and meaning in life). They both seek to make positive change at multiple levels, from individuals to relationships to organizations and cultures. They both have experienced an explosion of research in the last 15 years. And they both appeal to a wide range of people, including those working in clinical, social, educational, and business disciplines.

Yet despite these similarities, ACT and positive psychology have hardly referenced each other. In this book, we propose that these two areas are related and unification will lead to faster, more profound and enduring improvements to the human condition. The chapters in this book will illustrate how this integration can take place, with a focus on concrete ways to empower and change what practitioners do.

What Is Acceptance and Commitment Therapy?

Acceptance and Commitment Therapy (ACT) is a unique and creative approach to behavior change that alters the very ground rules of most Western psychotherapy. It is a mindfulness-based, values-oriented behavioral therapy that has many parallels to Buddhism, yet is not religious in any way. It is a modern scientific approach, a contextual behavioral therapy that is firmly based on the principles of applied behavioral analysis, and there are now over 60 randomized controlled trials to support its effectiveness.

ACT gets its name from one of its core messages: accept what is out of your personal control, and commit to action that improves and enriches your life. The aim of ACT is, quite simply, to maximize human potential for a rich, full, and meaningful life. ACT (which is pronounced as the word "act," not as the initials A.C.T.) does this by a) teaching you mindfulness skills to deal with your painful thoughts and feelings effectively—in such a way that they have much less impact and influence over you; and b) helping you to clarify your core values and use that knowledge to guide, inspire, and motivate committed action.

Mindfulness is a "hot topic" in Western psychology right now—increasingly recognized as a powerful intervention for everything from work stress to depression, to increasing emotional intelligence, to enhancing performance. Mindfulness basically means paying attention with openness, curiosity, and flexibility. In a state of mindfulness, difficult thoughts and feelings have much less impact and influence over behavior—so mindfulness is likely to be useful for everything from full-blown psychiatric illness to enhancing athletic or business performance.

ACT breaks mindfulness skills down into 3 categories:

1. defusion: distancing from, and letting go of, unhelpful thoughts, beliefs, and memories

2. acceptance: making room for painful feelings, urges, and sensations, and allowing them to come and go without a struggle

3. contact with the present moment: engaging fully with your here-and-now experience, with an attitude of openness and curiosity

In many models of coaching and therapy, mindfulness is taught primarily via meditation. However, in ACT, meditation is seen as only one way among hundreds of ways to learn these skills—and this is a good thing because most people are not willing to meditate! ACT gives you a vast range of tools to learn mindfulness skills—many of which require only a few minutes to master. In ACT, mindfulness serves two main purposes: to overcome psychological barriers that get in the way of acting on your core values and to help you engage fully in the experience when you are acting on your values.

Thus the outcome ACT aims for is mindful, values-guided action. In technical terms, this is known as "psychological flexibility," an ability that ACT sees as the very foundation of a rich, full, and meaningful life.

What Is Positive Psychology?

Instead of being viewed as a movement or a paradigm shift, positive psychology is best viewed as a mobilization of attention and financial resources to previously ignored topics (Duckworth, Steen, & Seligman, 2005). For decades, psychology has emphasized the reduction of distress and disorder. While this emphasis has led to efficacious treatments for a variety of psychological problems, the primary reasons for living have been ignored. Nobody lives to be merely free of distress and disorder, and the positive is not merely the absence of distress and disorder. There are other ingredients to a life well lived, and these ingredients have been the focus of positive psychology research and practice.

When first introduced to the world, Seligman and Csiksentmihalyi (2000) mapped out the terrain covered by positive psychology. The field of positive psychology at the subjective level is about valued experiences: well-being, contentment, and satisfaction (in the past); hope and optimism (for the future); and flow and happiness (in the present). At the personal level, it is about positive individual traits: the capacity for love and vocation, courage, interpersonal competence, perseverance, forgiveness, originality, future mindedness, spirituality, and wisdom. At the group level, it is about the civic virtues and institutions that move individuals toward better citizenship: responsibility, nurturance, altruism, civility, tolerance, and work ethic.

The working assumption of positive psychology is that the positive, healthy aspects of life are not simply the bipolar opposite of distress and disorder. This theme arises again in a special issue of the *Review of General Psychology* dedicated to positive psychology, where the editors claim that psychology has been effective at learning "how to bring people up from negative eight to zero, but not as good at understanding how people rise from zero to positive eight" (Gable & Haidt, 2005, p. 103). That is, the primary aim is to address and cultivate positive experiences, strengths and virtues, and the requirements for positive relationships and institutions.

In this description, positive psychology seems to push too far to the other extreme, focusing only on the positive, with a caveat that of course, pain and suffering are important as well. It is only in the last few years that researchers have advocated for the need to move beyond the superficial connection between the "positive" and "negative" dimensions of the human psyche (Sheldon, Kashdan, & Steger, 2011b). For instance, if you are attempting to teach children to be compassionate, you simply cannot ignore the negative, because it is built into the fiber of empathy, and perspective taking. Prominent positive psychologists often discourage a focus on weaknesses (because this is less efficient and profitable); (Buckingham & Clifton, 2001) and reinforce the notion that when it comes to positive experiences, strengths, or virtues, "more is better" (Peterson & Seligman, 2004). This idea has recently been overturned as extremist because evidence continues to emerge that depending on the context, there are tipping points and boundary conditions for the effective use of strengths (e.g., Biswas-Diener, Kashdan, & Minhas, 2011; Linley, 2008). Thus, the working assumptions of positive psychology continue to evolve, which we view as a sign of healthy progress.

In the current incarnation of positive psychology, the focus appears to be less on targets that are "positive" at the superficial, surface level and more on whatever elements lead to healthy living or well-being. In some cases, positive emotions and psychological strengths lead to suboptimal living, whereas emotions such as anxiety and guilt, and behaviors reflecting narcissism and quarrelsomeness, lead to the best possible outcomes. This more dynamic, nuanced approach to a well-lived life has much in common with the working assumptions of ACT.

A Bridge between Two Islands

Both ACT and positive psychology have experienced an explosion of research in the last decade. For example, the term "positive psychology" appeared as a keyword in only seven scientific articles in 2000. This number has exploded to over 100 per year since 2008. ACT has experienced a similar expansion, with "Acceptance and Commitment Therapy" appearing as a keyword less than 10 times a year before 2004, and then exploding to over 40 in 2009 and 2010 and then to 80 in 2011 (Scorpos search, April 5, 2011). Almost all of the over 58 randomized controlled trials in ACT have been published since 2008. Searching on the keywords "positive psychology" and "Acceptance and Commitment Therapy" is likely to vastly underestimate the influence of these fields, as it ignores many relevant keywords, such as "mindfulness," "acceptance," "strengths," and "upward spiral." Still, the numbers clearly indicate that positive psychology and ACT are growing and thriving as research disciplines.

The time has thus come to unify these exciting fields. They have the same goal, to promote human flourishing, but because they have worked independently from each other, they have come up with largely non-overlapping insights and approaches. They have both made great strides, and yet, we can't help but wonder what would happen if people from the two fields actually sat down and spoke to each other. Would this not accelerate progress? This book asks that question in every chapter, and in every case it returns a clear answer: Yes.

If we are going to sit down and talk, the first thing we need to do is develop a common language. Without that language, we will be confused with each other and grow frustrated. Indeed, this confusion is widespread in psychology. Every subdiscipline seems to create its own island of words and constructs. Positive psychology talks about the presence of a nearly universal list of 24 character strengths, ACT focuses on six core processes, personality researchers focus on the big five personality dimensions, and emotional intelligence researchers focus on the five (+-2) components. Each new researcher that comes upon the scene seems keen to create a new brand or at least a few new psychological terms that can be uniquely associated with him or her. Meanwhile, people on the front lines, such as therapists, coaches, and consultants, are drowning in a sea of jargon.

We propose there is a way to survive the flood and even navigate it effectively. Our solution is to identify a small set of basic factors (or foundations) from which we can build a wide range of larger psychological constructs, in much the same way that we can build complex physical compounds from simple primary elements (e.g., we can manufacture steel from iron and carbon). But how do we select these psychological foundations when there are so many options to choose from?

We decided to select a set of basic ingredients that can be arranged and rearranged into almost any strand of well-being. We selected our foundations on the basis of two key criteria: (1) they must be guided by the best available science, and (2) they must be of direct practical use for facilitating cognitive and behavioral change to improve well-being. Thus, we did not select brain regions or neuronal pathways as foundations, because although knowledge of these things is relevant to well-being, it does not provide a practitioner with direct ways of instigating positive behavioral change. Similarly, we did not select elements that are associated with well-being if the implications for intervention were unclear; a good example is the personality dimension of "extraversion."

At this point, let's note that although some positive psychology practitioners describe happiness as being synonymous with "well-being," the truth is that "happiness" is only a single strand of a multidimensional matrix (Kashdan, Biswas-Diener, & King, 2008). Beyond happiness, we can also consider meaning and purpose in life, love and connectedness, a sense of autonomy, a sense of competence, and optimal cognitive and physical functioning. This broadly defined view of well-being also includes anxiety and depression and other constructs that are frequently targeted by cognitive-behavioral interventions. Thus, our list of foundations had to be relevant to healthy functioning as well as to the amelioration of deficits or problems.

The foundations are presented in Table 1. They are assumed to mediate the relationship between specific interventions (e.g., mindfulness practice) and aspects of well-being (increased positive affect and meaning). Like psychological building blocks, one can rearrange any number of the seven foundations into increasingly complex dimensions. Similarly, one can deconstruct more complex dimensions into these seven foundations, and this can provide insight into the types of interventions that might be most useful separately or in unique combinations.

Table 1: The Seven Foundations of Well-Being

Foundations	Examples	Example interventions
1) Functional beliefs about the self, others, and the world	Do you believe you can overcome barriers and achieve goals (hope)? Do you view problems as a challenge or threat (problem-solving orientation)? Do you believe you have social worth (self-esteem)?	• Defusion: Undermining the power of unhelpful thoughts. (e.g., experiencing thoughts as passing events that don't have to dictate action) • Cognitive restructuring of beliefs

Foundations	Examples	Example interventions
2) Mindfulness and awareness	Are you aware of your emotions, actions, external stimuli, and mental processes? Can you label and clarify the exact mixture of emotions that you are feeling at a given point in time?	• Mindfulness practice directed at various domains • Improving emotion recognition and discrimination
3) Perspective taking	Can you take the perspective of others (empathy)? Can you take perspective on yourself (self-as-context)?	• Videotaped experiments to learn discrepancies between self-views, the views of others, and actual performance • Practice shifting perspectives and taking the view of an observer
4) Values	What do you care about (values, personal strivings)? Do other people's desires for you dominate your own (controlled versus autonomous motives)?	• Values clarification • Identifying personal strivings and motives behind them • Identifying implicit motives

5) Experiential acceptance	In order to live according to what you care about, are you willing to have private experiences such as distress and self-doubt (courage)?	• Creative hopelessness (connecting with unworkability of control) • Willingness practice (practice acting in valued way and opening up to feelings)
6) Behavioral control	Are you able to control what you say and do in a way that promotes your goals and values (self-regulation, willpower)? Do you persist (grit) and rebound from failure (resilience)? Are you able to modify feelings in an adaptive way?	• Linking behaviors to values • Goal setting, anticipating and planning for barriers, anticipating benefits from achieving goals • Music, biofeedback, distraction, and other strategies that change emotions and help regulate behavior
7) Cognitive skill	How well do you solve problems and reason (IQ)? How well do you shift attention and inhibit irrelevant stimuli (flexible mindset)?	• Improving intellectual functioning • Attentional training (e.g., practice controlling or altering attention)

Functional Beliefs

Functional beliefs are central to various forms of cognitive-behavioral therapy (Barlow, 2002; Beck, 1983; Ciarrochi & Bailey, 2008). For example, Beck's therapy focuses on core and intermediate beliefs (Beck, 1995), Young's therapy focuses on schema (Young, 1990), and Wells's therapy focuses on meta-beliefs about emotions and worry (Wells, 1997). ACT does not focus on specific beliefs but rather encourages the practitioner to a) identify when beliefs are dominating over other sources of information (other thoughts, the environment) and when beliefs are "unworkable" (i.e., acting on the belief does *not* work to make life rich, full, and meaningful)(Ciarrochi & Robb, 2005). ACT undermines the power of beliefs through the use of defusion (changing the context so that a person can experience their belief as nothing more or less than a passing thought, which they do not have to act on). Positive psychology seeks not so much to undermine unhelpful beliefs but rather to promote positive, functional beliefs such as hope, self-esteem, and a positive problem-solving orientation (Ciarrochi, Heaven, & Davies, 2007; Sheldon, Kashdan, & Steger, 2011a). However, plenty of models within positive psychology do advocate the active challenging and disputation of dysfunctional beliefs. Chapters 3 and 4 discuss beliefs related to love and self-compassion, and chapters 7, 8, and 10 discuss the issue of how beliefs are best modified.

Mindfulness

Mindfulness, broadly defined, means conscious awareness with an open, receptive attitude, of what is happening in the present moment (Bishop et al., 2004; Williams, 2008). Conscious awareness involves intentionally regulating attention toward what is happening here and now. We can describe a person as "gently observing" what is happening, as opposed to "judging" it. An "open, receptive attitude" reflects the quality of one's attention, characterized by curiosity, and a turning toward one's experience rather than away from it. For example, even when our thoughts and feelings are painful or difficult, in a state of mindfulness we are receptive to and curious about these psychological events instead of trying to avoid or get rid of them (Hayes, Luoma, Bond, Masuda, & Lillis, 2006). In and of itself, awareness of one's environment can be directionless. The quality of curiosity focuses one's attention and motivates a person to explore his or her environment with an appreciation of novelty, challenge, and uncertainty (Silvia & Kashdan, 2009). It is hardly surprising, then, that people who are predisposed to present-moment awareness, or trained to be mindful, show greater openness to experiences that challenge their personal beliefs (Niemiec et al., 2010)

Many practitioners of positive psychology construe mindfulness as a platform that facilitates other healthy skills, making them more likely to be used in a given situation for greater benefit. For instance, mindfulness skills can make it easier to repair negative moods, enhance positive moods, or increase the amount of positive appraisals about the self, world, and future.

In ACT, mindfulness is also used to facilitate other skills for healthy living and to increase the efficacy of those skills. However, in ACT, mindfulness would not be used to try to directly alter one's mood. Rather, mindfulness would be used to facilitate action in line with core values, enhance performance, increase engagement in the task at hand, and appreciate this moment of life, whether it be a moment of joy or of pain. (The reasons that ACT avoids targeting positive mood directly will be made clear in the experiential acceptance discussion below.) Chapter 2 covers this area in detail.

Perspective Taking

Many domains of psychology study perspective taking, and it goes by such labels as "psychological mindedness," "reflective functioning," "empathy," and "theory of mind" (Eisenberg, 2003; Eisenberg, Murphy, & Shepard, 1997). In positive psychology, researchers and practitioners have given minimal attention to perspective taking; they have generally classed it under character strengths as a merger of "personal intelligence" and "perspective" (Peterson & Seligman, 2004). ACT-related interventions and research focus heavily on perspective taking and empathy (Ciarrochi, Hayes, & Bailey, 2012; Hayes, Strosahl, & Wilson, 1999), and in particular on the development of an observer perspective, technically referred to as "self-as-context." This is a perspective from which all experience can be noticed and you are aware of your own flow of experiences but without any investment in or attachment to them. Chapters 5 and 8 cover this area in detail, and chapter 9 offers an approach to manipulate the perspective of both individuals and groups.

Values

We can define values in many ways, but generally we can think of them as verbal descriptions of what people are personally invested in, regard highly, and seek to uphold and defend. Recognizing and endorsing these cherished ideals is quite different from behaving in ways that are congruent with them (e.g., see section on behavioral control). Many researchers view values as central to a person's sense of self; they operate as standards that guide thought and action (Feather, 2002; Hitlin, 2003; Kristiansen & Zanna, 1994; Rohan, 2000; Schwartz & Bilsky, 1987). Positive psychologists discuss values in the form of personal strivings, goal setting, or personal philosophies for what is most important in life (Emmons, 1996; Schwartz & Bilsky, 1990). The distance between valued preferences and actual behavior can be vast, which can be a pivotal point of intervention.

ACT makes use of positive psychology literature but speaks of values in a specific way, as qualities of purposive action that can never be obtained as an object, but can be instantiated from moment to moment (Hayes, Strosahl, & Wilson, 2011). Thus, ACT sees values as desired global qualities of ongoing action (or, in layman's terms, "your heart's deepest desires for how you want to behave as a human being"). This definition is consistent with ACT's focus on behavior.

There is also a substantial literature on meaning and purpose in life that seems closely linked to values. Some researchers have defined purpose as a "central, self-organizing life aim" (McKnight & Kashdan, 2009; Steger, 2009). Others have fleshed out this definition by unifying principles from positive psychology and ACT (Kashdan & McKnight, 2009).

Purpose is central. Purpose is a predominant theme of a person's identity. If we envision a person positioning descriptors of his or her personality on a dartboard, purpose would be near the innermost circle.

Purpose is self-organizing. It provides a framework for systematic behavior patterns in everyday life. Self-organization should be evident in the goals people create, the effort devoted to these goals, and decision making when confronted with competing options of how to allocate finite resources such as time and energy. A purpose motivates a person to dedicate resources in particular directions and toward particular goals and not others. That is, terminal goals and projects are an outgrowth of a purpose.

Purpose cannot be achieved. It is a life aim, one that is regularly being directed to new targets. A purpose provides a foundation that allows a person to be more resilient to obstacles, stress, and strain. Persistence is easier with a life aim that resonates across time and context. It is easier to confront long-lasting, difficult challenges with the knowledge that there is a larger mission in the background. Moving in the direction of a life aim can facilitate other elements of well-being such as life satisfaction, serenity, and mindfulness (Wilson & Murrell, 2004; Wong & Fry, 1998). Chapters 6 and 11 provide a detailed discussion of these issues.

Experiential Acceptance

Experiential acceptance means embracing "private experiences" (e.g., thoughts, emotions, memories—experiences an individual has that no outside observer can directly see) and allowing these experiences to be present without trying to avoid or get rid of them. Willingness, a close ally of acceptance, involves allowing difficult private experiences to be present, in the service of a valued action (Ciarrochi & Bailey, 2008). Experiential avoidance—the ongoing attempt to avoid or get rid of unwanted private experiences—transforms the perfectly normal experience of pain to one of suffering and ineffective action (Ciarrochi, Kashdan, Leeson, Heaven, & Jordan, 2011; Kashdan, Barrios, Forsyth, & Steger, 2006). There are two major reasons for this. First, attempts to control or suppress feelings often result in an increase in those feelings, as when attempting to not feel anxious makes you more anxious. Second, emotions and values are often two sides of the same coin, and therefore to avoid one means to avoid the other. You cannot have loving relationships without risking vulnerability and all the painful thoughts and feelings that inevitably go with it. Positive psychology addresses the experiential avoidance component under the umbrella of mindfulness (Brown & Ryan, 2003) or effective emotion regulation (John & Gross, 2004).

13

ACT places a major emphasis on experiential acceptance but does not see it as a form of emotion regulation. Indeed, ACT seeks to minimize any attempt to directly modify private experience for fear that such attempts may reinforce experiential avoidance (Ciarrochi & Robb, 2005). Thus, ACT practitioners rarely seek to directly increase the frequency or intensity of pleasant thoughts or feelings. Rather, the ACT practitioner focuses on helping people to *be* with *all* their thoughts and feelings—both the pleasant and the painful—while *doing* what is important (i.e., acting on values). Chapters 2, 3, 4, and 10 deal with the issues of avoidance and acceptance.

Behavioral Control

Behavioral control refers to one's ability to regulate behavior in a way that is consistent with one's values. Positive psychology might label this component "perseverance," "self-regulation," or "willpower." Research in this area often focuses on identifying factors that promote goal success, such as mental contrasting (considering benefits and barriers related to goals) (Oettingen, Mayer, Sevincer, et al., 2009), implementation intentions (establishing if-then plans to deal with barriers to goals) (Gollwitzer & Schaal, 1998), and self-concordance of goals (the goals match your inner-most needs) (Koestner, Lekes, Powers, & Chicoine, 2002; Sheldon & Houser-Marko, 2001).

When effort is devoted to valued aims, ACT refers to this as "commitment." Generally, there is a tight link between values, purpose, and commitment, and these dimensions are not always easy to disentangle. Despite the difficulty level, we think it is pragmatic to separate values from commitment to highlight the difference between knowing what you want (values, purpose) and acting on what you want (behavioral control). Chapters 6, 10, and 11 tackle the issues of values, purpose, and commitment.

Cognitive Skill

Cognitive skill refers to components of intellectual functioning such as reasoning, problem solving, and attentional control. Both positive psychology and ACT are somewhat neutral with regard to this factor, except that they both agree it is good to have. Research increasingly suggests that cognitive skill is more modifiable than originally thought (Cassidy, Roche, & Hayes, 2011; Jaeggi, Buschkuehl, Jonides, & Perrig, 2008). This dimension is essential to any complete definition of well-being and indeed directly links to the other foundations. For example, values clarification has been shown to increase cognitive performance among stigmatized groups (Cohen, Gracia, Apfel, & Master, 2006). A certain level of cognitive skill is needed to be able to take perspective (McHugh et al., 2004). Finally, basic cognitive training in inhibition of responses increases behavioral control (Houben & Jansen, 2011). Chapter 12 covers this skill in great detail.

Linking the Seven Foundations to Strengths

Character strengths, often viewed as a centerpiece of positive psychology (Peterson & Seligman, 2004; Seligman, 2011) can be understood as a mixture of the foundations in Table 1. Strengths often have an element of valuing (e.g., "love of learning," "capacity for love," "fairness," "honesty," "humility," "spirituality," and "gratitude.") *Capacity for love* probably involves not only valuing loving relationships but also the ability to take perspective and believe you are worthy of love. *Leadership* involves valuing influence and probably requires all seven elements above (e.g., cognitive capacity, experiential acceptance of uncontrollable events, perspective taking). *Self-control* is one of those extremely broad strengths that involves elements of cognitive skill (inhibition), as well as experiential acceptance (e.g., not acting impulsively to get rid of urges), behavioral control, and functional beliefs (belief that you can achieve goals). *Self-compassion* can be seen as a combination of experiential acceptance (recognize that you will beat yourself up sometimes), mindfulness (be aware of this self-criticism), perspective taking (recognizing the similarity of your own suffering to that of others), and values (put self-kindness into play in your life).

Other areas of study in positive psychology can also be understood in terms of the seven foundations. *Spirituality* is a particularly potent yet understudied strength (Heaven, Ciarrochi, & Leeson, 2010; Heaven &

Ciarrochi, 2007). Spirituality generally includes values (connect with god or the universe), beliefs that could be functional or dysfunctional ("God gives me strength" versus "God is trying to punish me for being so shameful"), the observer perspective (a sense of a constant, unchanging self), and frequently, mindfulness (engaging in and appreciating the present moment and all it holds). *Moral emotions* such as shame can be seen, in some contexts, as involving dysfunctional beliefs about the self (I am completely worthless), as well as unhelpful attempts to escape the self (low experiential acceptance). Rather than bombard you with more examples, we invite you to take a few minutes before reading on to think about some other popular psychological constructs and see to what extent you can "deconstruct" them in terms of our seven foundations.

The Importance of Intervention Purpose

To truly integrate positive psychology and ACT, we must first look a little deeper at their purpose and philosophical assumptions. We shall see that as long as positive psychology and ACT adopt similar philosophical assumptions, they can work well together.

At this point, a warning to the reader: we have named the seven foundations as if they are real entities, like animals walking about in the world. However, in reality we view these foundations through a pragmatic philosophy. The foundations help us to organize a rather bewildering array of constructs. We make no assumption that they are real entities lying in the brain waiting to be discovered by some neurosurgeon.

Our pragmatic view stands in contrast to more mechanistic views. As a contrast to our approach, consider the following recent declaration by Seligman (2011):

> Well-being is a construct, and happiness is a thing.
> A "real thing" is a directly measurable entity.... [T]he elements
> of well-being are themselves different kinds of things. (p. 24)

By describing well-being in this way, Seligman implicitly takes a philosophical stance called elemental realism (formerly known as "mechanism") (Ciarrochi & Bailey, 2008; Hayes, Strosahl, & Wilson, 2011).

Elemental realism gets its name because it assumes that one can know the true nature of reality and objectively discover the elements of which it is composed. The elemental realist views the universe as a machine consisting of parts that interact. The goal of analysis is to model the universe accurately.

The key question for the elemental realist is, "What elements and forces make the model work?" Success is defined by how well a model is able to make predictions and establish meaningful, reliable causal patterns. Most forms of cognitive psychology are good examples of elemental realism, as are the information processing models found in positive psychology. There is of course, absolutely nothing wrong, outdated, or inferior with this philosophical stance. Acknowledging one's philosophical worldview simply means owning up to the improvable assumptions upon which one's work rests. Thus one philosophical worldview can never refute another.

The worldview adopted by ACT and some positive psychologists is functional contextualism (a form of pragmatism). Functional contextualism assumes we can never know the true nature of reality or the elements that comprise it; all we can do is observe how an aspect of the universe functions in a given context (and part of that context will always be the human mind itself). Functional contextualism focuses on something called the "act-in-context." "Context" means whatever comes before the act that influences it (antecedents) and whatever follows the act that reduces or increases the chance of its recurring (consequences). The "act" is whatever happens in between the antecedents and the consequences.

The key question in functional contextualism is, "How can we manipulate the antecedents and consequences to best achieve our goals?" The functional contextualist *will* divide an event into "elements" (e.g., antecedents and consequences) but does so purely for pragmatic purposes (i.e., Does the division help us achieve our goals?). The functional contextualist would make no assumption that this "division" uncovers or reveals something of the "true nature" of reality; it is nothing more or less than a useful strategy for achieving a specific goal.

The goal of functional analysis is to find ways to predict and influence behavior. Prediction in itself is not enough. Typical research in this tradition focuses on manipulating antecedents and consequences and observing how behavior changes as a result. A particular activity is "successful" if it helps to achieve stated goals. Applied Behavioral Analysis (ABA) and Acceptance and Commitment Therapy (ACT) are two examples of models based on functional contextualism.

Scientists and practitioners in positive psychology can take either an elemental realism viewpoint or a functional contextualist viewpoint, whereas ACT folks take only a functional contextualist viewpoint. Thus, for collaboration to occur, positive psychologists need to put on their functional contextualist hat. They can always remove it later and take up the perfectly valid elemental realist perspective.

If we all agree to wear the functional contextualist hat, we can begin our conversation across islands. We might start with the question: "What is the purpose of our constructs?" The answer is: they help us to classify and guide interventions. They help us focus the intervention (e.g., on experiential acceptance) and adopt the most appropriate measures that capture how well an intervention works (e.g., Does experiential acceptance improve, and does it lead to greater well-being?). This answer begets another more general question. What is the purpose of our interventions? There are at least two possible answers to this question, and the answer we choose will determine the appearance and function of the intervention:

1. The purpose is to promote psychological states with a predominance of pleasant thoughts and feelings

2. The purpose is to aid in the promotion of psychological flexibility: the capacity to live mindfully and act effectively in line with one's core values (see Kashdan and Rottenberg, 2010, for alternative definitions)

The first purpose directly emphasizes the importance of modifying the form and frequency of private experiences; the second purpose emphasizes changing the nature of one's relationship with private experiences—to one of mindfulness and acceptance—while directly modifying one's actions. ACT typically adopts the latter approach, whereas some positive psychologists typically adopt the former. However, these approaches do not have to be mutually incompatible; in many contexts, they can complement one another.

The way we conduct an intervention will vary enormously depending upon our purpose, intention, or ultimate goal. Consider mindfulness.

You could engage in a mindfulness practice to facilitate acceptance of painful emotions (ACT consistent), or you could engage in it with the purpose of inducing calm, relaxed, pleasant emotional states (Cormier & Cormier, 1998). If you have the former purpose in mind, then you might be anything but relaxed. You might be fully present to feelings of anxiety as you mindfully talk with a potential lover, or you might be fully aware and accepting of your racing heart and sweaty hands as you get up to give an important speech.

And obviously, the way you would frame the mindfulness intervention would also be quite different, depending on the purpose or end goal. If your focus is behavioral, you might frame a mindfulness practice in terms of anchoring in the present moment so that you can be less reactive to your feelings and engage fully in the task at hand, which is essential for peak performance. However, if your focus is on directly changing emotional states, you might describe the mindfulness exercise as an excellent way to relax and unwind after a difficult day. Furthermore, the specific purposes and end goals limit the applications of any given intervention. For example, if mindfulness is used primarily to facilitate acceptance of unpleasant feelings, then it can be used in any sort of fear-provoking situation, from public speaking to charging the enemy on a battlefield, whereas if mindfulness is used as a relaxation technique, then it can only be of use in situations where there is no genuine threat. (No relaxation technique known to humankind will reverse a fight-or-flight response in the face of a challenging stressful situation.)

We have discussed strategies that seek to change the valence of emotional state (e.g., from negative to positive). In addition to valence-change strategies, there are valence-neutral change strategies that are used by both ACT and positive psychology. For example, mindfulness might be used to increase a state of "equanimity" or "concentration." These states are not inherently positive or negative, and both can be used to promote the same purpose, namely, flexible, value-consistent behavior.

Are Strengths Inherently Positive?

Applying the word "strength" to a psychological trait makes it seem inherently positive. Who, after all, would not want more strength, resilience, or optimism? However, within a functional contextualist viewpoint, nothing is inherently good or bad. Rather, we evaluate the benefits of a trait (or pattern of behaving) by answering two questions: 1) What value is the behavior serving? and 2) How is that behavior working in a particular social context? For example, forgiveness has been defined in part as the behavior of giving people a second chance (Park, Peterson, & Seligman, 2004). To assess whether this behavior is useful, we need to first ask: What is "giving a second chance" in the service of? Let's assume that this behavior is intended to increase intimacy in a close relationship. The second question then is, how is it working? In a supportive romantic relationship, forgiveness may work quite well. However, in an abusive relationship, giving the abuser a second, third, and fourth chance may work very poorly.

Indeed, recent research supports this view. McNulty and Fincham (2011) have shown that the "positive" processes of forgiveness, optimistic expectations, positive thoughts, and kindness can be related to higher **or** lower well-being, depending on context. Specifically, in a longitudinal study, these processes predicted better relationship well-being among spouses in healthy marriages but worse relationship well-being in more troubled relationships. In another study, Baker and McNulty (2011) showed that self-compassion may sometimes be helpful or harmful to relationships, at least among men. Men high in self-compassion have better relationships only if they are conscientious and willing to correct interpersonal mistakes and engage in constructive problem solving. In contrast, men high in self-compassion have worse relationships if they are not motivated to correct their mistakes (low conscientiousness).

There has been substantial debate about whether optimistic illusions are good or bad. Some argue that they are fundamental to mental health (Taylor & Brown, 1988), whereas others suggest such illusions can be harmful to relationships (Norem, 2002), workplace effectiveness, academic performance, and physical health and longevity (Dunning, Heath, & Suls, 2004). This debate may be resolved by assuming that illusions are helpful in some contexts, but not in others, and proceeding to study illusions in context. Fredrickson and Losada (2005) recognize this issue when they talk about the importance of "appropriate negativity" and the possibility of having too high a ratio of positive to negative emotions.

The Big Questions

Our goal in this book is to build a more complete and integrative approach to improving the human condition. To facilitate integration, we posed a number of questions to our contributors. We describe them below, and we leave it to you to explore the book with curiosity and search for the answers.

When Is Experiential Control Most Likely to Work? When Will It Fail?

We know experiential avoidance is often a destructive coping strategy. Is there any danger that some positive psychology interventions might unintentionally promote unhelpful avoidance? What are contexts where emotional control might work to improve well-being (e.g., Is seeking pleasant emotional states the same as avoiding unpleasant ones)? When does it fail? Please note, by "emotional control," we mean control of internal states (thoughts, feelings, sensations, urges, images, memories), not control of the actions that occur simultaneously with these states. Humans can control their actions without having to control their internal states; we can feel furious, but act calmly; we can feel anxious, but act assertively.

When Is Cognitive Restructuring Most and Least Likely to Work?

ACT often seeks to minimize direct attempts at cognitive restructuring, in part because it might increase unhelpful language processes (e.g., reasoning about the future/worrying, believing that reasoning can solve everything, excessive dominance of symbols over experience). ACT emphasizes cognitive defusion, techniques that attempt to change one's relationship with thoughts, rather than trying to alter their form or frequency. For example, when we defuse from unhelpful thoughts, we are less likely to believe them or allow them to influence our action. With defusion as an alternative to restructuring, is there anything gained by cognitive restructuring? When is restructuring most likely to work? When is it least likely to work?

Are All Mindfulness Interventions Created Equally?

Does the purpose of the intervention and type of instruction matter? For example, does it make a difference if mindfulness is taught as a way to reduce stress or as a way to increase psychological flexibility?

Do We Need to Improve Self-Concepts?

ACT typically focuses on helping folks to let go of unhelpful self-concepts and spends less time seeking to directly improve self-concept. What are contexts where changing self-concept might be helpful? When might it be harmful? For example, it might be unhelpful to target hope or self-esteem without linking it to concrete behavior. If everybody is special no matter what they do, why do anything?

Values and Committed Action

Is happiness a value or a side effect of valued activity? Should we reinforce the valuing of pleasant emotions (e.g., creating contexts where pleasant emotions are more likely to occur)? Is directing people to pay attention to their pleasant feelings another way of directing them to what they value?

Can We Separate the Positive from the Negative?

To what extent is it possible to study the positive without the negative? Are these separations artificial? Oxygen and hydrogen form water, which has emergent qualities that cannot be inferred from hydrogen and oxygen. Can the same be said about positive and negative emotions? Is it sometimes unhelpful to talk about "positive" and "negative" emotions? Given that fear, sadness, and guilt are useful, life-enhancing emotions that play a major role in building a rich, meaningful life, is it fair to call them "negative"? Would we do better to talk about "pleasant" and "unpleasant" emotions rather than "positive" and "negative"?

Structuring the Book

The range of topics in this book will be as broad as the fields of ACT and positive psychology. To help the reader find order in this chaos, we wanted to list each of the seven foundations that are discussed in subsequent chapters. The check marks in the table below indicate the components given the greatest emphasis. This single visual provides insight into the variety of topics and angles explored by our distinguished authors.

	Chapter 2: Mindfulness Broadens Awareness and Builds Meaning at the Attention-Emotion Interface	Chapter 3: Love and the Human Condition	Chapter 4: Self-Compassion and ACT	Chapter 5: Perspective Taking	Chapter 6: Committed Action
Functional Beliefs	√		√	√	
Mindfulness and Awareness	√	√	√		
Perspective Taking			√	√	
Values		√			√
Experiential Acceptance	√	√	√		
Behavioral Control					√
Cognitive Skill				√	

Chapter 7: Positive Interventions	Chapter 8: On Making People More Positive and Rational	Chapter 9: Microculture as a Contextual Positive Psychology Intervention	Chapter 10: Accepting Guilt and Abandoning Shame	Chapter 11: Using the Science of Meaning to Invigorate Values-Congruent, Purpose-Driven Action	Chapter 12: Nurturing Genius
√	√		√	√	
√	√		√		
√	√	√	√		
√	√	√	√	√	
			√	√	
√		√	√	√	
		√			√

References

[Baker, L., & McNulty, J. (2011). Self-compassion and relationship maintenance: The moderating roles of conscientiousness and gender. *Journal of Personality and Social Psychology, 100,* 853-873.

Barlow, D. H. (2002). *Anxiety and its disorders: The nature and treatment of anxiety and panic* (2nd ed.). New York: Guilford Press.

Beck, A. T. (1983). Cognitive therapy of depression: New perspectives. In P. J. Clayton & J. E. Barrett (Eds.), *Treatment of depression: Old controversies and new approaches.* New York: Raven Press.

Beck, J. S. (1995). *Cognitive therapy: Basics and beyond:* New York: Guilford Press.

Bishop, S. R., Lau, M., Shapiro, S., Anderson, N., Carlson, L., Segal, Z. V., et al. (2004). Mindfulness: A proposed operational definition. *Clinical Psychology: Science and Practice, 11,* 230-241.

Biswas-Diener, R., Kashdan, T. B., & Minhas, G. (2011). A dynamic approach to psychological strength development and intervention. *Journal of Positive Psychology, 6,* 106-118.

Brown, K. W., & Ryan, R. M. (2003). The benefits of being present: Mindfulness and its role in psychological well-being. *Journal of Personality & Social Psychology, 84*(4), 822-848.

Buckingham, M., & Clifton, D. O. (2001). *Now, discover your strengths.* New York: The Free Press.

Cassidy, S., Roche, B., & Hayes, S. C. (2011). A relational frame training intervention to raise intelligence quotients: A pilot study. *Psychological Record, 61,* 173-198.

Ciarrochi, J., & Bailey, A. (2008). *A CBT-Practitioner's guide to ACT: How to bridge the gap between Cognitive Behavioral Therapy and Acceptance and Commitment Therapy.* Oakland, CA: New Harbinger Publications.

Ciarrochi, J., Hayes, L., & Bailey, A. (2012). *Get out of your mind and into your life: Teens.* Oakland, CA: New Harbinger.

Ciarrochi, J., Heaven, P. C., & Davies, F. (2007). The impact of hope, self-esteem, and attributional style on adolescents' school grades and emotional well-being: A longitudinal study. *Journal of Research in Personality, 41,* 1161-1178.

Ciarrochi, J., Kashdan, T. B., Leeson, P., Heaven, P., & Jordan, C. (2011). On being aware and accepting: A one-year longitudinal study into adolescent well-being. *Journal of Adolescence, 34*(4), 695-703.

Ciarrochi, J., & Robb, H. (2005). Letting a little nonverbal air into the room: Insights from acceptance and commitment therapy: Part 2: Applications. *Journal of Rational-Emotive & Cognitive Behavior Therapy, 23*(2), 107-130.

Cohen, G. L., Garcia, J., Apfel, N., & Master, A. (2006). Reducing the racial achievement gap: A social-psychological intervention. *Science, 313,* 1307-1310.

Cormier, L. S., & Cormier, W. H. (1998). *Interviewing strategies for helpers: Fundamental skills and cognitive behavioral interventions* (4th ed.). Pacific Grove, Calif.: Brooks/Cole.

Duckworth, A. L., Steen, T. A., & Seligman, M. E. P. (2005). Positive Psychology in clinical practice. *Annual Review of Clinical Psychology, 1*, 629–651.

Dunning, D., Heath, C., & Suls, M. (2004). Flawed self-assessment: Implications for health, education, and the workplace. *Psychological Science in the Public Interest, 5*, 69-106.

Eisenberg, N. (2003). Prosocial behavior, empathy, and sympathy. In M. H. Bornstein, L. Davidson, C .L. M. Keyes, & K. A. Moore, (Eds.), *Well-being: Positive development across the life course. Crosscurrents in contemporary psychology* (pp. 253-265). Mahwah, NJ: Lawrence Erlbaum.

Eisenberg, N., Murphy, B. C., & Shepard, S. (1997). The development of empathic accuracy. In W. J. Ickes (Ed.), *Empathic accuracy* (pp. 73-116).

Emmons, R. A. (1996). Striving and feeling: Personal goals and subjective well-being. In P. M. Gollwitzer, J. A. Bargh (Eds.), *The psychology of action: Linking cognition and motivation to behavior* (pp. 314-337). New York: Guilford Press.

Feather, N. T. (2002). Values and value dilemmas in relation to judgments concerning outcomes of an industrial conflict. *Personality and Social Psychology Bulletin, 28*, 446-459.

Fredrickson, B., & Losada, M. (2005). Positive affect and the complex dynamics of human flourishing. *American Psychologist, 60*, 678-686.

Gable, S. L., & Haidt, J. (2005). What (and why) is positive psychology. *Review of General Psychology, 9*, 103-110.

Gollwitzer, P. M., & Schaal, B. (1998). Metacognition in action: The importance of implementation intentions. *Personality and Social Psychology Review, 2*, 124-136.

Hayes, S. C., Luoma, J. B., Bond, F. W., Masuda, A., & Lillis, J. (2006). Acceptance and commitment therapy: Model, processes and outcomes. *Behavior Research and Therapy, 44*(1), 1-25.

Hayes, S. C., Strosahl, K., & Wilson, K. G. (1999). *Acceptance and Commitment Therapy: An experiential approach to behavior change.* New York: Guilford Press.

Hayes, S. C., Strosahl, K., & Wilson, K. G. (2011). *Acceptance and Commitment Therapy: The process and practice of mindful change* (2nd ed.). New York: Guilford Press.

Heaven, P., Ciarrochi, J., & Leeson, P. (2010). Parental styles and religious values among teenagers: A 3-year prospective analysis. *Journal of Genetic Psychology, 171*, 93-99.

Heaven, P. C. L., & Ciarrochi, J. (2007). Personality and religious values among adolescents: A three-wave longitudinal analysis. *British Journal of Psychology, 98*, 681-694.

Hitlin, S. (2003). Values as the core of personal identity: Drawing links between two theories of the self. *Social Psychology Quarterly, 66*, 118-137.

Hobbes, T. (1651/2009). *Leviathan, or the matter, forme, and power of a commonwealth, ecclesiasticall and civill.* Yale Uni: Project Guenberg Ebooks.

Houben, K., & Jansen, A. (2011). Training inhibitory control. A recipe for resisting sweet temptations. *Appetite, 56*, 345-349.

Jaeggi, S., Buschkuehl, M., Jonides, J., & Perrig, W. (2008). Improving fluid intelligence with training on working memory. *Proceedings from the National Academy of Sciences, 105,* 6829-6833.

John, O. P., & Gross, J. J. (2004). Healthy and unhealthy emotion regulation: Personality processes, individual differences, and life span development. *Journal of Personality, 72*(6), 1301-1333.

Kashdan, T. B., Barrios, V., Forsyth, J. P., & Steger, M. F. (2006). Experiential avoidance as a generalized psychological vulnerability: Comparisons with coping and emotion regulation strategies. *Behavior Research and Therapy, 44,* 1301-1320.

Kashdan, T. B., Biswas-Diener, & King, L. A. (2008). Reconsidering happiness: The costs of distinguishing between hedonics and eudaimonia. *Journal of Positive Psychology, 3,* 219-233.

Kashdan, T. B., & McKnight, P. E. (2009). Origins of purpose in life: Refining our understanding of a life well lived. *Psychological Topics, 18,* 303-316.

Kashdan, T. B., & Rottenberg, J. (2010). Psychological flexibility as a fundamental aspect of health. *Clinical Psychology Review, 30,* 865-878.

Koestner, R., Lekes, N., Powers, T., & Chicoine, E. (2002). Attaining personal goals: Self-concordance plus implementation intentions equals success. *Journal of Personality & Social Psychology, 83,* 231-244.

Kristiansen, C. M., & Zanna, M. P. (1994). The rhetorical use of values to justify social and intergroup attitudes. *Journal of Social Issues, 50,* 47-65.

Linley, A. (2008). *Average to A+: Realising strengths in yourself and others.* Coventry, UK: CAPP Press.

McHugh, M., McNab, J., Symth, C., Chalmers, J., Siminski, P., & Saunders, P. (2004). *The availability of foster carers: Main report.* Sydney: Social Policy Research Centre, University of New South Wales.

McKnight, P. E., & Kashdan, T. B. (2009). Purpose in life as a system that creates and sustains health and well-being: An integrative, testable theory. *Review of General Psychology, 13,* 241-251.

McNulty, J., & Fincham, F. (2012). Beyond positive psychology? Toward a contextual view of psychological processes and well-being. *American Psychologist, 67*(2), 101-110.

Niemiec, C. P., Brown, K. W., Kashdan, T. B., Cozzolino, P. J., Breen, W., Levesque, C., et al. (2010). Being present in the face of existential threat: the role of trait mindfulness in reducing defensive responses to mortality salience. *Journal of Personality & Social Psychology, 99,* 344-365.

Norem, J. K. (2002). Defensive self-deception and social adaptation among optimists. *Journal of Research in Personality, 36*(6), 549-555.

Oettingen, G., Mayer, D., Sevincer, T., Stephens, E. J., Pak, H.-J., & Hagenah, M. (2009). Mental contrasting and goal commitment: The mediating role of energization. *Personality and Social Psychology Bulletin, 35,* 608-622.

Park, N., Peterson, C., & Seligman, M. (2004). Strengths of character and well-being. *Journal of Social and Clinical Psychology, 23,* 603-619.

Peterson, C., & Seligman, M. E. (2004). *Character strengths and virtues: A handbook and classification*. Oxford: Oxford University Press.

Rohan, J. (2000). A rose by any name? The values construct. *Personality and Social Psychology Bulletin, 4*, 255-277.

Rousseau, J. J. (1783/1979). *Emile, or On Education* (A. Bloom, Trans.). New York: Basic Books.

Schwartz, S. H., & Bilsky, W. (1987). Toward a universal psychological structure of human values. *Journal of Personality and Social Psychology, 53*, 550-562.

Schwartz, S. H., & Bilsky, W. (1990). Toward a theory of the universal content and structure of values: Extensions and cross-cultural replications. *Journal of Personality and Social Psychology, 58*, 878-893.

Seligman, M. (2011). *Flourish: A visionary new understanding of happiness and well-being*. New York: Free Press.

Seligman, M. E., & Csikszentmihalyi, M. (2000). Positive psychology: An introduction. *American Psychologist, 55*(1), 5-14.

Sheldon, K., Kashdan, T. B., & Steger, M. F. (2011a). *Designing positive psychology*. Oxford: Oxford University Press.

Sheldon, K., Kashdan, T. B., & Steger, M. F. (2011b). *Designing positive psychology: Taking stock and moving forward*. New York: Oxford University Press.

Sheldon, K. M., & Houser-Marko, L. (2001). Self-concordance, goal attainment, and the pursuit of happiness: Can there be an upward spiral? *Journal of Personality and Social Psychology, 80*(1), 152-165.

Silvia, P. J., & Kashdan, T. B. (2009). Interesting things and curious people: Exploration and engagement as transient states and enduring strengths. *Social and Personality Psychology Compass, 3*, 785-797.

Steger, M. (2009). Meaning in life. In S. J. Lopez (Ed.), *Oxford handbook of positive psychology*. Oxford, UK: Oxford University Press.

Taylor, S., & Brown, J. (1988). Illusion and well-being: A social psychological perspective on mental health. *Psychological Bulletin, 103*, 193-210.

Wells, A. (1997). *Cognitive therapy of anxiety disorders: A practice manual and conceptual guide*. Hoboken, NJ: Wiley .

Williams, J. M. G. (2008). Mindfulness, depression and modes of mind. *Cognitive Therapy and Research, 32*, 721-733.

Wilson, K., & Murrell, A. (2004). Values work in acceptance and commitment therapy: Setting a course for behavioral treatment. In S. C. Hayes, V. Follette, & M. Linehan (Eds.), *Mindfulness and acceptance: Expanding the cognitive-behavioral tradition*. New York: Guilford Press.

Wong, P., & Fry, P. (1998). *The human quest for meaning: A handbook of psychological research and clinical application*. Mahwah, NJ: Erlbaum.

Young, J. E. (1990). *Cognitive therapy for personality disorders: A schema-focused approach*. Sarasota, FL: Professional Resource Exchange.

CHAPTER 2

Mindfulness Broadens Awareness and Builds Meaning at the Attention-Emotion Interface

Eric L. Garland

Florida State University

Barbara L. Fredrickson

University of North Carolina at Chapel Hill

The purpose of this chapter is to articulate linkages between the broaden-and-build theory of positive emotions (Fredrickson, 1998; Fredrickson, 2004) and key components of "Third Wave" psychotherapies such as mindfulness, acceptance, and commitment to valued action. We will use insights culled from cognitive and affective sciences to clarify a series of testable ideas that have direct bearing on clinical intervention. Although research and theory on Acceptance and Commitment Therapy (or ACT, Hayes, Strosahl, & Wilson, 1999) has blossomed over the past decade, comparatively little attention has been paid to positive psychological processes in the ACT literature. We contend that positive mental states, when harnessed intentionally, are keys to resilience that can propel one in the direction of living a more meaningful life.

We begin our discussion by describing the systemic, emergent, and self-maintaining nature of emotional states. Next, we detail the broaden-and-build theory of positive emotions and the body of empirical research that supports its premises. Then we discuss the interrelationship between emotion, attention, and meaning as the context for discussing three key components of a positive-emotion focused intervention strategy: mindfulness, reappraisal, and savoring. Lastly, we attempt to integrate this clinical approach within the overall framework of ACT.

Emotional Systems Can Spiral Upward or Downward

Contemporary affective science portrays emotions as constellations of subjective feeling states, physiological responses in brain and body, expressions evident on the face and in posture, and repertoires of thought and action. In other words, emotions are emergent, dynamic systems energized by the reciprocal causal links between the cognitive, behavioral, and somatic mechanisms through which emotions are instantiated. Thus, emotions can be seen as self-organizing systems that operate to maximize and maintain their own existence. Take, for example, the emotion of despair. Despair resulting from a loss may be accompanied by rumination and withdrawal behaviors coupled with a sense of fatigue. These constituents of despair may then interact dynamically to produce more despairing feelings, further rumination on loss, and increased withdrawal and fatigue. Despair becomes entrenched by generating emotion-consistent appraisals (i.e., the tendency to interpret new experiences in terms of the potential for loss and lack of control). This interpretational bias produces durable negative beliefs about self and world, which, when coupled with repeated experiences of despair and isolation stemming from withdrawal behaviors, foster narrowing, socially isolating thought-action tendencies. Over time, this process may spiral further downward into a self-destructive cycle, leading to social alienation, the relinquishing of commitments, and acts of desperation that fuel feelings of despair, hopelessness, and burdensomeness that are characteristic of depression.

We refer to such dynamic, self-perpetuating, negative emotional systems as *downward spirals*. In contrast, we refer to self-perpetuating cycles of positive emotions as *upward spirals*, given their associations with improved functioning and enhanced social affiliation. Upward spirals are evident in prospective studies where initial positive emotions predict future positive emotions, in part by increasing broad-minded thinking (Burns et al., 2008; Fredrickson & Joiner, 2002). In turn, having a broadened mindset predicts the occurrence of such a mindset in the future, in part by promoting cognitive coping strategies that increase positive emotions (Garland, Gaylord, & Fredrickson, 2011). When positive emotions expand people's mindsets, these cognitive effects may increase the frequency and intensity of positive emotions as one increasingly focuses attention on pleasurable, beautiful, rewarding, or meaningful events and encounters. By generating a greater awareness of positive experiences and perspectives, positive emotions tend to consolidate over time, leading to more frequent positive emotions in the future.

Upward spirals can be distinguished from downward spirals in the ways they influence behavior. Whereas downward spirals lead to excessive self-focused attention and rigid, stereotyped defensive behavior (i.e., pulling away from what matters most), upward spirals lead to greater openness to others and spontaneous or novel exploratory behaviors (i.e., a push toward what matters most). As such, upward spirals of positive emotion and broadened thought-action repertoires may be linchpins to resilience (Fredrickson, Tugade, Waugh, & Larkin, 2003; Tugade, Fredrickson, & Barrett, 2004), stress reduction (Garland et al., 2011), and the prevention of inertia that is often observed among people with clinical disorders (Garland et al., 2010).

Emotional spirals, like other systems, are preserved by feedback processes that operate to maintain the status quo—they change their structural configurations only as a result of being disturbed from an outside source. This raises the question of whether and how disturbances and difficulties can promote greater durability and healthy functioning (instead of dysfunction). The central thesis of the present chapter is that mindfulness might facilitate access to positive emotions with which a person can disrupt a downward spiral and, in turn, nudge the emotional balance toward sustainable positivity.

The Broaden-and-Build Theory of Positive Emotions

Downward spirals hinge on the capacity of negative emotions to narrow the scope of attention and cognition (Schmitz, De Rosa, & Anderson, 2009; Talarico, LaBar, & Rubin, 2004). Such cognitive narrowing is held to be an evolved adaptation that aided the survival of human ancestors in threatening circumstances (Frijda, 1988) insofar as it supported the quick enactment of bottom-up, habitual, defensive actions (e.g., fight, flight, freeze) that would otherwise be impeded by top-down, reflective thinking. For instance, in the brief time required to dodge the strike of a serpent, one could not engage in creative problem solving without getting a fang in the foot. Conversely, narrowly focused attention onto the head of the snake allows for the deployment of rapid, nonconscious coordinated muscular action to step backward and avoid the strike. Only with narrow, reflexive, mindless movements would a person survive the situation.

The broaden-and-build theory takes a complementary position and asserts that positive emotions broaden individuals' thought-action repertoires, enabling them to draw flexibly on higher-level associations and a wider-than-usual array of sensory information, ideas, and behaviors; in turn, broadened cognition engenders behavioral flexibility. As people become better able to flexibly adopt novel behaviors and familiar behaviors in new contexts, they develop more psychosocial resources such as resilience and affiliative bonds (Cohn, Fredrickson, Brown, Mikels, & Conway, 2009; Fredrickson, Cohn, Coffey, Pek, & Finkel, 2008; Waugh & Fredrickson, 2006). Our notion of broad thought-action repertoires, or flexibility, is similar to the ACT notion of psychological flexibility, which is the ability to contact the present moment and be sensitive to details of the situation (e.g., to contingencies of reinforcement), and the ability to persist in meaningful activity despite the presence of psychological or physical pain (Kashdan & Rottenberg, 2010).

Take, for example, the case of two different third graders in gym class, Edie and Max. When the gym teacher has the class play tee-ball for the first time, Edie meets the new challenge with curiosity. It's her first time playing tee-ball (or anything like it), so she's not very good. When

Edie steps up to bat and takes a swing at the ball on the tee, she misses with a resounding "whiff" of the bat through the air. When her class-mates laugh, instead of being embarrassed, she laughs along with them. Edie takes another swing, and this time, the ball stays in place while the bat flies out of her hand and lands a few feet away. Her peers laugh even harder, and she joins them in sharing the hilarity of the situation. She meets their smiles with her own and feels the glow of positive emotions. Consequently, she's more willing to give it another try. Just before her third swing, Edie notices that she's been holding her right elbow too high. She corrects her stance and smacks the ball down the field. Her peers cheer for her, and after class, they approach her to giggle about the crazy day at tee-ball. Sharing in a few more laughs, they become friends, and later decide to ask their parents to enroll them in an afterschool tee-ball team. In no time, Edie increases her athletic skills and cements lasting friendships that promote positive emotions in the future. Eventually, Edie goes on to play ball in high school and later decides to major in journalism to become a sports reporter. She eventually lands a high profile position on a major sports television network.

Conversely, Max is embarrassed by his inexperience with tee-ball. He tries to avoid the gaze of his gym teacher so he won't be picked to play in the class tee-ball game. When he is called up, he swings and misses, and focuses his attention on the laughing faces of his peers. He interprets their expressions as evidence that they are mocking him, and he feels ashamed and angry. He refuses to take a second swing and sits down disengaged on the sidelines. In so doing, he robs himself of the opportu-nity to experience positive emotions that might otherwise promote his engagement in new behaviors and relationships. He grows up believing "I'm no good at sports" and shuns any social interaction that centers on athletic events, a pattern of experiential avoidance that causes him to lead a circumscribed life well into adulthood.

Insofar as positive emotions broaden cognition and increase engage-ment in behaviors leading to increased social bonds, they conferred an evolutionary advantage to human ancestors, who may have been better equipped to survive by virtue of the development of such adaptive mind-sets, skills, and resources. Positive emotions, although fleeting, can have a long-lasting impact on functional outcomes by expanding people's mindsets in ways that lead to enhanced well-being and social connectedness.

The broaden-and-build theory has been tested in a wide range of observational, experimental, and clinical trial studies. The proposition that positive emotions broaden cognition has been demonstrated in experiments where putting people into positive emotional states leads to a more expansive ability to attend to what is happening as the present moment unfolds; discoveries, have been found using research methods as diverse as behavioral measures (Fredrickson & Branigan, 2005; Rowe, Hirsh, & Anderson, 2007), eye-tracking (Wadlinger & Isaacowitz, 2008), and brain imaging (Schmitz et al., 2009; Soto et al., 2009). Moreover, inducing positive emotions expands the range of behaviors in which one may be likely to engage (Fredrickson & Branigan, 2005) and facilitates creative problem solving (Isen, 1987; Rowe et al., 2007). Interpersonally, being in a positive emotional state increases trust in others (Dunn & Schweitzer, 2005) and the sense of connection between individuals (Aron, Norman, Aron, McKenna, & Heyman, 2000; Waugh & Fredrickson, 2006). Hence, positive emotions broaden cognition into upward spirals that have consequential impacts on the ability to successfully create healthy social interactions and relationships.

A number of prospective, observational studies provide evidence consistent with the proposition that positive emotions build durable personal resources (Cohn & Fredrickson, 2009; Cohn et al., 2009; Gable, Gonzaga, & Strachman, 2006; Stein, Folkman, Trabasso, & Richards, 1997). More conclusive evidence for the "build" hypothesis comes from a randomized controlled trial of loving-kindness meditation (LKM) (Fredrickson et al., 2008), an intervention selected to increase daily experience of positive emotions. This longitudinal study demonstrated that, relative to a waitlist control group, those randomly assigned to the 7-week LKM intervention over time reported increases in positive emotions. Over the course of the study, participants trained to induce positive emotions through LKM exhibited a 300% increase in the relationship between time spent in meditation and the resultant positive emotions. That is, the longer participants engaged in LKM practice, the more intense their experiences of positive emotions. These positive emotions appeared to be durable in that they persisted on days that participants did not meditate. In turn, the upward shifts in positive emotions induced by LKM produced increases in a wide range of personal resources, including having a sense of competence for handling life challenges, feeling meaningfully connected to other people, and having better resistance to illness (stronger immunological functioning)—gains that led to downstream increases in life satisfaction coupled with reductions in depressive symptoms (Fredrickson et al., 2008). These salutary effects of learning LKM persisted at one-year follow-up, providing evidence for enduring changes in trait positive affect (Cohn & Fredrickson, 2010).

These two propositions of the broaden-and-build theory—that positive emotions broaden awareness and build resources—may be further understood by examining the frequency of various emotions in everyday life. Fredrickson and Losada (2005) suggest that the affective quality of a person's life can be represented by his or her positivity ratio, defined as the ratio of positive to negative emotions experienced over time. Positivity ratios characteristic of optimal human functioning will surpass 1-to-1, given the operation of lawful asymmetries between positive and negative emotions: (a) *positivity offset* refers to the observation that the modal human experience is mild positive affect (Cacioppo, Gardner, & Berntson, 1999), and indeed, normal functioning has been characterized by positivity ratios of about 2-to-1 (Schwartz et al., 2002); (b) *negativity bias*, often summed up as "bad is stronger than good" (Baumeister, Bratslavsky, Finkenauer, & Vohs, 2001), implies that to correct for the sheer potency of negative emotions, positive emotions would need to outnumber them. Consistent with these well-documented asymmetries, Fredrickson and Losada identified 3-to-1 as the tipping point ratio, above which the broaden-and-build effects of positive emotions generate well-being. People who experience a proportion of positive to negative emotions in excess of 3-to-1 exhibit exemplary mental health and psychosocial function, a salutary state known as flourishing (Keyes, 2002). Below this ratio, people are thought to experience positive emotions in rates too low to support such optimal functioning and may instead show emotional distress, social alienation, or the lack of fulfillment that Keyes (2002) calls languishing.

A third proposition of the broaden-and-build theory asserts that positive emotions undo the psychophysiological consequences of negative emotions. Whereas negative emotions prepare the body and mind for specific defensive actions (e.g., fight, flight), positive emotions appear to dismantle or "undo" such preparation, an effect presumably linked to the broadened thought-action repertoires that accompany positive emotions. In a series of laboratory experiments, Fredrickson and colleagues tested the "undo effect" by first inducing negative emotions in participants who were then randomly assigned to one of three conditions in which they experienced subsequent positive, neutral, or negative emotions. Continuous measures of heart rate and blood pressure responding revealed that positive emotions sped cardiovascular recovery from anxiety and fear (Fredrickson & Levenson, 1998; Fredrickson, Mancuso, Branigan, & Tugade, 2000). This line of research indicates that positive emotions can be a potent means of counteracting the effects of negative emotional states.

If positive emotions exert consequential effects on well-being, it follows that they would facilitate resilience (Folkman & Moskowitz, 2000) (i.e., the ability to successfully adapt and cope with adversity). This higher incidence of positive emotions accounts for the greater ability of resilient people to rebound from adversity, undo cardiovascular reactivity, prevent the occurrence of depressive symptoms, and continue to flourish (Fredrickson et al., 2003; Ong, Bergeman, Bisconti, & Wallace, 2006; Tugade & Fredrickson, 2004). Further, biobehavioral research indicates that resilient people, who are better able to maintain their focus on the present moment and worry less about future negative contingencies than their less resilient counterparts, exhibit more situationally appropriate physiological activation in response to an emotional provocation, from which they are then able to efficiently recover (Waugh, Wager, Fredrickson, Noll, & Taylor, 2008). However, resilience is not merely innate; it can be trained (Cicchetti & Blender, 2006). For instance, a laboratory experiment showed that when healthy adults scoring low on measures of trait resilience are taught to positively reappraise a stressful situation as a challenge to be met and overcome, they exhibit the faster cardiovascular recovery that is a hallmark of resilience (Tugade & Fredrickson, 2004). In this study, the extent to which resilient people could find positive meaning in challenging life events was partially mediated by their experience of positive emotion in the face of those circumstances. In other words, people appear to spontaneously use positive emotions to find meaning within stressful situations. How then might positive emotions be intentionally cultivated to foster resilience in clinical populations? To answer this question, we must delve into the nature of attention, emotion, and meaning itself.

Meaning and the Attention-Emotion Interface

Human beings are meaning makers. Although at the core we experience the same primordial drives toward approach and avoidance as do all invertebrates and the same basic emotional states of joy, contentment, love, disgust, anger, and fear as our mammalian ancestors (Ekman, 1971, 1977; Plutchik, 1962, 1980), our capacity for *appraising* and *constructing* the meaning of our experiences creates a multifarious and ever-shifting palette of moods and affect. In other words, we *derive* our decidedly human emotional experience from these basic emotions through the processes of cognitive appraisal (Ellsworth & Scherer, 2002; Lazarus, 1991, 1999). We must look no further than the example of pleasure. For although pleasure is a primal and universal human experience (Kringelbach & Berridge, 2009), sources of pleasure vary to a near infinite extent. That people could experience pleasure from experiences as diverse as sky diving, fasting and kneeling on hard wooden pews, eating a Big Mac, sadomasochistic sex acts, the discovery of a new mathematical theorem, pulling weeds and pruning in a garden, a death metal concert, or focusing attention on the sensation of the breath is indicative of the relativistic nature of meaning making and its emotional consequences. Moreover, an event or behavior that is pleasurable in one context may be perceived as aversive in another. For instance, sprinting from a ravenous tiger bears a different hedonic tone than sprinting toward a finish line, even though both events involve the behavior of running as fast as possible.

What then governs how meaning and emotion are generated in the encounter between self and world? Although our everyday human experience can potentially access an infinitely complex universe, an individual can process only a limited set of data as information at any one moment. Thus human information processing is selective and involves attention, that is, the function by which certain subsets of data gain preeminence in the competitive processing of neural networks at the expense of other subsets of data (Desimone & Duncan, 1995). Thus, attended stimuli govern behavior, insofar as they receive preferential information processing. Attention can be driven by reflexive, stimulus-driven, bottom-up processes, or by reflective, strategic, top-down processes (Corbetta & Shulman, 2002). While basic stimulus properties such as brightness or contrast attract attention in a bottom-up fashion, the salience, goal-relevance, or higher-order meaning of the object can guide attention to select and distinguish it from the environmental matrix in which it is embedded (Koivisto & Revonsuo, 2007).

As William James asserted in an oft-cited quote, "My experience is what I agree to attend to" (1890). Yet, despite its centrality, attention exists in a reciprocal relationship with emotion. The object of attention elicits emotion, while emotion tunes and directs attention (Anderson, Siegel, Bliss-Moreau, & Barrett, 2011; Friedman & Forster, 2011; Lang & Bradley, 2011; Lang, Bradley, & Cuthbert, 1997). This attention-emotion interface is the psychological substratum that makes motivated goal achievement possible. Thus, the human mind is not merely a passive receptor of sensory information that reacts in an input-output fashion but, rather, an active agent that *selects* information and *appraises* this information for its contextual meaning or value. Emotion arises from these selection and appraisal processes. Bateson (1972) asserted that ordinary awareness often fails to capture the rich, interconnected complexity of the environment because our desires and goals limit our attention to small portions of data. Depending on how people attend to the components of their experience, different phenomenological realities are constructed. Consistent with this view, appraisal accounts of emotions (Ellsworth & Scherer, 2002; Lazarus, 1991) hold that the emotional quality of any given circumstance springs from what we attend to and how we subsequently interpret the objects of attention.

People interpret the meaning of the objects of attention by ascribing to them conceptual categories according to their memories of past experiences. The way we organize and categorize the influx of information from our senses creates our lived experience of "reality" (Keeney, 1983). Thus, there is no inherent meaning in these details of experience outside of the contexts in which they are observed. This observation reveals that the ubiquitous concepts—like "self," "world," and "causality"—derived from sense data and social feedback are in fact malleable and subject to contextual change.

The manner in which individuals ascribe meaning to an emotional stimulus relative to its context has been described by Relational Frame Theory (Hayes & Wilson, 1995), the foundation of ACT. According to this theory, humans use language and cognition to arbitrarily relate events to one another and to alter the functions of events based on their contexts (Hayes, Luoma, Bond, Masuda, & Lillis, 2006). Language and cognition encode these arbitrary relations between events. As such, behavioral responses derive not from events themselves but rather from the network of arbitrary relational rules established via a history of conditioning and reinforcement. By virtue of such *relational framing*, we make sense of events and appraise their emotional significance.

The drive to make sense or meaning of one's experiences is central to human existence (Frankl, 1959; Singer, 2004). Moreover, the need to make sense of experience and to regulate emotion in desired directions motivates changes in belief (Boden & Berenbaum, 2010). In turn, changes in emotion arise from the specific meaning appraisals made in a situation (Frijda, 1986). Appraisals are discrete and pertain to specific events; in contrast, beliefs often extend over time and scope, and therefore have the potential to influence many discrete situational appraisals (Boden & Berenbaum, 2010; Lazarus, 1991). For instance, for an individual who holds the belief "I must be perfect," receiving an A+ on a test will result in the appraisal "I am perfect" and consequent feelings of contentment, whereas receiving an A- results in the appraisal "I am a failure" coupled with sadness. Thus, beliefs serve as the lens through which situational appraisals are made, with attendant emotions.

In turn, emotions influence the content and conviction of beliefs. The interoceptive experience of an emotion provides a signal that tunes attention to the stimuli that elicited the emotion (Clore & Gasper, 2000). This emotional signal alerts the human information processing system to the presence of objects and events that are related to a given belief. Subsequently, stimuli that are mutually congruent with belief and the current emotional state are preferentially selected for further processing (Boden & Berenbaum, 2010). In addition, because emotion is directly experienced as self-evident (Clore & Gasper, 2000), it often serves as evidence that supports or disconfirms a given belief (Centerbar, Schnall, Clore, & Garvin, 2008). Put another way, emotions that are consistent with a given situational appraisal or belief tend to strengthen it, whereas explanation-inconsistent emotions tend to weaken that appraisal or belief. Moreover, emotional valence can influence the content of interpretations of ambiguous stimuli. For example, participants experiencing experimentally induced sadness reported greater self-blame for relationship conflicts in contrast to those experiencing induced happiness

(Forgas, 1994). Induction of anger and disgust result in more negative interpretations of neutral homophones (for example, hearing the word "tense" instead of "tents") (Barazzone & Davey, 2009; Davey, Bickerstaffe, & MacDonald, 2006), and people experiencing naturally occurring or experimentally induced fear interpret situations as riskier (Lerner & Keltner, 2001). Thus, emotional valence can bias meaning-making processes both in terms of the content of beliefs and the extent to which they are held to be true.

As appraisals and beliefs change in concert with changes in emotional state, so too do changing interpretations influence felt experiences. For instance, a person who has received a cancer diagnosis might first interpret this event as a catastrophe and feel crushing emotions of fear and despair. Later, this individual might come to view the diagnosis as an impetus to retire from an unsatisfying job and pursue a new life in a city where he or she had always dreamed of living, and feel emotions of contentment, gratitude, or even joy. This transformation of meaning, or reappraisal, is possible only due to the ambiguity of most life situations.

Life Is an Ambiguous Stimulus

In a very real sense, life is an ambiguous stimulus. Does survival of a heart attack indicate that death is imminent or that one has been given a new lease on life? Is falling in love an assurance of a lifelong partnership or the first sign of an inevitable heartbreak? Many human situations are complex and their meanings subtle. Thus, to make sense of and gain agency over our experiences, we engage in the process of self-reflection (Bandura, 2001).

Through self-reflection, people come to realize that their lives are filled with uncertainty about their own identities, their relationships with others, and their environmental circumstances (Olivares, 2010). Because living involves adaptation to irregular changes and perturbations from the environment, the process of self-reflection reveals the indeterminate nature of life. The uncertainty stemming from threatening stimuli whose nature is unknown or unpredictable evokes stress (Monat, Averill, & Lazarus, 1972) and a sense of loss of control (Folkman, 1984). In response to uncertainty, we are driven to make meaning of our experiences and in so doing to reduce that uncertainty (Olivares, 2010).

Indeed, a series of cunning experiments demonstrated that the sense of lacking control promotes illusory pattern perception in ambiguous situations (Whitson & Galinsky, 2008). Hence, people consciously or unconsciously attempt to regain a sense of control by projecting patterns onto the chaos of their lives. This meaning-making process is hinged on the appraisal of stressors and their meaningful integration into our autobiographical narratives.

Stress Appraisal and the Downward Spiral of Perseveration

A demanding encounter with the environment in and of itself does not carry any particular valence, and takes on positive or negative meaning only after its relevance for one's well-being has been appraised. While many taxing events may harm or threaten to harm the individual, other stimuli present a challenge that involves the possibility of benefit to the person. Using an earlier example, running reliably creates stress physiology, yet a person's experience of bodily changes differs depending on whether he or she is running from a predator or toward the finish line of a marathon. While in the former case, the organism is under definite threat, in the latter case the person stands to gain a sense of accomplishment for facing the challenge. Thus, the experience of stress is contextual; humans use context to appraise stimuli and establish their significance.

According to Lazarus and Folkman's transactional model of stress and coping (1984), stress results from a process that initiates with a primary appraisal of stimuli for their inherent threat value. These appraisals are often executed without conscious deliberation (Bargh & Chartrand, 1999); for example, appraisals of others' intentions are made, on average, in less than 30 seconds (Ambady & Rosenthal, 1992), and appraisals of threat (e.g., a person with a phobia of snakes detecting the presence of a snake) can be made in less than 50 milliseconds (Ohman, Carlsson, Lundqvist, & Ingvar, 2007). Such rapid and unconscious appraisals may use innate reflexes, nondeclarative memory, and implicit cognitive operations, in contrast to intentional appraisal processes that rely on declarative memory and propositional reasoning (Ellsworth & Scherer, 2002).

Subsequently, a cognitive process of secondary appraisal determines the sufficiency of available resources and coping options to meet the demands of the potential threat. If the stressor is appraised to be navigable, a sense of positive affect and self-efficacy will result. If the available resources are deemed insufficient to negotiate the challenge presented by the threatening stimulus, this appraisal will activate the stress reaction sequelae, from the extended amydgala to the hypothalamic-pituitary-adrenal axis, the locus coeruleus, and the autonomic nervous system. This pathway unleashes a neuroendocrine cascade of stress hormones, in which secretion of beta-endorphin and adrenocorticotropin lead to the release of cortisol from the adrenal cortex (Brosschot, Gerin, & Thayer, 2006). Cortisol promotes the processing of threat-related information and the encoding of fear memories by sensitizing neurotransmission between the amygdala and hippocampus (McEwen, 2007). Furthermore, stress appraisal activates a rapid "fight-or-flight response" (Cannon, 1929), mediated by the central autonomic network (Thayer & Lane, 2009), a system of neural circuits linking prefrontal cortex, amygdala, brainstem, sympathetic and parasympathetic nervous systems, viscera, and periphery. During the fight-or-flight response, the central autonomic network innervates muscle groups, drives and modulates the pacemaker of the heart, effects gastric contractions, stimulates sweat gland activity, and regulates shifts in body temperature (Janig, 2002).

This defensive response evolved as a means of adapting to immediate, life-threatening stressors, yet the context of modern, industrialized society rarely presents humans with such threats. In comparison with the ancestral environment of humans, today we often face stress from our attribution of symbolic meaning to events deemed exigent to well-being (Rosmond, 2005). For instance, our bodies react to a critical email from a supervisor in the same vein as we would to threats to physical safety. Although the acute stress response may be adaptive, chronic stress can be deleterious and is often maintained and prolonged through mental representations of the stressor. Humans often engage in perseverative cognition, a maladaptive process of fruitlessly maintaining a cognitive representation of the stressor even after it is no longer present (Brosschot et al., 2006). Perseverative cognitive styles such as catastrophizing (i.e., exaggeration of the threat value of a stimulus) or rumination (the experience of recurrent, intrusive negative thoughts about an event) result in a downward spiral of cognitive stress-appraisal processes, negative affect, and sustained activation of the autonomic nervous system.

In turn, protracted activation of physiologic systems subserving the stress response exacts a toll on multiple body systems known as allostatic load (McEwen & Wingfield, 2003), which, over time, can result in atrophy of brain tissue, hormonal and metabolic dysregulation, and susceptibility to physical and mental disorders (McEwen, 2003). Allostatic load is thought to dysregulate stress and reward neurocircuitry within the extended amygdala, moving the brain reward set point from its normal level and resulting in decreased sensitivity to reward and increased sensitivity to stress, punishment, or aversive states (Koob & Le Moal, 2001). Effects of this sensitization may be observed among persons suffering from depression and anxiety, who may be cognitively biased toward processing objects, persons, and events that they construe as disappointing, upsetting, or frightening, while neglecting what is beautiful, affirming, or pleasurable (Garland et al., 2010; Mathews & MacLeod, 2005). Such information processing biases maintain and reinforce dysphoria, fear, and self-loathing via downward spiral processes and an emotional balance tipped toward negativity.

Positive Reappraisal

Fortunately, the stress response is fluid and mutable; new data from the changing environment coupled with novel information about one's own reactions to the threat may initiate a reappraisal process, in which the original stress appraisal is changed as a result of the feedback. For example, a stimulus that was originally appraised as threatening may be reinterpreted as benign. Reappraisals modify the physiological, psychological, and social consequences of the stress reaction through dynamic feedback-feedforward mechanisms, which alter the informational value or meaning of the stimulus while calibrating the behavioral response to that stimulus.

Reappraisal may be one of the keys to resilience. In the face of adversity, people often believe that they have personally benefited or grown from dealing with the stressful event. This positive emotion–focused coping strategy, known as *positive reappraisal*, is the adaptive process through which stressful events are reconstrued as benign, beneficial, or meaningful (Lazarus & Folkman, 1984). Positive reappraisal, alternately conceptualized as benefit finding (Affleck & Tennen, 1996), is associated with reduced distress and improved mental health outcomes (Helgeson, Reynolds, & Tomich, 2006), and also appears to exert salutary influences on physiological parameters associated with stress (Bower, Low, Moskowitz, Sepah, & Epel, 2008; Carrico et al., 2006; Cruess et al., 2000; McGregor et al., 2004; Tugade & Fredrickson, 2004). Positive reappraisal is an active coping strategy (Folkman, 1997) involving contemplation of the stressor, its context, and its relevance for the individual. Moreover, positive reappraisal has a distinct physiological signature characterized by increases in parasympathetic nervous system activation (Witvliet, Knoll, Hinman, & DeYoung, 2010), which offers a critical step toward a willingness to reengage with the stressor. For instance, a person who has recovered from cancer might view survival as evidence of strength and resilience, and might decide to dedicate his or her life to helping others make similar recoveries. Hence, positive reappraisal is an adaptive and often approach-oriented strategy, one that may produce a sense of coherence (Antonovsky, 1987), which is critical to health and well-being.

In light of the body of research that suggests positive reappraisal is an adaptive form of coping and may be a crucial component in resilience, this cognitive strategy may hold significant therapeutic potential if intentionally harnessed. It is an open question how best to facilitate positive reappraisal in the clinical setting. This remains an understudied area, perhaps due to the emphasis of Second Wave cognitive therapies on positivism (the philosophical view that one can know Reality through information derived from the senses and the use of evidence to verify beliefs) and techniques designed to promote more logical thinking. It is not overtly logical to interpret a cancer diagnosis as a life-affirming blessing, and in fact, such reappraisals may actually run counter to the objective evidence often used in standard cognitive restructuring techniques. Yet, the Third Wave approach embodied by ACT is more constructivist than positivist, emphasizing functional contextualism and pragmatism over "truth."

The functional contextualism inherent in ACT urges us to abandon attempts to establish the veracity of beliefs and instead focus on the function of beliefs. Positive reappraisal is sensible from this functional contextualist view. Given that most situations in life are ambiguous with regard to their relevance for the individual, they may be appraised negatively or positively. Yet, negative appraisals spawn negative emotions and initiate habitual, mindless patterns of stereotypic, defensive behavior. In contrast, positive appraisals result in positive emotions, which broaden cognition and build personal resources through novel, exploratory, and creative problem-solving behaviors. Thus, the operative question is not "Is this belief correct?" but rather "What is the consequence of holding this belief?" (Ciarrochi & Bailey, 2008). As Hayes, Strosahl, and Wilson (1999) state, "The truth criterion of contextualism is successful working. Analyses are true only in terms of the accomplishment of particular goals" (p. 19). Insofar as positive reappraisal facilitates goal achievement by bolstering resilience and broadening thought-action repertoires via upward spiral processes, it satisfies this truth criterion. Hence, positive reappraisal may be especially relevant for a clinical approach marrying the Third Wave orientation with principles drawn from the broaden-and-build theory. The integration of these approaches hinges on the construct of mindfulness.

The Role of Mindfulness in Positive Reappraisal

We argue that the *state* of mindfulness allows for the possibility of positive reappraisal (Garland, Gaylord, & Park, 2009). This naturalistic state involves an attentive and nonjudgmental metacognitive monitoring of moment-by-moment cognition, emotion, perception, and sensation without fixation on thoughts of past and future (Garland, 2007; Lutz, Slagter, Dunne, & Davidson, 2008). Mindfulness is metacognitive in the sense that it involves a meta-level of awareness that monitors the content of consciousness while reflecting back upon the process of consciousness itself (Nelson, Stuart, Howard, & Crowley, 1999). Mindfulness is naturalistic in that it is a basic and inherent capacity of the human mind, although people differ in their ability and willingness to wield this ability (Brown, Ryan, & Creswell, 2007; Goldstein, 2002). As such, the innate function of mindfulness can be fostered by practice. The *practice* of mindfulness (which involves repeated placement of attention onto an object while alternately acknowledging and letting go of distracting thoughts and emotions) engenders the transitory state of mindfulness, which, when engaged repeatedly over time, may accrue into *trait* or *dispositional* mindfulness (Chambers, Gullone, & Allen, 2009), the propensity toward exhibiting nonjudgmental awareness in everyday life.

The metacognitive state of mindfulness can moderate the impact of potentially distressing psychological content through the mental operation of stepping back from thoughts, emotions, and sensations, known as *decentering* (Segal, Williams, & Teasdale, 2002) or *reperceiving* (Shapiro, Carlson, Astin, & Freedman, 2006). This set-shifting function may be a key link between appraisal and reappraisal, involving a shift in mental process rather than in contents (Hayes & Wilson, 2003). Shifting from the contents of consciousness to the process of consciousness is thought to lead to a lack of attachment to thoughts and emotions, liberating awareness from fixed or rigid narratives about self and world (Niemic et al., 2010; Shapiro et al., 2006). "Through reperceiving brought about by mindfulness, the stories (e.g. about who we are, what we like or dislike, our opinions about others, etc.) that were previously identified with so strongly become simply 'stories'" (Shapiro et al., 2006). The cognitive set-shifting process of reperceiving or decentering may afford a fundamental cognitive flexibility, facilitating the flexible selection of cognitive appraisals as "we become able to reflectively choose what has been previously reflexively adopted or conditioned" (Shapiro et al., 2006). Ultimately, decentering creates distance between thoughts and thinker, and thus, from socially conditioned narratives. This new distance or space enables the selection of values that are more congruent with individual goals.

Mindfulness is arguably the keystone in the arch of positive reappraisal. For a person to reconstrue his or her appraisal of a given event as positive, he or she must suspend the initial stress appraisal and disengage cognitive resources from it—in effect, "letting go" of the appraisal while viewing it from a metacognitive vantage point that attenuates semantic evaluations associated with the event. According to the mindful coping model (Garland et al., 2009), when a given event is viewed as a threat that exceeds one's capabilities, this stress appraisal results in perturbations to bodily homeostasis. In turn, feedback from the body is often interpolated as emotion (Friedman, 2011; James, 1890). As one becomes aware of the presence of negative emotions resulting from the stress appraisal, one can initiate an adaptive response by "stepping back," or decentering from this stress appraisal and its resultant emotions into the state of mindfulness. Operating from this mindful state results in increased capacity to reorient attention to novel stimuli (Jha, Krompinger, & Baime, 2007) as well as greater cognitive flexibility (Moore & Malinowski, 2009). As a result, individuals can access new data with which to reappraise their circumstances and reframe them as meaningful or even beneficial. Attending to what is benign, purposeful, or affirming in the situation may result in experiences of positive emotion, which mediate and further promote positive reappraisal (Tugade & Fredrickson, 2004). Hence, from the metacognitive vantage point afforded by mindfulness, positive features of the object, event, circumstance, or context that had been previously unattended now become accessible to consciousness as the "stuff" that reappraisals are made of.

While mindfulness may temporarily suspend evaluative language, because the human mind is embedded in narratives that reduce uncertainty and produce a coherent life story (Olivares, 2010), it is inevitable that one will reengage into a semantic-linguistic mode as one integrates the encounter with the stressor into one's autobiographical memory. As one returns to this narrative mode from the state of mindfulness, reappraisals may arise either through a conscious process of reflection or through more automatic processes, based on spontaneous insight. The result of such positive reappraisal is positive emotions such as hope, compassion, and love, and accepting attitudes such as trust, confidence, and equanimity, which reduce stress and in turn influence subsequent appraisal processes.

Ultimately, the repeated, intentional engagement of the metacognitive state of mindfulness may result in the development of trait mindfulness over time. Developing a more mindful disposition, in turn, leads to a heightened propensity toward making positive reappraisals in the face of distress as a cognitive coping style (see Figure 1). Recent evidence from our prospective observational study of adult participants of a mindfulness-based stress and pain management program supports this assertion; we found that increases in dispositional mindfulness were reciprocally linked with increases in positive reappraisal and that the stress-reductive effects of increases in dispositional mindfulness were mediated by increases in positive reappraisal (Garland et al., 2011). Similarly, findings from a quasi-experimental study comparing college students participating in a mindful communication course to those receiving a standard communications curriculum found that mindfulness training was associated with significant increases in dispositional mindfulness, which were correlated with increases in positive reappraisal (Huston, Garland, & Farb, in press). Unpublished data from our lab indicate that among populations of people recovering from severe addictive and mental health disorders, treatment-related increases in mindfulness and positive reappraisal are significantly correlated. Lastly, a recent study found that when compared to controls, meditators exhibited greater attenuation of negative emotions during reappraisal of stressful stimuli as evidenced by reduced brain activity in centro-parietal regions subserving attentional and emotional processing (Gootjes, Franken, & Van Strien, 2010). Convergent findings across these diverse samples suggest the presence of a fundamental psychological relation: positive reappraisal and mindfulness appear to serially and mutually enhance one another, creating the dynamics of an upward spiral that reduces distress and leads to flourishing.

Figure 1. Mindful Coping Model: Longitudinal View

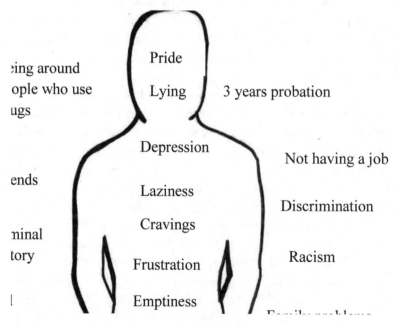

Appraisal Begets Attention and Savoring

The upward spiral of mindfulness and positive reappraisal does not terminate with the reframing of circumstances as benign, beneficial, or meaningful. As the process unfolds, attention becomes tuned in accordance with the new mental set and meaning imbued by the reappraisal. Accordingly, *what one attends to and ultimately sees is shaped by the newly established semantic frame.* This radical proposition is supported by findings from an elegant experiment conducted by Koivisto and Revonsuo (2007). Participants attended to pictures of furniture or animals in displays containing one of each type of picture as well as two filler pictures from other categories. On the third and fourth trials, an unexpected stimulus word (either *cat* or *sofa*) replaced the fixation cross at the center of the pictures. Subjects were randomly assigned to either attend to animals or furniture, with the stimulus word being either congruent or incongruent with the category of the attended pictures, and were asked to write down what objects they saw and whether they noticed something "new and additional that was not present in the previous trials." Results indicated that participants were significantly more likely to detect the presence of a word that was congruent with the attended picture category. In other words, the semantic relation between an observer's attentional set and the unexpected stimulus determine whether that stimulus will be seen. An unexpected stimulus that is related in meaning to the interests of the observer is more likely to be seen, whereas unexpected stimuli that are incongruent with the semantic frame of the observer are likely to be overlooked. These findings are complemented by those of a recent study in which neutral human faces paired with negative gossip were more likely to be seen, and seen for longer, than other neutral faces (Anderson et al., 2011). Hence, meaning influences attentional selection and may ultimately dictate whether one perceives a given feature, object, or event.

Given the significant influence of meaning on attentional selection, when a person positively reappraises his or her circumstances, he or she may begin to focus on and become aware of the beautiful, affirming, and rewarding elements of life. This intentional awareness of pleasant events in the present, or savoring (Bryant, Chadwick, & Kluwe, 2011), is one of the most powerful means of amplifying positive emotion (Quoidback,

Berry, Hansenne, & Mikolajczak, 2010). Indeed, selectively attending to positive stimuli is an effective form of positive emotion regulation (Wadlinger & Isaacowitz, 2008). As one savors, one attends not only to the most perceptually salient, conspicuous features of the event but also to its more subtle features, broadening the diversity and range of sensations and feelings. Yet, savoring is more than attention to pleasant stimuli. Savoring involves metacognition and self-reflection, in which one focuses awareness on both the pleasurable stimulus and the experiences of positive emotion that unfold from the stimulus (Frijda & Sundararajan, 2007). In other words, savoring contains an element of mindfulness. By virtue of mindfully attending not only to the pleasant object or event but also to the pleasurable state that arises from the encounter with that object or event, people can deepen or prolong the savored experience.

By instructing clients to mindfully focus attention on pleasurable objects and events (e.g., the sight of a beautiful sunset or the satisfying taste of a meal), mindfulness training may increase the perceived hedonic value of natural rewards and thereby counter the insensitivity to pleasurable objects, events, and experiences that results from chronic stress (Koob & Le Moal, 2001). Such exercises may amplify pleasure from perceptual and sensorimotor experience in a similar fashion to sensate-focus techniques (Albaugh & Kellogg-Spadt, 2002; Heiman & Meston, 1997; Masters & Johnson, 1970) and promote emotion regulation by generating positive attentional biases (Wadlinger & Isaacowitz, 2010). Controlled clinical trials of sensate focus training as a means of enhancing sexual pleasure and function demonstrate that individuals can learn to attend to the sensory quality of experiences to increase pleasure and improve response (Heiman & Meston, 1998). Similarly, increased attention to the sensory experience of eating has been shown to elevate consummatory pleasure (LeBel & Dubé, 2001). Given that attending to present-moment experience has been prospectively associated with happiness in time-lagged analyses (Killingsworth & Gilbert, 2010), it is plausible that learning to mindfully attend to and savor positive events may offset the anhedonia involved in downward spirals of psychopathology. In support of this hypothesis, a recent randomized controlled trial of Mindfulness-Based Cognitive Therapy with adults with residual depressive symptoms found that mindfulness training increased the experience of reward and positive emotion from pleasant daily life activities (Geschwind, Peeters, Drukker, van Os, & Wichers, 2011).

Furthermore, as one cultivates a self-reflexive awareness during the savoring process, one elaborates on the appraisal, triggering networks of wider associations and meanings to emerge during the temporally extended apprehension of the implications of the object of savoring (Frijda & Sundararajan, 2007). For example, consider the example of "David," a 60-year-old man who was recently diagnosed with a potentially life-threatening cancer. After undergoing treatment for cancer David might mindfully decenter from the stress appraisal "I'm doomed— I'm going to die" to attend to the fact of his present survival, leading to the reappraisal "I'm lucky to be alive" and a sense of relief or contentment. Savoring this emotion might lead to the association "I've had so much good fortune in my life," resulting in a broadening of attention to encompass other positive features of past and present circumstances, such as finding a loving partner, enjoying time with friends, experiencing successes at work, engaging in meaningful activities, and even appreciating the beautiful view from his window. Consequently, the reappraisal might mature into feelings of deep gratitude and joy coupled with the conviction that "I've been given a second chance so I can appreciate the blessings in my life and share them with others." Such elaborative processing of positive reappraisals and their attendant emotions, when punctuated by the self-reflexivity and absorption found in momentary states of mindfulness that occur during savoring, may allow for the emergence of holistic meaning and the "felt sense" that gives an experience its affective flavor (Teasdale, 1997). Thus, when savoring, pleasure evolves into meaning and, ultimately, into a way of being that further reinforces tendencies to positively reappraise until these tendencies consolidate into a new, more adaptive schema. In this way, mindfulness promotes a self-reinforcing cycle of positive reappraisal and savoring—the expanding gyre of an upward spiral that broadens awareness and builds meaning toward the development of sustainable well-being.

Implications for Clinical Practice

The network of concepts introduced above has direct importance for the clinical practitioner. According to Victor Frankl, the inventor of a seminal form of existential therapy known as logotherapy, the role of the psychotherapist "consists of widening and broadening the visual field of the patient so that the whole spectrum of potential meaning becomes conscious and visible to him" (Frankl, 1959). This broadening of the world of experience is a fundamental therapeutic process that makes possible cognitive techniques like restructuring and may represent a heretofore underspecified link between Second and Third Wave therapies.

This link may be the answer to the question posed by Longmore and Worrell (2007) in their highly controversial paper, "Do we need to challenge thoughts in cognitive behavior therapy?" After reviewing the literature, these authors conclude that there is a lack of empirical support for the notion that cognitive change is a causal factor in the clinical outcomes of cognitive behavior therapy (CBT), based on findings suggesting that (a) there is no significant difference between therapeutic efficacy of cognitive restructuring and behavioral activation, (b) adding cognitive interventions to behavioral treatments has little added value, and (c) there is limited evidence that cognitive processes mediate the treatment effect of CBT. Yet, the authors suggest that there may be common therapeutic change processes that underlie techniques like cognitive restructuring and behavioral experiments. Both of these techniques may involve decentering from previously held beliefs or appraisals into a broadened, metacognitive state, where one accesses a larger scope of information with which to construct a new appraisal and activate a more adaptive schematic model of the world. If implemented as procedures that promote new ways of behaving and experiencing, both of these techniques have the capacity to change the client's actual ways of being in the world.

Hence, clinicians can capitalize on the attention-emotion interface to help clients construct more meaningful narratives by providing them with training in *mindful reappraisal*.

Through explicit training in mindfulness skills coupled with cognitive restructuring techniques aimed at producing *functional*, rather than *realistic*, appraisals, the natural facilitation of positive reappraisals afforded by mindfulness practice may be further bolstered. We are not advocating for the adoption of unrealistic beliefs for the purpose of producing positive emotions; rather we are focusing on function over the lone motivation of truth seeking. Clinicians could promote reappraisal by teaching clients to first become aware of the presence of distressing thoughts or emotions in response to an activating event and then to engage in mindfulness of the breath to decenter from stress appraisals into the state of mindfulness. After the client has decentered from distressing mental content into the mindful state, the therapist could use Socratic questioning to generate positive reappraisals of the event (e.g., "How has dealing with this situation made you a stronger person? How can you learn something from this situation? Is there a blessing in disguise here?"). Then the therapist could employ a Socratic approach to direct the client's attention to previously unattended features of the activating event and its larger environmental context. From the perspective of functional contextualism or pragmatism, the therapist would be especially interested in focusing on those features that are life-affirming, meaningful, or valued by the client. Clearly, this is a lineal description of an iterative and recursive process that involves numerous cycles of mindful decentering and reappraisal within and across multiple treatment sessions, during which time clients are taught to oscillate between decentering and reappraisal until catastrophic appraisals abate and new, adaptive appraisals are more readily constructed, accepted, and integrated.

When the wider spectrum of potential meaning becomes "visible" to the client through this process, the therapist can then direct the client to savor these features and the positive mental states that arise from their contemplation. The savoring component of mindful coping should be conducted with intensity, as if it were the last time one would ever experience those positive events, or, as Carlos Castenada (1968) posed the challenge, like a warrior who always keeps death over his shoulder. By savoring with this degree of engagement, the hedonic value of experience is maximized (Higgins, 2006).

For instance, in the previous example, David might first appraise his experience of a grueling treatment regimen of chemotherapy and surgery as evidence that he is "doomed" and become afflicted with fear and despair. A therapist could guide David to initiate mindful breathing practice as a means of disengaging from this stress appraisal into the equanimous state of mindfulness. Once David mindfully attends to his breath, in letting go of feelings of worry and sadness he might become aware of the sense of being alive in the present moment. In so doing, he might generate the reappraisal "I'm lucky to be alive," and subsequently feel a sense of relief and gratitude.

The therapist could then ask David to focus his attention on the feeling of gratitude, and to notice what thoughts, emotions, images, or memories arise into awareness as he savors and contemplates the sense of being grateful. Consequently, he might experience a vivid image of the beautiful view out his apartment window overlooking a river at sunset, and feel a deep sense of appreciation and joy, which in turn might lead to the memory of playing with his adorable grandchildren and the thought, "I have so much I want to share with them." The therapist could then ask David to contemplate the realizations that he wishes to impart to his grandchildren, and how his cancer diagnosis and treatment have played a role in bringing him to this stage of his life. In the course of contemplating these issues, he might experience feelings of strength, resolution, and acceptance. The therapist could ask David to mindfully focus his awareness on these positive emotions, and in savoring them, he might come to believe, "Facing this cancer has made me a stronger person and has brought meaning to my life. I am grateful for it." The therapeutic process could be completed by helping David to commit to valued actions or behaviors that would support this new belief. The therapist could ask him, "As a person who has become stronger in facing cancer, what steps or actions can you take to continue to live the meaningful life you want to live?" The ultimate goal of this mindful reappraisal process (see Figure 2) would be to aid the client to reframe adverse circumstances in his or her life as opportunities for personal growth or sources of meaning.

Figure 2.   Mindful Reappraisal: An Expanded View of the Mindful Coping Model

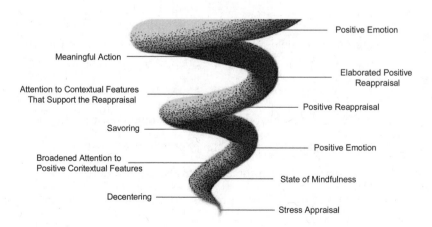

Although I (i.e., the first author) have implemented these therapeutic processes extensively and with success in private practice and agency settings with people suffering from depression, anxiety, addictive behaviors, and stress-related biobehavioral conditions, clinical trials are still needed to ascertain whether adding mindfulness and positive reappraisal training to cognitive-behavior therapy a) facilitates reappraisal; b) is an effective means of reducing distressing thoughts and emotions; and c) increases well-being, a sense of coherence, and resilience. We are in the midst of conducting controlled research for the purpose of answering these questions.

Clinical Recommendations

Provide mindfulness training as a means of increasing psychological flexibility and promoting positive reappraisal by encouraging clients to engage in formal mindfulness practice after the initial stress appraisal and prior to developing the reappraisal. This technique of "mindful reappraisal" is outlined below and further detailed elsewhere (Garland, forthcoming): ·

1. Help the client to become aware of what he/she is thinking and feeling in response to a challenging life event.

2. Remind the client that even if he/she feels upset, he/she still has a choice about how to think about and respond to the situation.

3. Instruct the client to practice a few minutes (3–5) of mindful breathing, to help him/her step back from distressing thoughts and feelings and become more open to new possible meanings.

4. Encourage the client to ask him/herself the following questions:

    a. What are some other ways that I could view this situation?

    b. How can I find personal meaning in this situation?

    c. How can I learn something from this situation?

    d. How can dealing with this situation make me a stronger person?

    e. Is there a blessing in disguise here?

5. Guide the client to focus on and savor these new meanings.

- Encourage clients to intentionally and mindfully savor pleasant, satisfying, or meaningful events and their positive emotional responses to those events.

- Use clients' experiences of positive emotion to promote the generation of more functional beliefs and foster commitment to valued action.

- Have clients complete weekly positive data logs (Padesky, 1994) as homework assignments to reinforce positive reappraisals and new adaptive schemas.

Conclusion: How Mindful Coping Can Be Integrated into Acceptance and Commitment Therapy

The mindful coping model that we articulate here raises an apparent paradox: mindfulness encourages nonevaluative contact with phenomenological experience and attenuates emotional distortions of the perceptual process (Hayes & Wilson, 2003), whereas positive reappraisal attributes a positively valenced, semantic meaning to experience. Hence, striving to reconstrue situations as positive would seem to be contrary to the ethic and quality of mindfulness. Indeed, the integration of mindfulness and positive reappraisal detailed here may seem incongruent with classic Buddhist literature (Kalupahana, 1987), which are often taken to frankly discourage attachment to or cultivation of positive experiences. Pursuit of positive experience inevitably results in emotional pain, this view holds, as the transience of events and objects leads to loss of what was pursued (Watts, 1957, 1961). On the other hand, Buddhism emphasizes the cultivation of the four noble states of mind known as the *Brahmaviharas*, or Four Immeasurables (lovingkindness, compassion, sympathetic joy, and equanimity), three of which are infused with positivity. Yet, Buddhist traditions emphasize equanimity (a construct closely linked with the notion of acceptance within ACT) as vital for keeping pursuit of the other three noble states from turning saccharine.

Some modern theorists conceptualize mindfulness as antithetical to reappraisal due to the supposition that reappraisal requires identification with and aversion toward the original stress appraisal (Chambers et al., 2009). Moreover, ACT may be apparently incompatible with reappraisal, given its focus on undermining emotion regulation efforts in favor of developing acceptance toward unwanted psychological experiences (Hayes et al., 1999). ACT's guiding theoretical framework posits that the attempt to alter or regulate undesirable thoughts and feelings promotes experiential avoidance, which in turn leads to distress, suffering, and compromised functioning. From this perspective, reappraisal as an emotion regulation strategy seems counterproductive at best and altogether incongruent with mindfulness.

A broader perspective is needed to resolve this paradox. We contend that the state of mindfulness is a key mechanism that makes reappraisal possible. Chambers et al. (2009) highlight a fundamental difference between mindfulness and reappraisal: reappraisal alters the content of consciousness, while mindfulness alters one's relationship to those contents. While we agree with this characterization, we contend that mindfulness and reappraisal are not diametrically opposed poles along a single continuum but rather represent different but complementary stages of an adaptive process. To reiterate, we hypothesize that mindfulness facilitates positive reappraisal in that it allows for a decentered mode of awareness in which thoughts and emotions are accepted. Mindfulness may therefore be seen as a precondition or initial phase in the reappraisal process but should not be considered synonymous with positive reappraisal itself. By accepting experiences instead of perseverating on them, cognitive resources are freed up, broadening the scope of attention to encompass pleasurable and meaningful events and building psychological flexibility.

Put another way, the accepting stance of mindfulness aids in decentering or undoing the perceived fusion between the initial cognitive appraisal and its correlated behavioral responses. In facilitating cognitive defusion, mindfulness opens a space in which the client can witness distressing thoughts and emotions as merely insubstantial events and not as truths or fixed determinants of action. Thus, the initial appraisal is deliteralized, that is, exposed for what it is, a relational framing of events rather than an experiential reality. Through deliteralization, the initial appraisal loses its power to determine the behavioral response. It is through the space afforded by decentering that the client can come into closer contact with a wider range of experiences, some of which may be reward or reinforce valued action. As Hayes, Strosahl, and Wilson (1999) state, "Cognitive defusion and openness to experience have the side effect of sensitizing the client to natural rather than verbally constructed contingencies, which in turn may allow the client to respond more effectively to environmental demands" (p. 237). Consequently, new cognitive appraisals of self and world can be made that advance the commitment to act in accordance with deeply held values. As such, mindfulness and acceptance may be key mechanisms that underlie the therapeutic influence of reappraisal on well-being, a notion supported by data showing that lower levels of experiential avoidance (i.e., greater acceptance) mediate the relationship of cognitive reappraisal and positive psychological outcomes (Kashdan, Barrios, Forsyth, & Steger, 2006). Further, the capacity to accept experiences rather than avoid them moderates the effect of traumatic life events on meaning in life and posttraumatic growth (Kashdan & Kane, 2011), a construct closely linked with positive reappraisal. Thus, we argue that mindful acceptance is the fulcrum on which reappraisals can be leveraged in service of living a more meaningful life.

The aim of this process is not to regulate thoughts and emotions "away" by suppressing, denying, or avoiding them but, rather, to foster committed action and imbue life with value. Ultimately, mindfulness imparts the individual with the freedom and, therefore, the responsibility for constructing a more purposeful and meaningful existence.

References

Affleck, G., & Tennen, H. (1996). Construing benefits from adversity: Adaptational significance and dispositional underpinnings. *Journal of Personality, 64*(4), 899-922.

Albaugh, J. A., & Kellogg-Spadt, S. (2002). Sensate focus and its role in treating sexual dysfunction. *Urologic Nursing, 22*(6), 402-403.

Ambady, N., & Rosenthal, R. (1992). Thin slices of expressive behavior as predictors of interpersonal consequences: A meta-analysis. *Psychological Bulletin, 111*, 256-274.

Anderson, E., Siegel, E. H., Bliss-Moreau, E., & Barrett, L. F. (2011). The visual impact of gossip. *Science, 332*(6036), 1446-1448.

Antonovsky, A. (1987). *Unraveling the mystery of health*. San Francisco: Jossey-Bass.

Aron, A., Norman, C. C., Aron, E. N., McKenna, C., & Heyman, R. E. (2000). Couples' shared participation in novel and arousing activities and experienced relationship quality. *Journal of Personality and Social Psychology, 78*, 273–284.

Bandura, A. (2001). Social cognitive theory: An agentic perspective. *Annual Review of Psychology, 52*, 1-26.

Barazzone, N., & Davey, G. C. (2009). Anger potentiates the reporting of threatening interpretations: An experimental study. *Journal of Anxiety Disorders, 23*(4), 489-495.

Bargh, J. A., & Chartrand, T. L. (1999). The unbearable automaticity of being. *American Psychologist, 54*(7), 462-479.

Bateson, G. (1972). *Steps to an ecology of mind*. Chicago: The University of Chicago Press.

Baumeister, R. F., Bratslavsky, E., Finkenauer, C., & Vohs, K. D. (2001). Bad is stronger than good. *Review of General Psychology, 5*(4), 323-370.

Boden, M. T., & Berenbaum, H. (2010). The bidirectional relations between affect and belief. *Review of General Psychology, 14*(3), 227-239.

Bower, J., Low, C., Moskowitz, J., Sepah, S., & Epel, E. (2008). Benefit finding and physical health: Positive psychological changes and enhanced allostasis. *Social and Personality Psychology Compass, 2*(1), 223-244.

Brosschot, J. F., Gerin, W., & Thayer, J. F. (2006). The perseverative cognition hypothesis: A review of worry, prolonged stress-related physiological activation, and health. *Journal of Psychosomatic Research, 60*(2), 113-124.

Brown, K. W., Ryan, R. M., & Creswell, J. D. (2007). Mindfulness: Theoretical foundations and evidence for its salutary effects. *Psychological Inquiry, 18*(4), 211-237.

Bryant, F. B., Chadwick, E. D., & Kluwe, K. (2011). Understanding the processes that regulate positive emotional experience: Unsolved problems and future directions for theory and research on savoring. *International Journal of Wellbeing, 1*(1), 107-126.

Burns, A. B., Brown, J. S., Sachs-Ericsson, N., Plant, E. A., Curtis, J. T., Fredrickson, B. L., et al. (2008). Upward spirals of positive emotion and coping: Replication, extension, and initial exploration of neurochemical substrates. *Personality and Individual Differences, 44*, 360-370.

Cacioppo, J. T., Gardner, W. L., & Berntson, G. G. (1999). The affect system has parallel and integrative processing components: Form follows function. *Journal of Personality and Social Psychology, 76*(5), 839-855.

Cannon, W. B. (1929). Organization of physiological homeostasis. *Physiology Review, 9*, 399-431.

Carrico, A. W., Ironson, G., Antoni, M. H., Lechner, S. C., Duran, R. E., Kumar, M., et al. (2006). A path model of the effects of spirituality on depressive symptoms and 24-h urinary-free cortisol in HIV-positive persons. *Journal of Psychosomatic Research, 61*(1), 51-58.

Castaneda, C. (1968). *The teachings of Don Juan: A Yaqui way of knowledge*. Berkeley: University of California Press.

Centerbar, D. B., Schnall, S., Clore, G. L., & Garvin, E. D. (2008). Affective incoherence: When affective concepts and embodied reactions clash. *Journal of Personality and Social Psychology, 94*(4), 560-578.

Chambers, R., Gullone, E., & Allen, N. B. (2009). Mindful emotion regulation: An integrative review. *Clinical Psychology Review, 29*(6), 560-572.

Ciarrochi, J., & Bailey, A. (2008). *A CBT practitioner's guide to ACT*. Oakland, CA: New Harbinger.

Cicchetti, D., & Blender, J. A. (2006). A multiple-levels-of-analysis perspective on resilience: Implications for the developing brain, neural plasticity, and preventive interventions. *Annals of the New York Academy of Sciences, 1094*, 248-258.

Clore, G. L., & Gasper, K. (2000). Feeling is believing: Some affective influences on belief. In N. H. Frijda, A. S. R. Manstead, & S. Bem (Eds.), *Emotions and belief: How feelings influence thoughts* (pp. 10-44). Cambridge, England: Cambridge University Press.

Cohn, M. A., & Fredrickson, B. L. (2010). In search of durable positive psychology interventions: Predictors and consequences of long-term positive behavior change.

Cohn, M. A., Fredrickson, B. L., Brown, S. L., Mikels, J. A., & Conway, A. M. (2009). Happiness unpacked: Positive emotions increase life satisfaction by building resilience. *Emotion, 9*(3), 361-368.

Corbetta, M., & Shulman, G. L. (2002). Control of goal-directed and stimulus-driven attention in the brain. *Nature Reviews: Neuroscience, 3*(3), 201-215.

Cruess, D. G., Antoni, M. H., McGregor, B. A., Kilbourn, K. M., Boyers, A. E., Alferi, S. M., et al. (2000). Cognitive-behavioral stress management reduces serum cortisol by enhancing benefit finding among women being treated for early stage breast cancer. *Psychosomatic Medicine, 62*(3), 304-308.

Davey, G. C., Bickerstaffe, S., & MacDonald, B. A. (2006). Experienced disgust causes a negative interpretation bias: A causal role for disgust in anxious psychopathology. *Behavior Research and Therapy, 44*(10), 1375-1384.

Desimone, R., & Duncan, J. (1995). Neural mechanisms of selective visual attention. *Annual Review of Neuroscience, 18*, 193-222.

Dunn, J. R., & Schweitzer, M. E. (2005). Feeling and believing: The influence of emotion on trust. *Journal of Personality and Social Psychology, 88*(5), 736-748.

Ekman, P. (1971). Universals and cultural differences in facial expressions of emotions. In J. Cole (Ed.), *Nebraska symposium on motivation* (pp. 207-283). Lincoln: University of Nebraska Press.

Ekman, P. (1977). Biological and cultural contributions to body and facial movement. In J. Blacking (Ed.), *A.S.A. Monograph 15, the anthropology of the body* (pp. 39-84). London: Academic Press.

Ellsworth, P. C., & Scherer, K. R. (2002). Appraisal processes in emotion. In R. J. Davidson (Ed.), *Handbook of affective sciences* (pp. 572-595). New York: Oxford University Press.

Folkman, S. (1984). Personal control and stress and coping processes: A theoretical analysis. *Journal of Personality and Social Psychology, 46*(4), 839-852.

Folkman, S. (1997). Positive psychological states and coping with severe stress. *Social Science & Medicine, 45*(8), 1207-1221.

Folkman, S., & Moskowitz, J. T. (2000). Positive affect and the other side of coping. *American Psychologist, 55*(6), 647-654.

Forgas, J. P. (1994). Sad and guilty? Affective influences on the explanation of conflict in relationships. *Journal of Personality and Social Psychology, 66*, 56-68.

Frankl, V. E. (1959). *Man's search for meaning.* New York: Simon & Schuster.

Fredrickson, B. L. (1998). What good are positive emotions? *Review of General Psychology, 2*(3), 300-319.

Fredrickson, B. L. (2004). The broaden-and-build theory of positive emotions. *Philosophical Transactions of the Royal Society of London B Biological Sciences, 359*(1449), 1367-1378.

Fredrickson, B. L., & Branigan, C. (2005). Positive emotions broaden the scope of attention and thought-action repertoires. *Cognition and Emotion, 19*(3), 313-332.

Fredrickson, B. L., Cohn, M. A., Coffey, K. A., Pek, J., & Finkel, S. M. (2008). Open hearts build lives: Positive emotions, induced through loving-kindness meditation, build consequential personal resources. *Journal of Personality and Social Psychology, 95*(5), 1045-1062.

Fredrickson, B. L., & Joiner, T. (2002). Positive emotions trigger upward spirals toward emotional well-being. *Psychological Science, 13*(2), 172-175.

Fredrickson, B. L., & Levenson, R. W. (1998). Positive emotions speed recovery from the cardiovascular sequelae of negative emotions. *Cognition and Emotion, 12*, 191-220.

Fredrickson, B. L., & Losada, M. F. (2005). Positive affect and the complex dynamics of human flourishing. *American Psychologist, 60*(7), 678-686.

Fredrickson, B. L., Mancuso, R. A., Branigan, C., & Tugade, M. M. (2000). The undoing effect of positive emotions. *Motivation and Emotion, 24*, 237-258.

Fredrickson, B. L., Tugade, M. M., Waugh, C. E., & Larkin, G. R. (2003). What good are positive emotions in crises? A prospective study of resilience and emotions following the terrorist attacks on the United States on September 11th, 2001. *Journal of Personality and Social Psychology, 84*(2), 365-376.

Friedman, B. H. (2011). Feelings and the body: The Jamesian perspective on autonomic specificity of emotion. *Biological Psychology, 84*(3), 383-393.

Friedman, R. S., & Forster, J. (2011). Implicit affective cues and attentional tuning: An integrative review. *Psychological Bulletin, 136*(5), 875-893.

Frijda, N. H. (1986). *The emotions.* Cambridge, England: Cambridge University Press.

Frijda, N. H. (1988). The laws of emotion. *American Psychologist, 43*(5), 349-358.

Frijda, N. H., & Sundararajan, L. (2007). Emotion refinement: A theory inspired by Chinese poetics. *Perspectives on Psychological Science, 2*(3), 227-241.

Gable, S. L., Gonzaga, G. C., & Strachman, A. (2006). Will you be there for me when things go right? Supportive responses to positive event disclosures. *Journal of Personality and Social Psychology, 91*(5), 904-917.

Garland, E. L. (2007). The meaning of mindfulness: A second-order cybernetics of stress, metacognition, and coping. *Complementary Health Practice Review, 12*(1), 15-30.

Garland, E. L. (forthcoming). *Mindfulness-oriented recovery enhancement: Reclaiming a meaningful life from addiction, stress, and pain.* Washington, DC: NASW Press.

Garland, E. L., Fredrickson, B. L., Kring, A. M., Johnson, D. P., Meyer, P. S., & Penn, D. L. (2010). Upward spirals of positive emotions counter downward spirals of negativity: Insights from the broaden-and-build theory and affective neuroscience on the treatment of emotion dysfunctions and deficits in psychopathology. *Clinical Psychology Review, 30*, 849-864.

Garland, E. L., Gaylord, S. A., & Fredrickson, B. L. (2011). Positive reappraisal coping mediates the stress-reductive effect of mindfulness: An upward spiral process. *Mindfulness, 2*(1), 59-67.

Garland, E. L., Gaylord, S. A., & Park, J. (2009). The role of mindfulness in positive reappraisal. *Explore (NY), 5*(1), 37-44.

Geschwind, N., Peeters, F., Drukker, M., van Os, J., & Wichers, M. (2011). Mindfulness training increases momentary positive emotions and reward experience in adults vulnerable to depression: A randomized controlled trial. *Journal of Consulting and Clinical Psychology, 79*, 618-628.

Goldstein, J. (2002). *One Dharma: The emerging western Buddhism.* San Francisco: Harper San Francisco.

Gootjes, L., Franken, I. H., & Van Strien, J. W. (2010). Cognitive emotion regulation in yogic meditative practitioners: Sustained modulation of electrical brain potentials. *Journal of Psychophysiology, 25*(2), 87-94.

Hayes, S. C., Luoma, J. B., Bond, F. W., Masuda, A., & Lillis, J. (2006). Acceptance and Commitment Therapy: Model, processes and outcomes. *Behavior Research and Therapy, 44*(1), 1-25.

Hayes, S. C., Strosahl, K. D., & Wilson, K. G. (1999). *Acceptance and Commitment Therapy: An experiential approach to behavior change.* New York: Guilford Press.

Hayes, S. C., & Wilson, K. G. (1995). The role of cognition in complex human behavior: A contextualistic perspective. *Journal of Behavior Therapy and Experimental Psychiatry, 26*(3), 241-248.

Hayes, S. C., & Wilson, K. G. (2003). Mindfulness: Method and process. *Clinical Psychology: Science and Practice, 10*(2), 161-165.

Heiman J. R., & Meston C. M. (1998). Empirically validated treatments for sexual dysfunction. In K.S. Dobson, K.D. Craig (Eds.), *Empirically Supported Therapies: Best Practice in Professional Psychology.* New York: Sage Publications.

Hejmadi, A., Waugh, C. E., Otake, K., & Fredrickson, B. L. (manuscript in preparation). Cross-cultural evidence that positive emotions broaden views of self to include close others.

Helgeson, V. S., Reynolds, K. A., & Tomich, P. L. (2006). A meta-analytic review of benefit finding and growth. *Journal of Consulting and Clinical Psychology, 74*(5), 797-816.

Higgins, E. T. (2006). Value from hedonic experience and engagement. *Psychological Review, 113*(3), 439-460.

Huston, D., Garland, E. L., & Farb, N. A. (2011). Mechanisms of mindfulness in communications training. *Journal of Applied Communication Research, 39*(4), 406-421.

Isen, A. M. (1987). Positive affect, cognitive processes, and social behavior. *Advances in Experimental Social Psychology, 20*, 203-253.

James, W. (1890). *The principles of psychology.* New York: Henry Holt & Co.

Janig, W. (2002). The autonomic nervous system and its coordination by the brain. In R. J. Davidson (Ed.), *Handbook of affective sciences* (pp. 135-186). New York: Oxford University Press.

Jha, A., Krompinger, J., & Baime, M. (2007). Mindfulness training modifies subsystems of attention. *Cognitive, Affective, and Behavioral Neuroscience, 7*(2), 109-119.

Kalisch, R. (2009). The functional neuroanatomy of reappraisal: Time matters. *Neuroscience & Biobehavioral Reviews, 33*(8), 1215-1226.

Kalupahana, D. J. (1987). *The principles of Buddhist psychology.* Albany: State University of New York Press.

Kashdan, T. B., Barrios, V., Forsyth, J. P., & Steger, M. F. (2006). Experiential avoidance as a generalized psychological vulnerability: Comparisons with coping and emotion regulation strategies. *Behavior Research and Therapy, 44*(9), 1301-1320.

Kashdan, T. B., & Kane, J. Q. (2011). Posttraumatic distress and the presence of posttraumatic growth and meaning in life: Experiential avoidance as a moderator. *Personality and Individual Differences, 50*(1), 84-89.

Kashdan, T. B., & Rottenberg, J. (2010). Psychological flexibility as a fundamental aspect of health. *Clinical Psychology Review, 30*, 865-878.

Keeney, B. P. (1983). *Aesthetics of change.* New York: Guilford Press.

Keyes, C. L. (2002). The mental health continuum: From languishing to flourishing in life. *Journal of Health and Social Behavior, 43*(2), 207-222.

Killingsworth, M. A., & Gilbert, D. T. (2010). A wandering mind is an unhappy mind. *Science, 330*(6006), 932.

Koivisto, M., & Revonsuo, A. (2007). How meaning shapes seeing. *Psychological Science, 18*(10), 845-849.

Koob, G. F., & Le Moal, M. (2001). Drug addiction, dysregulation of reward, and allostasis. *Neuropsychopharmacology, 24*(2), 97-129.

Kringelbach, M. L., & Berridge, K. C. (2009). Towards a functional neuroanatomy of pleasure and happiness. *Trends in Cognitive Science, 13*(11), 479-487.

Lang, P. J., & Bradley, M. M. (2011). Emotion and the motivational brain. *Biological Psychology, 84*(3), 437-450.

Lang, P. J., Bradley, M. M., & Cuthbert, B. N. (1997). *Motivated attention: Affect, activation, and action.* New Jersey: Lawrence Erlbaum Associates, Inc.

Lazarus, R. (1991). *Emotion and adaptation.* New York: Oxford University Press.

Lazarus, R. (1999). *Stress and emotion: A new synthesis.* New York: Springer.

Lazarus, R., & Folkman, S. (1984). *Stress, appraisal, and coping.* New York: Springer.

LeBel, J. L., & Dubé, L. (2001). The impact of sensory knowledge and attentional focus on pleasure and on behavioral responses to hedonic stimuli, 13th Annual American Psychological Society Convention. Toronto, Ontario.

Lerner, J. S., & Keltner, D. (2001). Fear, anger, and risk. *Journal of Personality and Social Psychology, 81*(1), 146-159.

Longmore, R. J., & Worrell, M. (2007). Do we need to challenge thoughts in cognitive behavior therapy? *Clinical Psychological Review, 27*(2), 173-187.

Lutz, A., Slagter, H. A., Dunne, J. D., & Davidson, R. J. (2008). Attention regulation and monitoring in meditation. *Trends in Cognitive Science, 12*(4), 163-169.

Masters, W. H., & Johnson, V. E. (1970). *Human sexual inadequacy.* Boston: Little & Brown.

Mathews, A., & MacLeod, C. (2005). Cognitive vulnerability to emotional disorders. *Annual Review of Clinical Psychology, 1*, 167-195.

McEwen, B. S. (2003). Mood disorders and allostatic load. *Biological Psychiatry, 54*(3), 200-207.

McEwen, B. S. (2007). Physiology and neurobiology of stress and adaptation: central role of the brain. *Physiological Reviews, 87*(3), 873-904.

McEwen, B. S., & Wingfield, J. C. (2003). The concept of allostasis in biology and biomedicine. *Hormones and Behavior, 43*(1), 2-15.

McGregor, B. A., Antoni, M. H., Boyers, A., Alferi, S. M., Blomberg, B. B., & Carver, C. S. (2004). Cognitive-behavioral stress management increases benefit finding and immune function among women with early-stage breast cancer. *Journal of Psychosomatic Research, 56*(1), 1-8.

Monat, A., Averill, J. R., & Lazarus, R. S. (1972). Anticipatory stress and coping reactions under various conditions of uncertainty. *Journal of Personality and Social Psychology, 24*(2), 237-253.

Moore, A., & Malinowski, P. (2009). Meditation, mindfulness and cognitive flexibility. *Consciousness and Cognition, 18*(1), 176-186.

Nelson, T. O., Stuart, R. B., Howard, C., & Crowley, M. (1999). Metacognition and clinical psychology: A preliminary framework for research and practice. *Clinical Psychology and Psychotherapy, 6*, 73-79.

Niemiec, C. P., Brown, K. W., Kashdan, T. B., Cozzolino, P. J., Breen, W., Levesque, C., & Ryan, R. M. (2010). Being present in the face of existential threat: The role of trait mindfulness in reducing defensive responses to mortality salience. *Journal of Personality and Social Psychology, 99*, 344-365.

Ohman, A., Carlsson, K., Lundqvist, D., & Ingvar, M. (2007). On the unconscious subcortical origin of human fear. *Physiology & Behavior, 92*(1-2), 180-185.

Olivares, O. J. (2010). Meaning making, uncertainty reduction, and the functions of autobiographical memory: A relational framework. *Review of General Psychology, 14*(3), 204-211.

Ong, A. D., Bergeman, C. S., Bisconti, T. L., & Wallace, K. A. (2006). Psychological resilience, positive emotions, and successful adaptation to stress in later life. *Journal of Personality and Social Psychology, 91*(4), 730-749.

Padesky, C. (1994). Schema change processes in cognitive therapy. *Clinical Psychology and Psychotherapy, 1,* 267-278.

Plutchik, R. (1962). *The emotions: Facts, theories, and a new model.* New York: Random House.

Plutchik, R. (1980). *Emotion: A psychoevolutionary synthesis.* New York: Harper & Row.

Quoidback, J., Berry, E. V., Hansenne, M., & Mikolajczak, M. (2010). Positive emotion regulation and well-being: Comparing the impact of eight savoring and dampening strategies. *Personality and Individual Differences, 49*(5), 368-373.

Rosmond, R. (2005). Role of stress in the pathogenesis of the metabolic syndrome. *Psychoneuroendocrinology, 30*(1), 1-10.

Rowe, G., Hirsh, J. B., & Anderson, A. K. (2007). Positive affect increases the breadth of attentional selection. *Proceedings of the National Academy of Sciences USA, 104*(1), 383-388.

Schmitz, T. W., De Rosa, E., & Anderson, A. K. (2009). Opposing influences of affective state valence on visual cortical encoding. *The Journal of Neuroscience, 29*(22), 7199-7207.

Schwartz, R. M., Reynolds, C. F., Thase, M. E., Frank, E., Fasiczka, A. L., & Haaga, D. A. (2002). Optimal and normal affect balance in psychotherapy of major depression: Evaluation of the balanced states of mind model. *Behavioural and Cognitive Psychotherapy, 30*(4), 439-450.

Segal, Z., Williams, J. M., & Teasdale, J. D. (2002). *Mindfulness-based cognitive therapy for depression.* New York: Guilford Press.

Shapiro, S. L., Carlson, L. E., Astin, J. A., & Freedman, B. (2006). Mechanisms of mindfulness. *Journal of Clinical Psychology, 62*(3), 373-386.

Singer, J. A. (2004). Narrative identity and meaning making across the adult life-span: An introduction. *Journal of Personality, 72,* 437-459.

Soto, D., Funes, M. J., Guzman-Garcia, A., Warbrick, T., Rothstein, P., & Humphreys, G. W. (2009). Pleasant music overcomes the loss of awareness in patients with visual neglect. *Proceedings of the National Academy of Sciences USA, 106*(14), 6011-6016.

Stein, N., Folkman, S., Trabasso, T., & Richards, T. A. (1997). Appraisal and goal processes as predictors of psychological well-being in bereaved caregivers. *Journal of Personality and Social Psychology, 72*(4), 872-884.

Sterling, P., & Eyer, J. (1988). Allostasis: A new paradigm to explain arousal pathology. In S. Fisher & J. Reason (Eds.), *Handbook of life stress, cognition, and health.* New York: John Wiley & Sons.

Talarico, J. M., LaBar, K. S., & Rubin, D. C. (2004). Emotional intensity predicts autobiographical memory experience. *Memory & Cognition, 32*(7), 1118-1132.

Teasdale, J. D. (1997). The transformation of meaning: The interacting cognitive subsystems approach. In M. Power & C. R. Brewin (Eds.), *The transformation of meaning in psychological therapies* (pp. 141-156). Chichester: Wiley.

Teasdale, J. D., Segal, Z., & Williams, J. M. (1995). How does cognitive therapy prevent depressive relapse and why should attentional control (mindfulness) training help? *Behavior Research and Therapy, 33*(1), 25-39.

Thayer, J. F., & Lane, R. D. (2009). Claude Bernard and the heart-brain connection: Further elaboration of a model of neurovisceral integration. *Neuroscience and Biobehavioral Reviews, 33*(2), 81-88.

Tugade, M. M., & Fredrickson, B. L. (2004). Resilient individuals use positive emotions to bounce back from negative emotional experiences. *Journal of Personality and Social Psychology, 86*(2), 320-333.

Tugade, M. M., Fredrickson, B. L., & Barrett, L. F. (2004). Psychological resilience and positive emotional granularity: Examining the benefits of positive emotions on coping and health. *Journal of Personality, 72*(6), 1161-1190.

Wadlinger, H. A., & Isaacowitz, D. M. (2008). Looking happy: The experimental manipulation of a positive visual attention bias. *Emotion, 8*(1), 121-126.

Wadlinger, H. A., & Isaacowitz, D. M. (2010). Fixing our focus: Training attention to regulate emotion. *Personality and Social Psychological Review, 15*(1), 75-102.

Watts, A. (1957). *The way of Zen.* New York: Pantheon Books.

Watts, A. (1961). *Psychotherapy East & West.* New York: Random House.

Waugh, C. E., & Fredrickson, B. L. (2006). Nice to know you: Positive emotions, self-other overlap, and complex understanding in the formation of a new relationship. *The Journal of Positive Psychology, 1*(2), 93-106.

Waugh, C. E., Wager, T. D., Fredrickson, B. L., Noll, D. C., & Taylor, S. F. (2008). The neural correlates of trait resilience when anticipating and recovering from threat. *Social Cognitive and Affective Neuroscience, 3*(4), 322-332.

Whitson, J. A., & Galinsky, A. D. (2008). Lacking control increases illusory pattern perception. *Science, 322*, 115-117.

Witvliet, C. V., Knoll, R. W., Hinman, N. G., & DeYoung, P. A. (2010). Compassion-focused reappraisal, benefit-focused reappraisal, and rumination after an interpersonal offense: Emotion-regulation implications for subjective emotion, linguistic responses, and physiology. *The Journal of Positive Psychology, 5*(3), 226-242.

CHAPTER 3

Love and the Human Condition

Robyn D. Walser

National Center for PTSD and TL Consultation Services; California

Being human includes feeling, acting, and, most notably, thinking in ways that distinguish us from other animals. Humans are able to act and think in ways that develop and grow knowledge. We reflect upon ourselves, our pasts, and our futures, and we are able to create. This unique capacity brings with it many wonderful things: advances in technology, beautiful literature, communication and connection, and awareness of the self. However, this kind of unique capacity also brings suffering. We know, for instance, that we will one day die. We can compare ourselves to an imagined ideal and feel worse for it; we can evaluate and categorize in ways that are painful even if untrue. Knowledge plays a rich and powerful part in the human experience; however, it also has a shadowy nature. Just as we have the capacity to reflect on joy, we also have the capacity to reflect on pain and fear, and sometimes we do so in such a way as to be afflicted in long-standing ways.

Since its inception, the field of psychology has been dedicated to ameliorating the human suffering born out of emotional and psychological pain. Much effort has been focused on how to fix psychological problems and relieve sets of symptoms while also addressing the underlying explanations that might be causing the same. Psychology has pursued and tested theories and interventions that have sought to eliminate suffering caused by unfulfilled stages of growth and development, cold and rejecting mothers and absent fathers, improper internalization of objects, hidden drives and forces, barren and broken environments, and dysfunctional and irrational minds, to name a few. Each approach has been created in the service of understanding human behavior and the problems that lead to suffering.

Positive psychology has largely turned away from such problem-focused concepts and instead turned toward an understanding of positive emotions and personal psychological strengths and virtues (Seligman, 2002). Seligman describes well-being as engaging personal positive characteristics that occur across time and that lead to good feelings and a sense of gratification. He notes that focusing and acting on these positive traits will bring a sense of authentic happiness, a general sense of positive well-being. The goal in positive psychology is to thrive, even under difficult circumstances, and also to find fulfillment in everyday life (Compton, 2005; Seligman & Csiksentmihalyi, 2000).

Acceptance and Commitment Therapy (ACT; Hayes, Strosahl & Wilson, 2012) has also stepped away from typical models of psychopathology, radically rethinking how human beings work. Rather than holding negative internal experiences as problematic events to be solved, ACT seeks to understand the individual's relationship to these experiences, with a focus on their function rather than on the events themselves. ACT uses mindfulness and engenders *willingness to experience* in the service of engaging personal values to create a meaningful and vital life. Well-being is found in the openness to experience while participating in chosen activities that instantiate values. This personal work, done in the service of well-being, does not necessarily seek happiness as a final outcome. Rather it is focused on being present to all internal experience while simultaneously engaging, as an ongoing process, values-guided behavior.

In both ACT and positive psychology, there are assumptions about the role and influence of behavioral and cognitive theories, in addition to separate notions about mechanisms of change. However, each approach, in parallel fashion, is looking to values, or similarly named virtues, as an alternative to a focus on symptoms reduction and elimination. This is a significant development in psychology and allows great movement and freedom in the course of an individual's life.

The *full* range of emotional and psychological experiences that we encounter in the course of a life is at the heart of what it means to be human. We will encounter joy and pleasure, as well as anxieties, sadness, and disappointments. I argue, as have many before me (see Chodron, 1991; Hanh, 1976; Hayes et al., 2012; Kabat-Zinn, 1994, to name only a few) that there is no relief from this existential truth. To truly encounter the human condition means to experience great happiness, but it also means to touch immeasurable pain, the power of fear, the sorrow of loneliness, the angst of death, and all else that comes from the depths of experience related to the tenderness of the "heart." Knowing the latter, however, means knowing that humans not only flee these experiences but also that they have been taught that they *should* flee.

Human beings have learned to categorize and judge their emotions and thoughts. Internal experience is sorted into columns of good and bad and then responded to in similar fashion. That is, whole parts of our internal world are labeled as negative and then treated as a problem. These kinds of problems are to be eliminated or escaped; we must flee them and pursue internal experiences categorized as good. And indeed, sometimes that is the best thing to do. Yet, in doing so, humans are taught to leave behind the very experience of being. Nevertheless, it is these same conditions that require us to stand firm, to persevere, to stay *with* self and others in moments of pain—with full compassion and presence. When we are experiencing immeasurable pain, fear, and sorrow, when we are vulnerable and tender, that is the very time to turn toward experience rather than to escape it. It is the very time when we most need acceptance; when we most need love. To love then, as it is meant here, is to remain fully present, with self and others, when difficult internal conditions arise.

Love also means to *stay with* under other conditions too. It means remaining psychologically present under conditions of joy, happiness, and excitement and all else that *lifts* the heart. Generally speaking, we are not taught to leave these conditions behind. We are instead taught to seek these things. The general goal of life is to pursue "happiness." And while I agree that happiness is wonderful to experience and I quite like it myself, it often times remains elusive, is found unexpectedly, or rises and falls, and the moment of happiness is just that. Here lies the conundrum for so many of us. Life contains pain. And when it does, love can seem to disappear. But it needn't be that way.

There are many things in the world that lead to the experience of pain. Loss of a loved one, loss of a relationship, fear of rejection, fear of vulnerability, or loss of freedom, each leading us down a path that perhaps can be captured in a few words but is often lived inside of one: fear. Fear, on the one hand, is essential to our existence. It is the very thing that can keep us alive. On the other hand, when we extend our knowledge of fear and all that is related to it and begin to respond to it in ways that have nothing to do with survival, we come to think of fear itself as dangerous, something to be feared. We begin to relate to fear in ways that are not actually in the present moment (see Hayes, Barnes-Holmes, & Roche, 2001). Fearing the future, fearing the past, fearing what is out of our control, we lose bits and pieces of our lives to get control back, to try to not be fearful.

Our relationship with fear can rule our day-to-day activities and can even come to define our existence. We get caught up in fear in ways that stretch from our relationships with ourselves to our partnerships, to our families, to cultures, and to nations. And in this, fear separates, especially when held and evaluated as a grave and terrible experience, and when held as weak and wholly unwelcome. We shrink away from what is unwanted. We can watch fear and separation unfold, starting with the smallest moment of relationship to the self and growing into fear of others. It is in this separation from self and others that love is lost.

Fear has great power and can eat to the bone of all who live inside of it. We can see it in some of the painful stories that we meet in our lives. A client in therapy reveals that he has sexual thoughts about his same gender and is so thoroughly fearful, repulsed, and ashamed that he seethes in constant anger at his own experience and seeks to eliminate his own thoughts through years of substance abuse, isolation, and ultimately suicide. A daughter standing at the bedside of her dying mother watches in anguish as her mother slowly slips away. Somebody tells the daughter she should "be happy" because her mother "is in a better place now." Fear of death and powerful emotions have instigated the comment. However, the feeling of separation and aloneness grow as the comment sinks into the daughter's already broken heart; she does not feel happy. There is the story of a partnership separated by years of silence and disparate lives, a partner afraid of being rejected and one jealous of the other. The fear of abandonment grows, yet neither feels able to reach the other.

And on it goes … a family torn by tyranny, a community immersed in poverty, a culture steeped in violence and war. Each of these experiences possesses its own measure of sorrow. But each also contains the possibility of love, a possibility that is born in the *awareness* to the experience of pain and fear and is lived out in a choice to respond that is open, accepting, present, and compassionate.

However, our least fear to our greatest can interfere with our ability to be present and accepting of ourselves and others. When we work to escape the experience of fear by trying to make sense of it so it can be sorted and solved so that we will no longer have it, it seems we will then be freed to love. In this process, however, we "leave" our experience, we move away rather than stay, and we live in our minds with the *idea* of fear (not the actual fear itself) along with all that it seems to say about us: that we are weak, unlovable, broken. Our minds, in their vast capacity to construct futures and visit the past, extend beyond the sensations, thoughts, and emotions of fear, telling us that we are flawed and that we should separate from ourselves and others until we are no longer fearful. The cost to this separation, however, is too high. We are no longer open and compassionate; we give up the possibility of love, waiting to feel better first.

One goal in ameliorating human suffering then might be to assist ourselves in turning back toward love—letting go of engaging escape and staying with ourselves and others when it is most needed, instead. And as I personally think about it, perhaps, in the end, turning toward love is the only goal. This process, however, is difficult, as it may require questioning our own systems of what it means to be human. It may mean that values and virtues trump feeling good. Engaging the value of being loving here involves deep listening and awareness to one's own and another's innermost places and making connection with them in a place that includes, but is also beyond, our verbal understanding. Love involves *being with* in places that are uncomfortable, not easily shared, tainted with shame, humiliation, or embarrassment, and perhaps filled with pain and fear. How do we open ourselves to these darkest of places and stay present? We first need to recognize the ubiquity of human pain. In this, we can cease to hide from our own anger, doubts, and fears. We begin to see that these experiences also exist in the other. Second, we need to be aware, to be fully conscious of experience. When we look at the outcome of fear responded to without awareness, it looks reactionary; we pull away rapidly like a hand accidentally touching a flame. Responding to pain and fear with openness and awareness, however, can create the space needed to allow the fear to come and go … and come and go again. Allowing—being with—is the key to this process; allowing fear does not make one broken, it makes one human.

Knowing the World

There are at least two ways of knowing our world as humans: verbally and experientially (Hayes et al., 2012). We come to interact with the world, ourselves, and others from what we know with our minds and what we know with experience. We have learned great amounts of verbal knowledge; we have full and active minds. We have learned how to problem solve, think, write, organize, weigh decisions, evaluate, and judge. We also verbally define love and tuck the words of it into our interactions and lives. Love is defined in dictionaries and is characterized in stories, fables, books, and media. It is lauded in romance. In a thousand ways our world teaches us to "know" love with our verbal minds. Broadly speaking, love can be described as a strong emotion of personal affection and strong attachment (*Merriam-Webster Collegiate Dictionary*, 2000). Love can also be defined as a *virtue* that involves kindness and compassion and represents all of human benevolence and goodwill toward others.

Experiential knowledge is gained in the experience of *being* human. This kind of knowledge cannot be captured in words. No matter how great an effort I might make to describe experience, it can be "known" only in the actual experience itself. It is a felt sense that words will fail to clarify. We come to know the experience of love in the moment, in being fully engaged in the here and now. Love then, arises in moments, such as when a mother looks into her infant's eyes and in silence they remain together in locked gaze. It might come in a moment of intimacy between partners or in the stark recognition of loss. It might come in battle when a soldier comes face-to-face with his "enemy" and *sees*, instead, a fellow human being. In an expansive sense, love might come in a moment of intense presence to the pain and suffering of another … in the sensed recognition of fundamental humanness.

Both verbal knowledge and experiential knowledge are important, and the distinction between knowing verbally and knowing experientially is what each allows. A verbal understanding of love allows us to clarify it as a value, a chosen direction designed to give meaning to our lives. An experiential understanding allows us to be present to all that we feel and sense so that we may be aware and connected while choosing to remain present— under all diversity of thought and emotion. An experiential sense of self allows us to simply be present to our changing inner occurrences with no need to escape or understand in order to be with ourselves or another.

Finding the Experiencer

Both positive psychology and ACT share approaches that deserve a broader review than can be done in this chapter. However, each engages in work that guides the individual back to his here and now experience—to the experiencer. This can be broadly defined as mindfulness, or present moment awareness. And each has its own way of exploring these processes. For instance, positive psychology might support clients in *savoring* the moment (Seligman, 2002). *Savoring* is defined by Bryant and Veroff (2007) as the deliberate and conscious attention to the experience of pleasure and includes such techniques as sharing with others the value of the moment, being totally absorbed in a particular activity, and focusing on particular elements of sensation by sharpening perception in the moment. Savoring, as defined here, can bring us into moments of loving when pleasurable experiences are at hand.

ACT (Hayes et al., 2012) helps clients to defuse in the service of personal values. The work here involves teaching the client to disentangle from the literal mind. Clients are taught to gently observe mind, noticing it for what it is: an ongoing flow of thinking experience. Here clients can observe their minds, without being fused. Verbal knowledge, which can be the harbinger of doom, is no longer held as literally true, freeing the client to engage in loving action as defined by personal values, without any part of the mind needing to be changed first.

Both positive psychology and ACT also share mindfulness as an avenue to well-being. Mindfulness in each tradition is about fully connecting to the present moment, being in a place of consciousness itself. The outcome of mindfulness may be different in positive psychology and ACT. Positive psychology uses mindfulness to amplify joys and pleasures, increasing well-being. Clients are encouraged to engage in use of the skill—as that is where a "pleasant life is to be found" (Seligman, 2002, p. 111). Mindfulness in ACT is used to focus on all aspects of the present moment, the joys and the sorrows. Being fully aware is explored through a number of processes, including willingness or openness to experience, practice of present moment awareness, and a sense of self that is conscious of experience (self-as-context). The outcome is also well-being. The difference between ACT and positive psychology lies, perhaps, in the definition of well-being. Well-being for positive psychology is about the creation of happiness and meaning through engaging talents and strengths, and building on these results to create a more gratifying life. Well-being in ACT is found in lived values and life functioning—in engaging valued behavior even if the ultimate outcome is not happiness but vitality and purpose. Regardless, each fundamentally supports the power of connection to the here and now.

Conscious Awareness and Love

As we practice awareness of the moment, we begin to recognize the freedom of openness (Kasl, 2001). Being able to connect to consciousness itself, being *in* awareness, not only allows us to be mindful of the body, breathing, sound, sensation, and the mind, it also allows us to be aware of our relationship to ourselves and others. It is in this awareness that we can begin to loosen the tenacious hold of reactionary and self-protective behaviors related to fear or other negatively evaluated emotions. We can begin to observe when we are fused with mind, loosening the grip of thoughts and beliefs, shifting gently to the process, sitting more fully in an open and willing stance. It is here that we can make choices to engage in behaviors that are linked to values.

Furthermore, through conscious awareness of our attachments, we learn how it is that we try to control ourselves and others. We can examine the workability of control and explore whether it leads us down a path that is virtuous and meaningful or down a path of fear and separation. We can become aware of the experiences of pain and fear, and, with dispassionate observation, recognize the dynamic and nondangerous quality of these states. It is this nonjudgmental presence to our experiences that allows us to stop self-destructive and reactionary behaviors. When open and mindful, we no longer need to flee the evaluated, conjured, and false differences that lead to separation. The need to flee is relinquished; the choice to stay arrives. It is in this place, if we are fully aware, that we experience harming another as harming ourselves. There is no separation. Rather, we can sit in recognition of "oneness" and awareness of experience, choosing the relationship with self, others, community, and culture over the need to control, escape, avoid, or be other than what it means to be human. It is also in this place that we may find that the separation between us and all those we might fear and want to control are false—we will "see" that we and others are the same.

It is in mindful awareness that opening to fear can lessen defense and lead to those most tender moments of pain and joy. Being present in the here and now can help us notice the predictable ways in which we respond to our emotional experiences, while providing us with the chance and choice to respond differently. It is in this place that a values-consistent chosen action can occur, that love can be experienced in its completeness, both toward self and others.

Being Loving

In the end, we are left with what we choose. When we truly see the human condition, we come to know that we are not really alone. When we contact experience, we understand, in a place that is beyond words, that pain and fear are shared. When we truly know what it means to be human, when we are fully awake and aware, we simultaneously see our needs and fears in others and in ourselves. We recognize the human condition. And it is inside of this recognition that it is good to have fear and pain—when we no longer see fear and pain as an enemy. Our fear can tell us what is good and virtuous. If we fear loss, then we seek togetherness, if we fear loneliness then we seek connection, and if we fear death, then life is here for us to boldly live. All that we might choose for ourselves—fortitude, sufferance, appreciation, gratitude, grit, tolerance, strength, or grace—include their own measure of sorrow … and all are part of love.

Pointing to our humanness is not a call to pessimism. It is quite the opposite. This is a call to put forth; it is a request to move through, with awareness, the tribulations that seem to easily hold us back. It is here that our ability to *stay with* is most needed. To be able to freely look into the hearts of self and others and remain open and accepting in moments of great despair is the foundation of love. Inside of awareness, love can be felt as a clear and deep emotion, it can be experienced outside of words, it can lead to a change in the relationship we have with ourselves and others, purging separation. Love too, can be considered a virtue, an extension of us in a selfless act of compassion and kindness. Indeed, it can include an expansive reach of benevolent mattering to all humans and beyond.

Perhaps this is where ACT and positive psychology are taking the lead. Each is invested in turning toward a more vital life rather than the difficult process of eliminating pain and fear. Each reaches to include self, partnership, family, community, culture, and nation in the reduction of suffering, while opening to fundamental human wholeness, including both joy and suffering. Each is optimistic, looking to the values and virtues that humans engage to support and sustain meaning and purpose. If we were to weave a thread through all that ACT and positive psychology are attempting to do, it would come down to *love*. And what meaning and purpose is there but that?

References

Bryant, F. B., & Veroff, J. (2007). *Savoring: A new model of positive experience*. United Kingdom: Emerald Group Publishing Limited.

Compton, W. C. (2005). *Introduction to positive psychology*. Thomson-Wadsworth: Australia.

Chodron, P. (1991). *The wisdom of no escape and the path of loving-kindness*. Boston: Shambhala.

Hanh, T. N. (1976). *The miracle of mindfulness*. Boston: Beacon Press.

Hayes, S. C., Barnes-Holmes, D., & Roche, B. (Eds.). (2001). *Relational Frame Theory: A Post-Skinnerian account of human language and cognition*. New York: Plenum Press.

Hayes, S. C., Strosahl, K., & Wilson, K. G. (2012). *Acceptance and Commitment Therapy: The process and practice of mindful change*. 2nd ed. New York: Guilford Press.

Kabat-Zinn, J. (1994). *Wherever you go there you are: Mindfulness meditation in everyday life*. New York: Hyperion.

Kasl, C. (2001). *If the Buddha married: Creating enduring relationships on a spiritual path*. New York: Penguin Books.

Merriam-Webster Collegiate Dictionary. (2000). Merriam-Webster.com. Retrieved March 27, http://www.merriam-webster.com/cgi-bin/book.pl?c11.htm&1

Seligman, M. E. P. (2002). *Authentic happiness: Using the new positive psychology to realize your potential for lasting fulfillment*. New York: Free Press.

Seligman, M. E. P., & Csikszentmihalyi, M. (2000). Positive psychology: An introduction. *American Psychologist, 55*, 5-14.

CHAPTER 4

Self-Compassion and ACT

Kristin Neff

University of Texas at Austin

Dennis Tirch

Weill-Cornell Medical College,
American Institute for Cognitive Therapy

One of the central goals of therapy is to relieve suffering—to help clients escape the dark hole of self-loathing, anxiety, and depression they often find themselves in. But what's the best way to achieve this goal? Approaches such as Acceptance and Commitment Therapy (ACT) (Hayes, Strosahl, & Wilson, 1999) argue that it's important to help clients broaden their repertoire of overt and private behaviors (such as thinking and feeling), even in the presence of difficult emotions and stressful circumstances. ACT techniques, which emphasize psychological flexibility, encourage clients to change their relationship to emotions and cognitions by cultivating mindfulness—a present-moment, nonjudgmental form of awareness. The current chapter will examine a construct that is closely linked to mindfulness—self-compassion. We will try to demonstrate ways in which elements of the ACT model of psychological wellness are related to the experience of self-compassion and how certain processes involved in ACT are essential to the roots of self-compassion (Hayes, 2008). First, however, more in-depth understanding of what we mean by "self-compassion" is needed.

What Is Self-Compassion?

Compassion involves sensitivity to the experience of suffering, coupled with a deep desire to alleviate that suffering (Goertz, Keltner, & Simon-Thomas, 2010). Self-compassion is simply compassion directed inward. Drawing on the writings of various Buddhist teachers (e.g., Salzberg 1997), Neff (2003b) has operationalized self-compassion as consisting of three main elements: kindness, a sense of common humanity, and mindfulness. These components combine and mutually interact to create a self-compassionate frame of mind. Self-compassion is relevant when considering personal inadequacies, mistakes, and failures, as well as when confronting painful life situations that are outside of our control.

Self-kindness. Western culture places great emphasis on being kind to our friends, family, and neighbors who are struggling. Not so when it comes to ourselves. When we make a mistake or fail in some way, we may be more likely to beat ourselves up than put a supportive arm around our own shoulder. And even when our problems stem from forces beyond our control, such as an accident or traumatic event, we often focus more on fixing the problem than calming and comforting ourselves. Western culture often sends the message that strong individuals should be like John Wayne—stoic and silent toward their own suffering. Unfortunately, these attitudes rob us of one of our most powerful coping mechanisms when dealing with the difficulties of life—the ability to comfort ourselves when we're hurting and in need of care.

Self-kindness refers to the tendency to be supportive and sympathetic toward ourselves when noticing personal shortcomings rather than being harshly critical. It entails relating to our mistakes and failings with tolerance and understanding, and recognizing that perfection is unattainable. Self-compassion is expressed in internal dialogues that are benevolent and encouraging rather than cruel or disparaging. Instead of berating ourselves for being inadequate, we offer ourselves warmth and unconditional acceptance. Instead of getting fixated in a problem-solving mode and ignoring our own suffering, we pause to emotionally comfort ourselves when confronting painful situations. With self-kindness, we make a peace offering of warmth, gentleness, and sympathy from ourselves to ourselves so that true healing can occur.

Common humanity. All humans are flawed works in progress; everyone fails, makes mistakes, and engages in dysfunctional behavior. All of us reach for things we cannot have and must remain in the presence of difficult experiences that we desperately want to avoid. Just as the Buddha realized, some 2,600 years ago, all of us suffer. Often, however, we feel isolated and cut off from others when considering our struggles and personal shortcomings, irrationally reacting as if failure and pain were aberrations. This isn't a logical process but a kind of tunnel vision in which we lose sight of the larger human picture and focus primarily on our own seemingly feeble and worthless selves. Similarly, when things go wrong in our external lives through no fault of our own, we often assume that other people are having an easier time of it, that our own situation is abnormal or unfair. We feel cut off and separate from other people who are presumably leading "normal," happy lives.

With self-compassion, however, we take the stance of a compassionate "other" toward ourselves. Through this act of perspective taking, our outlook becomes broad and inclusive, recognizing that life's challenges and personal failures are simply part of being human. Self-compassion helps us to feel more connected and less isolated when we are in pain. More than that, it helps put our own situation into context. Perhaps a situation that seemed like the end of the world at first, being fired from a job, for instance, doesn't seem quite as terrible when considering that other people lose their homes or their loved ones. When we remember the shared nature of suffering it not only makes us feel less isolated, it also reminds us that things could be worse.

Recognition of common humanity also reframes what it means to be a self. When we condemn ourselves for our inadequacies, we are assuming that there is in fact a separate, clearly bounded entity called "me" that can be pinpointed and blamed for failing. But is this really true? We always exist in a present moment context, and the range of our behavioral responses is informed by our individual histories (Hayes, 1984). Let's say you criticize yourself for having an anger issue. What are the causes and conditions that led you to be so angry? Perhaps in-born genetics plays a role. But did you choose your genes before entering this world?

Or maybe you grew up in a conflict-filled household in which shouting and anger were the only ways to get heard. But did you choose for your family to be this way? If we closely examine our "personal" failings, it soon becomes clear that they are not entirely personal. We are the expression of millions of prior circumstances that have all come together to shape us in the present moment. Our economic and social backgrounds, our past associations and relationships, our family histories, our genetics—they've all had a profound role in creating the person we are today. And thus we can have greater acceptance and understanding for why we aren't the perfect people we want to be.

Mindfulness. Mindfulness involves being aware of present moment experience in a clear and balanced manner (Brown & Ryan, 2003). Mindful acceptance involves being "experientially open" to the reality of the present moment, allowing all thoughts, emotions, and sensations to enter awareness without judgment, avoidance, or repression (Bishop et al., 2004). Why is mindfulness an essential component of self-compassion? First, it is necessary to recognize you're suffering in order to give yourself compassion. While it might seem that suffering is obvious, many people don't acknowledge how much pain they're in, especially when that pain stems from their own inner self-critic. Or when confronted with life challenges, people often get fixated in problem solving such that they don't consider how much they are struggling in the moment. While the tendency to suppress or ignore pain is very human, an avoidant style of coping with negative emotions can lead to dysfunctional and ultimately ineffective strategies such as substance misuse, binge eating, or social withdrawal (Holahan & Moos, 1987). Mindfulness counters the tendency to avoid painful thoughts and emotions, allowing us to hold the truth of our experiences even when unpleasant.

At the same time, being mindful means that we don't become "over-identified" (Neff, 2003b) with negative thoughts or feelings so that we are caught up and swept away by our aversive reactions (Bishop et al., 2004). This type of rumination narrows our focus and exaggerates implications for self-worth (Nolen-Hoeksema, 1991). Not only did I fail, "I AM A FAILURE." Not only am I disappointed, "MY LIFE IS DISAPPOINTING." Overidentification means that we reify our moment to moment experiences, perceiving transitory events as definitive and permanent. When we observe our pain mindfully, however, new behaviors become possible. Like a clear, still pool without ripples, mindfulness mirrors what's occurring, without distortion. This allows us to take a wiser and more objective perspective on ourselves and our lives.

Self-Compassion and Well-Being

Gilbert and Irons (2005) suggest that self-compassion enhances well-being primarily because it deactivates the threat system (associated with self-criticism, insecure attachment, and defensiveness) and activates the self-soothing system (associated with secure attachment, safety, and the oxytocin-opiate system). By increasing feelings of safety and interconnectedness and reducing feelings of threat and isolation, self-compassion fosters greater emotional balance. The body of research literature on self-compassion—which has grown dramatically over the past decade—supports its psychological benefits.

The majority of studies on self-compassion have been correlational, using a self-report measure called the Self-Compassion Scale (Neff, 2003a). However, more recent research has started to examine self-compassion using experimental manipulations or interventions (e.g., Adams & Leary, 2007; Kelly, Zuroff, Foa, & Gilbert, 2009; Shapira & Mongrain, 2010). One of the most consistent findings is that greater self-compassion is linked to less anxiety, stress, and depression (see a recent meta-analysis by MacBeth & Gumley, 2010). For instance, Neff, Kirkpatrick, and Rude (2007) asked participants to take part in a mock job interview in which they were asked to "describe their greatest weakness." Even though self-compassionate people used as many negative self-descriptors as those low in self-compassion, they were less likely to experience anxiety as a result of the task. There may be physiological processes underlying the negative association between self-compassion, anxiety, stress, and depression. Rockcliff et al. (2008) found that an exercise designed to increase feelings of self-compassion was associated with reduced levels of the stress hormone cortisol. It also increased heart-rate variability, which activates the parasympathetic nervous system and is associated with a greater ability to regulate emotions so that they are responsive to situational demands (e.g., self-soothing when stressed) (Porges, 2007).

One easy way to help clients soothe and comfort themselves when they're feeling emotional distress is to encourage them to give themselves a gentle hug or caress, or simply put their hand on their heart and feel its warmth. What's important is to make a clear gesture that conveys feelings of love, care, and tenderness. If other people are around, it's possible to fold one's arms in a nonobvious way, gently squeezing in a comforting manner. Research indicates that soothing touch releases oxytocin, provides a sense of security, soothes distressing emotions, and calms cardiovascular stress (Goetz et al., 2010).

While self-compassion protects against maladaptive emotional states, it also helps to foster psychological strengths. For instance, self-compassion is associated with greater perspective-taking skills (Neff & Pommier, 2012), less dogmatism, and more cognitive flexibility (Martin, Staggers & Anderson, 2011), meaning that self-compassionate individuals tend to be more openminded and have a greater ability to switch cognitive and behavioral responses according to the context of the situation. Because self-compassion involves mentally stepping outside of oneself to consider the shared human experience and offer oneself kindness, findings suggest that general perspective-taking capacities may be central to compassionately understanding the experiences of both self and others.

Another important strength provided by self-compassion is the ability to cope effectively. This is illustrated in a recent study that examined the role self-compassion plays in adjustment to marital separation (Sbarra, Smith & Mehl, 2012). Researchers had divorcing adults complete a 4-minute stream-of-consciousness recording about their separation experience, and independent judges rated how self-compassionate their dialogues were. Those who displayed greater self-compassion when thinking about their breakup not only evidenced better psychological adjustment at the time, but this effect persisted over nine months. Findings were significant even after accounting for competing predictors such as the number of positive/negative emotions initially expressed in the dialogues, trait attachment anxiety or avoidance, depression, self-esteem, and optimism. In fact, self-compassion was the strongest predictor of adjustment outcomes. This research suggests that therapists should target self-compassion when helping clients adjust to divorce or other stressful life situations.

While self-compassion helps lessen the hold of negativity, it's important to remember that self-compassion does not involve pushing negative emotions away. Indeed, negative emotions are a prerequisite for self-compassion. This point could be confusing, because the conventional wisdom in popular culture suggests that we should think positively rather than negatively. The problem, however, is that if you try to eliminate the negative, it's going to backfire. A great deal of research shows any attempt to suppress unwanted thoughts causes them to emerge into conscious awareness more strongly and more frequently than if they were given attention in the first place (Wenzlaff & Wegner, 2000). This is a particularly important area of common ground among ACT research and self-compassion research, as will be discussed below. Research shows that people with greater self-compassion are less likely to suppress unwanted thoughts and emotions (Neff, 2003a). Similarly, they're more willing to experience difficult feelings and to acknowledge that their emotions are valid and important (Neff, Kirkpatrick, & Rude, 2007). This allows the pain to just be there, no more, no less, so that unhelpful "add-on" suffering is minimized.

Instead of replacing negative feelings with positive ones, new positive emotions are generated by *embracing* the negative. Feelings of care, belonging, and tranquility are engendered when we approach our suffering with kindness, a sense of common humanity, and mindfulness. These feelings are experienced alongside the negative. Not surprisingly then, greater self-compassion has been linked to positive emotions such as happiness, curiosity, enthusiasm, interest, inspiration, and excitement (Hollis-Walker & Colosimo, 2011; Neff, Rude, & Kirkpatrick, 2007). By wrapping one's pain in the warm embrace of self-compassion, positive states are generated that help balance the negative ones. The positive affect generated by the kind, connected, and accepting mindset of self-compassion may help us break free of fear and greatly improve the quality of our lives. Barbara Fredrickson's broaden-and-build theory (see chapter 2) suggests that positive emotions allow people to take advantage of opportunities rather than merely avoid dangers, which may help explain the role that self-compassion plays in motivation.

Self-Compassion and Motivation

Many people think that self-compassion runs counter to motivation. They believe that self-criticism is necessary to motivate themselves and that if they're too self-compassionate they'll be lazy and self-indulgent. But is this true? A good analogy can be found in how good parents motivate their children. A compassionate mother wouldn't ruthlessly criticize her son when he messes up, telling him he's a failure. Instead, she would reassure her child that it's only human to make mistakes and that she'll offer whatever support needed to help him do his best. Her child will be much more motivated to try to attain his goals in life when he can count on his mother's encouragement and acceptance when he fails rather than being belittled and labeled as unworthy.

It is easy to see this when thinking about healthy parenting, but it's not so easy to apply this same logic to ourselves. We're deeply attached to our self-criticism, and at some level we probably think the pain is helpful. To the extent that self-criticism does work as a motivator, it's because we're driven to succeed in order to avoid self-judgment when we fail. But if we know that failure will be met with a barrage of self-criticism, sometimes it can be too frightening to even try (Powers, Koestner, & Zuroff, 2007). We also use self-criticism as a means of shaming ourselves into action when confronting personal weaknesses. However, this approach backfires if weaknesses remain unacknowledged in an attempt to avoid self-censure (Horney, 1950). For instance, if you have a jealousy problem but continually blame things on your partner because you can't face up to the truth about yourself, how are you ever going to achieve a more harmonious relationship? With self-compassion, we are motivated toward achievement for a different reason—because we care. If we truly want to be kind to ourselves and don't want to suffer, we'll do things to help us reach our full potential, such as taking on challenging new projects or learning new skills. Because self-compassion gives us the safety needed to acknowledge our weaknesses, we're in a better position to change them for the better.

Research supports the idea that self-compassion enhances motivation rather than self-indulgence. For instance, while self-compassion has no association with the level of performance standards adopted for the self, it is negatively related to maladaptive perfectionism (Neff, 2003a). In other words, self-compassionate people aim just as high as those who lack self-compassion but don't become as distressed and frustrated when they can't meet their goals. Research shows that self-compassionate people are less afraid of failure (Neff, Hsieh, & Dejitterat, 2005) because they know they won't face a barrage of self-criticism if they do fail. They are also more likely to reengage in new goals after failure, meaning they're better able to pick themselves up and try again (Neely, Schallert, Mohammed, Roberts & Chen, 2009). In a series of four experimental studies, Breines and Chen (2012) used mood inductions to engender feelings of self-compassion for personal weaknesses, failures, and past moral transgressions. Compared to various control conditions, self-compassion resulted in more motivation to change for the better, try harder to learn, and avoid repeating past mistakes. Self-compassion has also been linked to greater personal growth initiative (Neff, Rude, & Kirkpatrick, 2007), which Robitschek (1998) defines as being actively involved in making changes needed for a more productive and fulfilling life.

Self-compassion has been found to promote health-related behaviors such as sticking to a diet (Adams & Leary, 2007), smoking cessation (Kelly et al., 2009), and starting a physical fitness regimen (Magnus, Kowalski, & McHugh, 2010). In addition, self-compassionate individuals demonstrate a greater ability to adjust and cope effectively with persistent musculoskeletal pain (Wren et al., 2012). Thus, self-compassion appears to enhance both physical and mental well-being.

In the two-chair dialogue studied by Gestalt therapist Leslie Greenberg, clients sit in different chairs to help get in touch with conflicting parts of themselves, experiencing how each aspect feels in the present moment. A variation on this technique can be used to increase self-compassion. To begin, put out three empty chairs, preferably in a triangular arrangement. Next, ask the client to think about an issue that troubles him or her and often elicits harsh self-judgment. Designate one chair for the voice of the inner critic, one chair for the part that feels judged, and one chair for the voice of a wise, compassionate observer. The client will be role-playing all three parts of him- or herself. After the dialogue finishes, you can help clients reflect upon what just happened. Do they have any new insights into how to treat themselves, how to motivate themselves with kindness rather than self-criticism, or other ways of thinking about the situation that are more productive and supportive?

Self-Compassion versus Self-Esteem

It's important to distinguish self-compassion from self-esteem, with which it might be easily confused. Self-esteem refers to the degree to which we evaluate ourselves positively and is often based on comparisons with others (Harter, 1999). In American culture, having high self-esteem means standing out in a crowd—being special and above average. There are potential problems with self-esteem, however, not in terms of having it, but in terms of how we get it. Research shows that people may engage in dysfunctional behaviors to obtain a sense of high self-worth (Crocker & Park, 2004), such as putting others down and inflating their own sense of self-worth as a way to feel better about themselves (Tesser, 1999). Self-esteem also tends to be contingent on perceived competence in various life domains (Harter, 1999), meaning that it can be unstable, fluctuating up and down according to our latest success or failure (Kernis, Paradise, Whitaker, Wheatman, & Goldman, 2000).

In contrast, self-compassion is not based on positive judgments or evaluations—it is a way of positively relating to ourselves. People feel compassion for themselves because they are human beings, not because they are special or above average, and thus it emphasizes interconnection rather than separateness. Self-compassion offers more emotional stability than self-esteem because it exists regardless of whether things are going well or poorly. For instance, it's associated with less anxiety and self-consciousness than self-esteem when considering personal weaknesses (Leary, Tate, Adams, Allen, & Hancock, 2007; Neff, Kirkpatrick et al., 2007), and is linked with more stable and less contingent feelings of self-worth (Neff & Vonk, 2009). Self-compassion is associated with less social comparison, public self-consciousness, and ego-defensiveness when receiving unflattering personal feedback than is self-esteem (Leary et al., 2007; Neff & Vonk, 2009). Moreover, while trait self-esteem evidences a substantial overlap with narcissism, self-compassion has not been found to be associated with narcissism (Neff, 2003a; Neff & Vonk, 2009). Thus, self-compassion appears to entail many of the benefits of high self-esteem with fewer of its drawbacks.

This distinction between self-compassion and self-esteem is important when dealing with clients who suffer from shame or low self-worth. Trying to help people to judge themselves more positively may increase the tendency to form global self-evaluations rather than focus on specific

87

maladaptive behaviors, making change more difficult. This is partly because people with low self-esteem often prefer to verify and maintain their identity rather than engage in the positive self-illusions that are common among those high in self-esteem (Swann, 1996). It may be more possible to raise people's levels of self-compassion, given that it requires them to merely acknowledge and accept their human limitations with kindness rather than change their self-evaluations from negative to positive.

Self-Compassion and Interpersonal Functioning

While there is evidence that self-compassion psychologically benefits the individual, there is also evidence that self-compassion enhances interpersonal relationships (Yarnell & Neff, 2012). In a study of heterosexual couples (Neff & Beretvas, 2012), for example, self-compassionate individuals were described by their partners as being more emotionally connected, accepting, and autonomy supporting while being less detached, controlling, and verbally or physically aggressive in their relationship than those lacking self-compassion. Not surprisingly, the partners of self-compassionate individuals also reported being more satisfied with their relationship. Because self-compassionate people meet many of their own needs for care and support, they have more emotional resources available to give compassion to relationship partners. Because they accept and validate themselves, they don't need to gain approval from others to maintain a sense of self-worth. This suggests that teaching skills of self-compassion when working with couples experiencing relationship difficulties would be an effective way to break patterns of emotional neediness, anger, control, and ego-defensiveness. It would also be a means to enhance intimacy and mutual support among couples.

An interesting question concerns whether self-compassionate people are more compassionate toward others. In one of the few studies on the topic, Neff and Pommier (2012) examined the link between self-compassion and empathy, personal distress, and forgiveness among college undergraduates, an older community sample, and individuals practicing Buddhist meditation. Among all three groups, self-compassionate people were less likely to experience personal distress when considering others' pain, meaning they were more able to confront suffering without being overwhelmed. This suggests that self-compassion may be an important skill to teach to caregivers and health professionals (Barnard & Curry, 2012), who often experience burnout from over-exposure to others' trauma. In addition, self-compassion was significantly associated with forgiveness. Forgiving others requires understanding the vast web of causes and conditions that lead people to act as they do (Worthington et al., 2005). The ability to forgive and accept one's flawed humanity, therefore, appears to be linked to the ability to forgive and accept others' transgressions.

The study also found that self-compassion was significantly linked to empathetic concern for others among community adults and Buddhists, but not undergraduates. This may be because young adults often struggle to recognize the shared aspects of their life experience, overestimating their distinctiveness from others (Lapsley, FitzGerald, Rice, & Jackson, 1989). Thus, young adults' schemas for why they are deserving of care and why others are deserving of care may be poorly integrated, so that their treatment of themselves and others is relatively unrelated. The strength of the association between self-compassion and other-focused concern tended to be the greatest among meditators, likely reflecting meditation practices that intentionally cultivate compassion for both self and others, and aim to recognize that all beings suffer and want release from suffering (see Hofmann, Grossman & Hinton, 2011 for a review). This research suggests that when working with youths there should be an explicit emphasis on connecting the experiences of oneself and others, and that meditation may be one way to facilitate this connection.

Origins of Self-Compassion

While research on this topic is new, there is some evidence to support Gilbert and Iron's (2005) contention that self-compassion is associated with the care-giving system. In a study of adolescents and young adults, Neff and McGehee (2010) found that maternal support was associated with significantly greater self-compassion, while maternal criticism was linked to less self-compassion. Self-compassion levels were also significantly predicted by degree of family functioning more generally.

Individuals from harmonious, close families were more self-compassionate, whereas those from stressful, conflict-filled homes were less self-compassionate. The study also found that self-compassion was linked to attachment style, with secure attachment linked to greater self-compassion. This suggests that individuals who did not receive warmth and support from their parents as children may not have the solid emotional foundation needed to give themselves compassion later in life. Similarly, Vettese, Dyer, Li, and Wekerle (2011) found that youths who were maltreated as children had significantly lower self-compassion, and this lack of self-compassion mediated the link between degree of maltreatment and later emotional regulation difficulties, psychopathology, and drug and alcohol dependence. Findings such as these highlight the need for clinical interventions that can enhance self-compassion to help individuals with problematic family histories cope effectively as adults.

Self-Compassion and Clinical Interventions

There is some evidence to suggest that self-compassion may be an important process in psychotherapeutic change. For example, increased self-compassion has been found to be a key mechanism in the effectiveness of mindfulness-based interventions such as Mindfulness-Based Cognitive Therapy (MBCT) and Mindfulness-Based Stress Reduction (MBSR; Baer, 2010). Jon Kabat-Zinn (1991) originally developed MBSR in the late 1970s, and it is probably the most common mindfulness intervention program offered worldwide. MBSR is an experiential learning program that includes weekly group sessions, regular home practice, and a core curriculum of formal and informal mindfulness practices. This core curriculum was later incorporated into MBCT as an adaptation for preventing depressive relapse (Segal, Williams, & Teasdale, 2001), and additional psycho-education and exercises specific to depression were included. Meta-analyses indicate that MBSR and MBCT are related to improved outcomes in participants dealing with a variety of stressors and health problems (Grossman, Niemann, Schmidt, & Walach, 2004).

Shapiro, Astin, Bishop, and Cordova (2005) found that health care professionals who took an MBSR program reported significantly increased self-compassion and reduced stress levels compared to a wait-list control group. They also found that increases in self-compassion mediated the reductions in stress associated with the program. Similarly, Kuyken et al. (2010) examined the effect of MBCT compared to maintenance antidepressants on relapse in depressive symptoms. They found that increases in mindfulness and self-compassion following MBCT participation mediated the link between MBCT and depressive symptoms at 15-month follow-up. It was also found that MBCT reduced the link between cognitive reactivity (i.e., the tendency to react to sad emotions with depressive thinking styles) and depressive relapse, and that increased self-compassion (but not mindfulness) mediated this association. This suggests that self-compassion skills may be an important key to changing habitual thought patterns so that depressive episodes are not retriggered.

Because self-compassion appears to be a major therapeutic factor in mindfulness-based interventions, people have recently been starting to develop ways to teach self-compassion. Paul Gilbert (2010b) developed a general therapeutic approach termed compassion-focused therapy (CFT) that helps clients develop the skills and attributes of a self-compassionate mind, especially when their more habitual form of self-to-self relating involves shame and self-attack. CFT increases awareness and understanding of automatic emotional reactions such as self-criticism that have evolved in humans over time, and how these patterns are often reinforced in early childhood. The key principles of CFT involve motivating people to care for their own well-being, to become sensitive to their own needs and distress, and to extend warmth and understanding toward themselves. CFT techniques include mindfulness training, visualizations, compassionate cognitive responding, and engaging in self-compassionate overt behaviors and habits. This takes place through a systematic process known as compassionate mind training (CMT). This program is currently being used with apparent success to treat eating disorders, anxiety disorders, bipolar disorders, smoking cessation, shame, and other forms of suffering (Gilbert, 2010a; Gilbert & Procter, 2006; Kelly, Zuroff, Foa, & Gilbert, 2009).

Kristin Neff and Chris Germer (2012) have developed a self-compassion training program suitable for nonclinical populations called mindful self-compassion (MSC). The term "mindful" is included in the name of the program because it also teaches basic mindfulness skills, which—as discussed above—are crucial to the ability to give oneself compassion. The structure of MSC is modeled on MBSR, with participants meeting for two hours once a week over the course of eight weeks, and also meeting for a half-day "mini retreat." The program uses discussion, experiential exercises, and contemplative meditations designed to increase awareness of self-compassion and how to practice it in daily life. Note that MSC mainly focuses on teaching self-compassion skills and includes mindfulness as a secondary emphasis (only one session in the eight-week course is exclusively devoted to mindfulness). In contrast, programs such as MBSR and MBCT mainly teach mindfulness skills and have an implicit rather than explicit focus on self-compassion. This suggests that the MSC program is complementary to mindfulness-based programs rather than being in competition with them.

A randomized controlled study of the MSC program was recently conducted that compared outcomes for a treatment group to those who were randomized to a waitlist control group (Neff & Germer, 2012). Compared to controls, MSC participants demonstrated a large and significant increase in their self-compassion levels (43%). To provide comparative insight into the size of this increase, three studies on MBSR (Birnie, Speca, Carlson, 2010; Shapiro, Astin, Bishop, & Cordova, 2005; Shapiro, Brown, & Biegel, 2007) yielded on average a 19% increase on the SCS, while three MBCT studies (Kuyken et al., 2010; Lee & Bang, 2010; Rimes & Wingrove, 2011) yielded an average increase of 9%. This suggests that the specific targeting of self-compassion in the MSC program is particularly effective. MSC participants also significantly increased in mindfulness (19%), compassion for others (7%) and life satisfaction (24%), while decreasing in depression (24%), anxiety (20%), stress (10%), and emotional avoidance (16%). All significant gains in study outcomes were maintained at six months and one-year follow-up. In fact, life satisfaction actually increased significantly from the time of program completion to the one-year follow-up, suggesting that the continued practice of self-compassion continues to enhance one's quality of life over time. The study also explored whether enhanced well-being was primarily explained by increases in self-compassion or whether it was also explained by increased mindfulness. It was found that while most of the gains in well-being were explained by increased self-compassion, mindfulness explained additional variance in terms of happiness, stress, and emotional avoidance. This suggests that both self-compassion and mindfulness are key benefits of the MSC program.

Advances in our understanding of the value of developing self-compassion as a change process in psychotherapy may also be applied to existing, evidence-based psychotherapies. ACT is a therapy that is particularly well suited to the integration of self compassion–focused interventions. As we will see, many of the key elements of the ACT process model are consistent with Neff's conceptualization of self-compassion, even if some of the language used may be different. Beyond the existing relationship between ACT practice and the development of self-compassion, ACT practitioners may benefit from targeting self-compassion as a process more directly. For example, John Forsyth and Georg Eifert (2008) have included compassion-focused techniques in their ACT protocol and self-help book for anxiety. The effectiveness of this self-help book is currently being examined in randomized controlled trials, and preliminary findings indicated that self-compassion many serve as an important process and outcome variable in this ACT intervention (Van Dam, Sheppard, Forsyth, & Earleywine, 2011). As theoretical and practical integration continues, self-compassion may more clearly emerge as an active psychotherapeutic process within the ACT model.

Self-Compassion from an ACT Perspective

ACT practitioners and researchers have been exploring the role of self-compassion in psychotherapy for some time now, though self-compassion has yet to be integrated as a formal component of the ACT process model (Forsyth & Eifert, 2008; Hayes, 2008; Luoma, Kohlenberg, Hayes, & Fletcher, 2012; Tirch, 2010; Van Dam et al., 2011).

In order to approach an understanding of self-compassion from an ACT perspective, we need to spend some time examining relational frame theory (RFT), the underlying theory of cognition that ACT is derived from. Among many other mental phenomena, RFT describes the processes of mindfulness, self-development, and perspective taking. It provides a behavioral account of language and cognition that can provide a useful way of considering how humans may develop a sense of self and a sense of others, and how we experience ourselves as situated in time and space (Barnes-Holmes, Hayes, Dymond, 2001; Törneke, 2010). All of this has relevance for understanding the emergence of self-compassion. An RFT account of self-compassion can help us understand how self-compassion functions and how we can develop methods to predict and influence self-compassionate behaviors.

In RFT theory, our ability to adopt a broader sense of self involves our ability to flexibly shift perspective. Our learned capacity for flexible perspective taking is also involved in our experience of empathy (Vilardaga, 2009), as well as our related experience of compassion. In order to understand self-compassion, therefore, it's useful to consider the "self" that is the focus of compassion, from an RFT perspective. The way we think about being a "self" and having a "self" and the way we use verbal functioning to experience the "self" are all dimensions of human experience that can be explored as ongoing verbal, behavioral processes rather than as static constructs (Vilardaga, 2009).

In RFT terms, the experience of "self" emerges from the type of verbal learning that establishes a perspective. A perspective means a point of view that is situated in time and space, relative to other points of view. We can symbolically represent this perspective in a number of ways. For example, we can imagine our perspective relative to another perspective: "How would she feel if she were in my shoes?" We can also imagine our perspective relative to all other perspectives: "I feel like I'm the only person in the world who feels this way!"

Using the language of behavior analysis, RFT posits that these verbal relations, known as "deictic relations," are trained relational operant behaviors, shaped by ongoing social interactions (Barnes-Holmes, Hayes, & Dymond, 2001). Deictic relations are building blocks of how we experience the world, ourselves, and the flow of time. Verbal relations that involve "I-You," "Here-There," and "Then-Now" involve perspective taking. For the concept "I" to have any meaning, there must be a "You" involved. For "Here" to have meaning as a point of view, there must be a "There." Our sense of a self emerges from perspective taking.

When people ask us who we are, we might respond by telling some form of "life story." Responses like "My name is Fred, I'm from Texas, and I'm an attorney" make perfect sense. From an ACT perspective, this sense of self is known as "self-as-content." However, mindfulness and self-compassion can allow for an experience of a different sort of self. This self exists as a sort of observer, a silent "you" who has been watching your experience, moment by moment, for a very long time. This is sometimes referred to as "the observing self," or a "transcendent self" but is most often referred to in ACT as "self as context" (Hayes, Strosahl, & Wilson, 1999).

How is it that this "observer self," distinct from an experiencing self, arises? In order to understand this, let's turn again to ACT's roots in research on human language and cognition, RFT. Part of human relational responding involves trained capacities for perspective taking. Through these processes, our experience of being involves a sense of ourselves as a perspective before which the entirety of our experience unfolds, throughout our whole lives. This sense of ourselves as an observer is referred to as self as context in ACT because this experiential sense of self serves as the context within which our experiences are contained (Hayes, Strosahl, & Wilson, 1999). This sense of an "observing self" is important because while this observer can notice the contents of consciousness, it is not those contents themselves. We have a thought, but we are more than that experience, just in the way that we have arms, but we are more than just our arms. Emotions don't feel themselves, thoughts don't observe themselves, and physical pain doesn't experience itself. Throughout our lives, we can notice the presence of an "observing self," before which all of our experiences arise, exist, and disappear in time.

Upon considering the relationship between self-as-context and self-compassion, we can note that returning to an awareness of self-as-context offers us a nonattached and disidentified relationship to our experiences. This allows the habitual stimulus functions of our painful private events and stories to hold less influence over us. From the perspective of the I-Here-Nowness of being, I can view my own suffering as I might view the suffering of another and be touched by the pain in that experience, without the dominant interference of my verbal learning history, with its potential for shaming self-evaluations (Vilardaga, 2009; Hayes, 2008).

Steven Hayes (2008) has suggested that compassion may be the only value that is inherent in the ACT model of psychological well-being. According to him, we may find the roots of self-compassion and compassion emerging from six core processes described in the ACT model of psychotherapeutic change, sometimes known as "hexaflex" processes (Hayes, Luoma, Bond, Masuda, & Lillis, 2006). These six processes work together in an interactive way to:

- bring us into direct experiential contact with our present moment experiences

- disrupt a literalized experience of mental events that narrows our range of available behaviors

- promote experiential acceptance

- help us to let go of overidentification with our narrative sense of "self"

- assist us in the process of values authorship

- facilitate our commitment to valued directions in our lives

Dahl, Plumb, Stewart, & Lundgren (2009) have outlined how these hexaflex processes directly affect compassion for self and others. According to their model, self-compassion involves our ability to willingly experience difficult emotions; to mindfully observe our self-evaluative, distressing, and shaming thoughts without allowing them to dominate our behavior or our states of mind; to engage more fully in our life's pursuits with self-kindness and self-validation; and to flexibly shift our perspective toward a broader, transcendent sense of self (Hayes, 2008).

Hexaflex processes are seen as fundamental elements of the ACT model of psychological well-being, which is known as "psychological flexibility" (Hayes et al., 2006). Psychological flexibility may be defined as "the ability to contact the present moment more fully as a conscious human being, and based on what the situation affords, to change or persist in behavior in order to serve valued ends" (Luoma, Hayes, & Walser, 2007, p. 17). Like self-compassion, psychological flexibility is strongly negatively correlated with depression, anxiety, and psychopathology and is highly positively correlated with quality of life (Kashdan & Rottenberg, 2010).

Evolutionary Basis of Compassion

Gilbert (2009) emphasizes that self-compassion is an evolved human capacity that emerges from the human behavioral systems involving attachment and affiliation, an argument supported by empirical research.

Seeking proximity and soothing from caregivers to provide a secure base for operation in the world is a mammalian behavior that predates the human ability for derived relational responding, deictic relational framing, and the kind of observational capacity that arises in mindfulness training.

Nevertheless, the unique evolutionary advantage that we humans have in our capacity for derived relational responding has resulted in our particularly human quality of self-awareness, the ability to base our behavior on abstract thought and imagination, including our ability to be sensitive and moved by suffering we witness and our ability to be aware of our awareness (e.g., mindfulness). According to Wilson, Hayes, Biglan, and Embry (in press), this human capacity for symbolic thought affords us an "inheritance system" with a capacity for combinatorial diversity similar to that of recombinant DNA. In this way, both our genetic and psycholinguistic evolution have led us to be soothed by the experience of self-compassion and, for that experience of soothing and ensuing courage, to afford us with greater psychological flexibility and a secure base for functioning in the world.

Wang (2005) hypothesizes that human compassion emerges from an evolutionarily determined "species-preservative" neurophysiological system. This system is hypothesized as evolving in a relatively recent evolutionary time frame compared to the older "self-preservative" system. This "species-preservative" system is based on an "inclusive sense of self and promotes awareness of our interconnectedness to others" (Wang, 2005, p. 75). Relative to some other animals, human infants and children may seem defenseless, requiring, as they do, a great deal of care and protection in their early lives. As a result, particular brain structures and other elements of the nervous and hormonal systems have evolved that promote nurturing behaviors, which involve protection of and care for others. Basic examples of this evolutionary progression can be observed by contrasting the parenting behaviors of reptiles and amphibians, for example, to that of mammalian species; the former lack even the most basic nurturing behaviors toward their own young, while mammalian species (rats, for example) can be observed to display a wide range of caretaking behaviors.

Moving higher on the evolutionary ladder, Wang's review of the relevant literature suggests that the human prefrontal cortex, cingulate cortex, and ventral vagal complex are involved in the activation of this "species-preservative" system (Wang, 2005). These structures are all involved in the development of healthy attachment bonds and self-compassion. The development of both individually adaptive and group adaptive behavioral systems for dealing with threats can be viewed as an example of multilevel selection theory (Wilson, Van Vugt, & O'Gorman, 2008) and reflects how our evolutionary history informs our verbal relational network in ways that connect us to one another, and our place as an emergent species in the flow of life. Such an evolutionary perspective is intrinsically contextual in nature and reflects a potential area for multidisciplinary theoretical integration in the developing science of self-compassion.

Interplay of Mindfulness, Self-Compassion, and Psychological Flexibility

The elements of common humanity, kindness, and mindfulness are involved in each of the hexaflex processes elaborated upon by ACT theory, yet self-compassion also involves an intentional turning of these processes decidedly toward the alleviation of human suffering. Accordingly, self-compassion may account for more of the variance in psychopathology than mindfulness alone (Kuyken et al., 2010). Recently, Van Dam and colleagues (2011) found that self-compassion accounted for as much as 10 times more unique variance in psychological health than a measure of mindfulness did in a large community sample. When we consider the role of self-compassion in ACT, there is a temptation to find a way to fit self-compassion into the hexaflex model. It is important to remember that the hexaflex concepts are meant to be clinically applicable, midlevel terms, which describe the underlying principles of RFT in relatively everyday language. The hexaflex components are useful descriptors, but they do not need to represent all and everything that is involved in human well-being and psychological flexibility. What distinguishes contextual behavioral science (CBS) is the application of fundamental behavioral principles to account for the prediction and influence of human behavior. As we will describe, further CBS research may help us to work in more effective ways with the powerful psychotherapy process variable that we find in self-compassion. Similarly, compassion-focused techniques may expand the technical base of ACT in theoretically consistent ways, much as techniques from Gestalt psychotherapy, other forms of CBT, and from the human potential movement have.

Conclusion

ACT is consistent with Neff's conceptualization of self-compassion in multiple ways, and each approach to understanding psychological resilience has something to offer the other. Although ACT's client protocols are generally presented in user-friendly language, the underlying behavioral theory and clinician literature that ACT is based upon can be challenging for therapists who are not coming from the behavior analytic tradition. Many find that RFT has a rather steep learning curve, given the range of new terms and concepts. ACT practitioners may benefit from the straightforward, direct, and understandable language and conceptual explanations that have emerged from the self-compassion literature. Also, interventions based upon theories of self-compassion and compassion such as the MSC program (Neff & Germer, 2012) and CFT (Gilbert, 2010b) might provide ACT clinicians with a range of effective, ACT-consistent procedures that involve the movement of common psychotherapy change processes.

Similarly, research on self-compassion may benefit from examining ways in which self-compassion is associated with ACT constructs such as acceptance, perspective taking, and psychological flexibility. The ACT-consistent goals of prediction and influence of human behavior, and precision, depth, and scope in functional analysis are scientifically healthy complements to the growing body of research on self-compassion.

Obviously, ongoing clinically relevant research on all of the emergent mindfulness- and compassion-informed psychotherapies is needed. In particular, there is a need for further randomized controlled trials that are designed with an awareness of the importance of mediational analyses for psychotherapy process variables. This is true for ACT, CFT, and MSC. By employing mediational analyses we might examine the degree to which psychological flexibility and self-compassion serve as active process variables in these therapies. Component analyses of ACT interventions, which examine the relative contribution of different hexaflex processes and self-compassion are recommended. Such analyses might compare an ACT therapy condition with an added unit of self-compassion to an ACT intervention without overt self-compassion references.

As concepts are integrated, we are confronted with the question of what exactly is being measured when we use measures of psychological flexibility and self-compassion such as the AAQ-II (Bond et al., in press) and the SCS (Neff, 2003a). A strong link between these measures appears to exist, although research on this topic is very new. For example, in a study of 51 parents of autistic children, Neff (unpublished data) found a .65 zero-order correlation between the SCS and AAQ. Teasing out the differences in the AAQ and SCS, as well as the underlying hypothesized processes, will prove to be an important future step. Importantly, measurement of self-compassion, compassion for others, fear of compassion, and shame could all be integrated into the study of perspective taking, deictic framing, and theory of mind tasks. In this way, emotionally charged perspective-taking exercises could be deployed to examine the dynamics of compassion across training in enhanced perspective taking, further exploring the role of self-as-context in the experience of mindfulness, compassion, and empathy.

Clinically, ACT practitioners may find that there are a wide range of ACT-consistent techniques and intervention strategies found among compassion-informed therapies such as CFT and MSC. Beyond this, a range of Buddhist-derived exercises that use attention and visualization to enhance compassion and self-compassion are available. Psychotherapists might find it advisable to integrate these methods into their existing psychotherapy technique repertoires. Additionally, writings on the science and practice of compassion and self-compassion may be a useful resource for the authorship of valued directions, for both therapist and patient alike.

Practitioners of CFT or MSC may find a range of techniques within the ACT literature that may help patients to broaden their behavioral repertoires. Defusion techniques, values authorship techniques, and targeting willingness in compassionate exposure are just a few ACT psychotherapeutic moves that are consistent with these compassion-focused approaches. Additionally, the underlying psychological flexibility process model of psychotherapy that forms the basis of ACT can provide a useful context within which to explore how a science of behavioral dynamics can account for and describe the experience of self-compassion.

From a less technical and theory-bound perspective, clinicians and clients who have encountered the experiential and contemplative techniques of either ACT or self compassion–based methods have had a shared experience, however it may be labeled. This experience involves more than adjustments of concepts and ideas. ACT and MSC methods allow people the space and time to step into the present moment, encountering themselves in a mindful, compassionate, and wholly accepting way. Perhaps this moment of radical acceptance and love is the greatest common ground between self-compassion psychology and ACT.

References

Adams, C. E., & Leary, M. R. (2007). Promoting self-compassionate attitudes toward eating among restrictive and guilty eaters. *Journal of Social and Clinical Psychology, 26*, 1120-1144.

Baer, R. A. (2010). Self-compassion as a mechanism of change in mindfulness- and acceptance-based treatments. In R. A. Baer (Ed.), *Assessing mindfulness and acceptance processes in clients: Illuminating the theory and practice of change* (pp. 135-153). Oakland, CA: New Harbinger Publications.

Barnard, L. K., & Curry, J. F. (2012). The relationship of clergy burnout to self-compassion and other personality dimensions. *Pastoral Psychology, 61,* 149–163.

Barnes-Holmes, D., Hayes, S. C., & Dymond, S. (2001). Self and self-directed rules. In S. C. Hayes, D. Barnes-Holmes, & B. Roche (Eds.), *Relational frame theory: A post-Skinnerian account of human language and cognition* (pp. 119-139). New York: Plenum.

Birnie, K., Speca, M., Carlson, L. E. (2010). Exploring Self-compassion and Empathy in the Context of Mindfulness-based Stress Reduction (MBSR). *Stress and Health, 26*, 359-371.

Bishop, S. R., Lau, M., Shapiro, S., Carlson, L., Anderson, N. D., Carmody, J., ... Devins, G. (2004). Mindfulness: A proposed operational definition. *Clinical Psychology: Science and Practice, 11*(3), 230-241.

Bond, F. W., Hayes, S. C., Baer, R. A., Carpenter, K. M., Guenole, N., Orcutt, H. K., Waltz, T., & Zettle, R. D. (in press). Preliminary psychometric properties of the Acceptance and Action Questionnaire—II: A revised measure of psychological flexibility and experiential avoidance. *Behavior Therapy.*

Brown, K. W., & Ryan, R. M. (2003). The benefits of being present: Mindfulness and its role in psychological well-being. *Journal of Personality and Social Psychology, 84*, 822-848.

Crocker, J., & Park, L. E. (2004). The costly pursuit of self-esteem. *Psychological Bulletin, 130*, 392-414.

Dahl, J. C., Plumb, J. C., Stewart, I., & Lundgren, T. (2009). *The art and science of valuing in psychotherapy: Helping clients discover, explore, and commit to valued action using acceptance and commitment therapy.* Oakland, CA: New Harbinger.

Forsyth, J. P., & Eifert, G. H. (2008). *The mindfulness & acceptance workbook for anxiety: A guide to breaking free from anxiety, phobias, and worry using Acceptance and Commitment Therapy.* Oakland, CA: New Harbinger.

Gilbert, P. (2009). The compassionate mind. London: Constable.

Gilbert, P. (2010a). An introduction to compassion focused therapy in cognitive behavior therapy. *International Journal of Cognitive Therapy, 3*(2), 97-112.

Gilbert, P. (2010b). Compassion focused therapy: Distinctive features. New York: Routledge.

Gilbert, P. & Irons, C. (2005). Focused therapies and compassionate mind training for shame and self-attacking. In P. Gilbert, (Ed.), *Compassion: Conceptualisations, research and use in psychotherapy.* London: Routledge.

Gilbert, P., & Procter, S. (2006). Compassionate mind training for people with high shame and self-criticism: Overview and pilot study of a group therapy approach. *Clinical Psychology & Psychotherapy, 13,* 353-379.

Goetz, J. L., Keltner, D., & Simon-Thomas, E. (2010). Compassion: An evolutionary analysis and empirical review. *Psychological Bulletin, 136,* 351-374.

Grossman, P., Niemann, L., Schmidt, S., & Walach, H. (2004). Mindfulness-based stress reduction and health benefits: A meta-analysis. *Journal of Psychosomatic Research, 57*(1), 35-43.

Harter, S. (1999). *The construction of the self: A developmental perspective.* New York: Guilford Press.

Hayes, S.C., Strosahl, K.D., & Wilson, K.G. (1999). *Acceptance and Commitment Therapy: An experiential approach to behavior change.* New York: Guilford Press.

Hayes, S. C., Barnes-Holmes, D., & Roche, B. T. (2001). *Relational frame theory: A post-Skinnerian account of human language and cognition.* New York: Plenum.

Hayes, S. C., Luoma, J., Bond, F., Masuda, A., & Lillis, J. (2006). Acceptance and Commitment Therapy: Model, processes, and outcomes. *Behaviour Research and Therapy, 44*(1), 1-25.

Hayes, S. C. (1984). Making sense of spirituality. *Behaviorism, 12,* 99-110.

Hayes, S. C. (2008a). The roots of compassion. Keynote address presented at the fourth Acceptance and Commitment Therapy Summer Institute, Chicago, IL. http://www.globalpres.com/mediasite/Viewer/?peid=017fe6ef4b1544279d8cf27adbe92a51

Hofmann, S. G., Grossman, P., Hinton, D. E. (2011). Loving-kindness and compassion meditation: Potential for psychological interventions. *Clinical Psychology Review, 31,* 1126-1132.

Holahan, C. J., & Moos, R. H. (1987). Personal and contextual determinants of coping strategies. *Journal of Personality and Social Psychology, 52*(5), 946-955.

Hollis-Walker, L., & Colosimo, K. (2011). Mindfulness, self-compassion, and happiness in non-meditators: A theoretical and empirical examination. *Personality and Individual Differences, 50*(2), 222-227.

Horney, K. (1950). *Neurosis and human growth: The struggle toward self-realization.* New York: Norton.

Kabat-Zinn, J. (1991). *Full catastrophe living: Using the wisdom of your body and mind to face stress, pain, and illness.* New York: Dell.

Kashdan, T. B., & Rottenberg, J. (2010). Psychological flexibility as a fundamental aspect of health. *Clinical Psychology Review, 30,* 865-878.

Kelly, A. C., Zuroff, D. C., Foa, C. L., & Gilbert, P. (2010). Who benefits from training in self-compassionate self-regulation? A study of smoking reduction. *Journal of Social and Clinical Psychology, 29,* 727-755.

Kernis, M. H., Paradise, A. W., Whitaker, D. J., Wheatman, S. R., & Goldman, B. N. (2000). Master of one's psychological domain? Not likely if one's self-esteem is unstable. *Personality and Social Psychology Bulletin, 26,* 1297-1305.

Kuyken, W., Watkins, E., Holden, E., White, K., Taylor, R. S., Byford, S., ... Dalgleish, T. (2010). How does mindfulness-based cognitive therapy work? *Behavior Research and Therapy, 48,* 1105-1112.

Lapsley, D. K., FitzGerald, D. P., Rice, K. G., & Jackson, S. (1989). Separation-individuation and the "New Look" at the imaginary audience and personal fable: A test of an integrative model. *Journal of Adolescent Research, 4,* 483-505.

Leary, M. R., Tate, E. B., Adams, C. E., Allen, A. B., & Hancock, J. (2007). Self-compassion and reactions to unpleasant self-relevant events: The implications of treating oneself kindly. *Journal of Personality and Social Psychology, 92,* 887- 904.

Lee, W. K. & Bang, H. L. (2010) Effects of mindfulness-based group intervention on the mental health of middle-aged Korean women in community. *Stress and Health, 26,* 341–348.

Luoma, J. B., Hayes, S. C., & Walser, R. D. (2007). *Learning ACT: An Acceptance & Commitment Therapy skills-training manual for therapists.* Oakland, CA: New Harbinger.

Luoma, J. B., Kohlenberg, B. S., Hayes, S. C., & Fletcher, L. (2012). Slow and steady wins the race: A randomized clinical trial of acceptance and commitment therapy targeting shame in substance use disorders. *Journal of Consulting and Clinical Psychology, 80,* 43-53.

MacBeth, A., & Gumley, A. (2012). Exploring compassion: A meta-analysis of the association between self-compassion and psychopathology. *Clinical Psychology Review, 32,* 545-552.

Magnus, C. M. R., Kowalski, K. C., & McHugh, T.-L. F. (2010). The role of self-compassion in women's self-determined motives to exercise and exercise-related outcomes. *Self and Identity, 9,* 363-382.

Martin, M. M., Staggers, S. M., & Anderson, C. M. (2011). The relationships between cognitive flexibility with dogmatism, intellectual flexibility, preference for consistency, and self-compassion. *Communication Research Reports, 28,* 275-280.

Neely, M. E., Schallert, D. L., Mohammed, S. S., Roberts, R. M., & Chen, Y. (2009). Self-kindness when facing stress: The role of self-compassion, goal regulation, and support in college students' well-being. *Motivation and Emotion, 33*(1), 88-97.

Neff, K. D. (2003a). Development and validation of a scale to measure self-compassion. *Self and Identity, 2,* 223-250.

Neff, K. D. (2003b). Self-compassion: An alternative conceptualization of a healthy attitude toward oneself. *Self and Identity, 2,* 85-102.

Neff, K. D. (2009). Self-compassion. In M. R. Leary & R. H. Hoyle (Eds.), *Handbook of individual differences in social behavior* (pp. 561-573). New York: Guilford Press.

Neff, K. D., & Beretvas, S. N. (2012). The role of self-compassion in romantic relationships. *Self and Identity.* DOI:10.1080/15298868.2011.639548

Neff, K. D., & Germer, C. K. (2012). A pilot study and randomized controlled trial of the Mindful Self-Compassion Program. *Journal of Clinical Psychology.* DOI: 10.1002/jclp.21923

Neff, K. D., Hsieh, Y., & Dejitterat, K. (2005). Self-compassion, achievement goals, and coping with academic failure. *Self and Identity, 4,* 263-287.

Neff, K. D., Kirkpatrick, K., & Rude, S. S. (2007). Self-compassion and its link to adaptive psychological functioning. *Journal of Research in Personality, 41,* 139-154.

Neff, K. D. & McGehee, P. (2010). Self-compassion and psychological resilience among adolescents and young adults. *Self and Identity, 9,* 225-240.

Neff, K. D., & Pommier, E. (2012). The relationship between self-compassion and other-focused concern among college undergraduates, community adults, and practicing meditators. *Self and Identity.* DOI:10.1080/15298868.2011.649546

Neff, K. D., Rude, S. S., & Kirkpatrick, K. (2007). An examination of self-compassion in relation to positive psychological functioning and personality traits. *Journal of Research in Personality, 41,* 908-916.

Neff, K. D., & Vonk, R. (2009). Self-compassion versus global self-esteem: Two different ways of relating to oneself. *Journal of Personality, 77,* 23-50.

Nolen-Hoeksema, S. (1991). Responses to depression and their effects on the duration of depressive episodes. *Journal of Abnormal Psychology, 100,* 569–582.

Porges, S. W. (2007). The polyvagal perspective. *Biological Psychology, 74,* 116-143.

Powers, T., Koestner, R., & Zuroff, D. C. (2007). Self-criticism, goal motivation, and goal progress. *Journal of Social and Clinical Psychology, 25,* 826-840.

Rimes, K. A., & Wingrove, J. (2011). Pilot study of Mindfulness-Based Cognitive Therapy for trainee clinical psychologists. *Behavioural and Cognitive Psychotherapy, 39,* 235-241.

Robins, C. J., Keng, S., Ekblad, A. G., & Brantley, J. G. (2012). Effects of mindfulness-based stress reduction on emotional experience and expression: A randomized controlled trial. *Journal of Clinical Psychology, 68,* 117-131.

Robitschek, C. (1998). Personal growth initiative: The construct and its measure. *Measurement and Evaluation in Counseling and Development, 30,* 183–198.

Rockcliff et al. (2008). A pilot exploration of heart rate variability and salivary cortisol responses to compassion-focused imagery. *Clinical Neuropsychiatry, 5,* 132-139.

Salzberg, S. (1997). *A heart as wide as the world.* Boston: Shambhala.

Sbarra, D. A., Smith, H. L., & Mehl, M. R. (2012). When leaving your ex, love yourself: Observational ratings of self-compassion predict the course of emotional recovery following marital separation. *Psychological Science, 23,* 261-269.

Segal, Z. V., Williams, J. M. G., & Teasdale, J. D. (2001). *Mindfulness-based Cognitive Therapy for Depression: A New Approach to Preventing Relapse.* New York: Guilford Press.

Shapira, L. B., & Mongrain, M. (2010). The benefits of self-compassion and optimism exercises for individuals vulnerable to depression. *The Journal of Positive Psychology, 5*(5), 377-389.

Shapiro, S. L., Astin, J. A., Bishop, S. R., & Cordova, M. (2005). Mindfulness-based stress reduction for health care professionals: Results from a randomized trial. *International Journal of Stress Management, 12,* 164-176.

Shapiro, S. L., Brown, K. W., & Biegel, G. M (2007). Teaching self-care to caregivers: Effects of mindfulness-based stress reduction on the mental health of therapists in training. *Training and Education in Professional Psychology, 1,* 105-115.

Shapiro, S. L., Brown, K., Thoresen, C., & Plante, T. G. (2011). The moderation of mindfulness-based stress reduction effects by trait mindfulness: Results from a randomized controlled trial. *Journal of Clinical Psychology, 67,* 267-277.

Swann, W. B. (1996). *Self-traps: The elusive quest for higher self-esteem.* New York: W. H. Freeman.

Tesser, A. (1999). Toward a self-evaluation maintenance model of social behavior. In R. F. Baumeister (Ed.), *The self in social psychology* (pp. 446-460). New York: Psychology Press.

Tirch, D. (2010). Mindfulness as a context for the cultivation for compassion. *International Journal of Cognitive Psychotherapy. 3,* 113-123.

Törneke, N. (2010). *Learning RFT: An introduction to relational frame theory and its clinical applications.* Oakland, CA: New Harbinger.

Van Dam, N., Sheppard, S. C., Forsyth, J. C., & Earleywine, M. (2011). Self-compassion is a better predictor than mindfulness of symptom severity and quality of life in mixed anxiety and depression. *Journal of Anxiety Disorders, 25,* 123–130.

Vettese, L. C., Dyer, C. E., Li, W. L., & Wekerle, C. (2011). Does self-compassion mitigate the association between childhood maltreatment and later emotional regulation difficulties? A preliminary investigation. *International Journal of Mental Health and Addiction, 9,* 480-491.

Vilardaga, R. (2009). A relational frame theory account of empathy. *The International Journal of Behavioral Consultation and Therapy, 5,* 178-184.

Wang, S. (2005). A conceptual framework for integrating research related to the physiology of compassion and the wisdom of Buddhist teachings. In P. Gilbert

(Ed.), *Compassion: Conceptualizations, research and use in psychotherapy*. New York: Routledge.

Wenzlaff, R. M., & Wegner, D. M. (2000). Thought suppression. In S. T. Fiske (Ed.), *Annual review of psychology* (Vol. 51, pp. 59-91). Palo Alto, CA: Annual Reviews.

Wilson, D. S., Hayes, S. C., Biglan, A., & Embry, D. (in press). Evolving the future: toward a science of intentional change. *Behavioral and Brain Sciences*.

Wilson, D. S., Van Vugt, M., & O'Gorman, R. (2008). Multilevel selection theory and major evolutionary transitions: Implications for psychological science. *Current Directions in Psychological Science*.

Worthington, E. L., O'Connor, L. E., Berry, J. W., Sharp, C., Murray, R., & Yi, E. (2005). Compassion and forgiveness: Implications for psychotherapy. In P. Gilbert (Ed.), *Compassion: Conceptualizations, research and use in psychotherapy* (pp. 168-192). New York: Routledge.

Wren, A. A., Somers, T. J., Wright, M. A., Goetz, M. C., Leary, M. R., Fras, A. M., Huh, B. K., & Rogers, L. L. (2012). Self-compassion in patients with persistent musculoskeletal pain: Relationship of self-compassion to adjustment to persistent pain. *Journal of Pain and Symptom Management, 43*, 759-770.

Yarnell, L. M., Neff, K. D. (2012). Self-compassion, interpersonal conflict resolutions, and wellbeing. *Self and Identity*. DOI:10.1080/15298868.2011.649545.

CHAPTER 5

Perspective Taking

Ian Stewart

National University of Ireland, Galway

Louise McHugh

University College Dublin

Throughout the world, teachers, sociologists, policymakers and parents are discovering that empathy may be the single most important quality that must be nurtured to give peace a fighting chance.

—Arundhati Ray

Introduction

Perspective taking is seen as a crucially important social skill that starts in early infancy and develops throughout childhood and beyond (e.g., Baron-Cohen, 1994). In positive psychology, perspective taking and related phenomena are allotted key theoretical importance. For example, perspective taking itself is one of the 24 key characteristics listed in Peterson and Seligman (2004) and seems related to others including open mindedness, kindness, social intelligence, forgiveness, fairness, and self-control.

But what exactly is perspective taking and how do we cultivate it? Relational frame theory (RFT), a contextual behavioral approach to understanding and influencing language and cognitive processes, can provide new insight into these questions. RFT views perspective taking as a key language-based skill that develops from early ages and underpins the development of several important phenomena including empathy, a sophisticated sense of self, and transcendence. In this chapter, we will discuss RFT research on the development of perspective taking in children and adults, and why it sometimes fails to develop. We will then use a three-level guide to training empathy in the therapeutic context to examine the key role of perspective taking in the development of empathy, the construction of self and other, and the achievement of psychological "transcendence," which functions to maintain empathy in the face of psychological barriers. In doing so, we will explore how RFT can shed light on the development of what are seen by positive psychologists as key personality characteristics and can thus point the way toward a wide variety of positive interventions.

A Relational Frame Approach to Perspective Taking

Until recently most psychological research on perspective taking had been conducted under the rubric of theory of mind (ToM). ToM suggests that perspective taking is based on an ability to mentally represent the mind (e.g., beliefs, desires, intentions, emotions, etc.) of another (e.g., Howlin, Baron-Cohen, & Hadwin, 1999). However, there are fundamental issues that this approach does not address. For instance, questions remain over the functional processes (i.e., those involving environment–behavior contingencies) that make up perspective taking. For example, how does exposure to everyday language allow children to learn to answer and ask questions about their own perspective in relation to that of others?

In contrast with ToM, one of the fundamental assumptions of the RFT approach is the importance of achieving both prediction and influence via the explanation of behavior. The latter requires the specification of manipulable processes as a sine qua non, which affords RFT an advantage at the level of intervention. In what follows, we will briefly introduce RFT as a functional analytic account of key forms of complex human behavior and then describe its conceptualization of perspective taking.

Relational Frame Theory

Relational frame theorists argue, based on several decades of research, that complex human behavior, including language and cognition, can be understood in terms of the learned capacity to relate stimuli under "arbitrary contextual control," referred to as relational framing (see Hayes, Barnes-Holmes, & Roche, 2001). To understand the meaning of arbitrary contextual control, consider this example. Someone tells a child who has never met either of the authors that "Ian is taller than Louise," and when the child is then asked who is shorter she answers "Louise." Her reply is based not on physical relations (she has never met us) but on the arbitrary (based on social convention) contextual cue "taller." She has previously learned to "relationally frame" stimuli in accordance with the relation of comparison in the presence of this cue, and thus when she hears it, she frames Ian and Louise this way and derives that Louise is shorter.

RFT argues that humans learn to relationally frame based on exposure to contingencies of reinforcement in the socioverbal community. In the case of the comparative frame described above, for example, they might initially learn to choose between different physical lengths when asked which is taller or shorter, and eventually this response generalizes so that the contextual cues alone control the response pattern and they can answer appropriately when asked a question such as that involving Ian and Louise. Other relational frames, including same, different, opposite, and so on, are learned in a similar way.

RFT researchers have provided an increasing quantity of empirical evidence showing the diversity of patterns of framing as well as how they can be established and influenced (e.g., Dymond, Roche, DeHouwer, in press). Despite this diversity, all forms of framing have the following three characteristics: mutual entailment (the fundamental bidirectionality of relational responding; for example, if "tall" means "lofty" then "lofty" means "tall"), combinatorial entailment (the combination of already known relations to generate novel relations; for example, if Ian is taller than Louise and Louise is taller than Joe then Ian is taller than Joe and Joe is shorter than Ian), and transformation of stimulus functions (transformation of psychologically relevant functions of a stimulus in accordance with the underlying relation in a given context; for example, if Ian is taller than Joe and I need another basketball player then I might pick Ian over Joe).

From an RFT perspective, once the individual begins to relationally frame through her interactions with the socioverbal community, she will thereafter continue to elaborate the network of objects, words, events, and concepts that are framed for her both overtly (e.g., in conversation with others) and covertly (e.g., in thinking), and the psychological qualities of her environment will be transformed in increasingly complex and diverse ways. Naturally, her own behavior and that of others are a very important part of her world, and thus they also become part of this network of relationally transformed stimuli and indeed become a critically influential part of it. From the RFT point of view, this is the beginning of the repertoire of perspective taking.

RFT and Perspective Taking

Perspective-taking skills are based on "deictic" relational framing, which specifies a relation in terms of the perspective of the speaker (McHugh, Barnes-Holmes, & Barnes-Holmes, 2004). The three frames most important in this regard are I-YOU, HERE-THERE, and NOW-THEN. Acquisition of these frames means learning to differentiate my behavior ("I") from that of others ("YOU") and learning that my current responding is always in this location ("HERE") rather than some other location ("THERE") and always at this time ("NOW") rather than some other time ("THEN").

Deictic frames differ from other frames in at least one important way. As mentioned earlier, other frames have formal or nonarbitrary counterparts that support their development. However, for deictic frames, there are no such easily identifiable nonarbitrary relations available. In this case, the relationship between the individual and other events serves as the constant variable upon which framing is based. For this reason, deictic frames must be taught through demonstration and multiple exemplars of the relational pattern. According to Barnes-Holmes, Hayes, and Dymond (2001, 122), "Abstraction of an individual's perspective on the world, and that of others, requires a combination of a sufficiently well-developed relational repertoire and an extensive history of multiple exemplars that takes advantage of that repertoire." In interactions with the verbal community, the child gradually learns to appropriately respond to and ask questions such as the following: "What are you doing here?" "What am I doing now?" "What will you do there?" The physical environment in which such questions are asked and answered differs across exemplars, but the required relational patterns of I-YOU, HERE-THERE and NOW-THEN are consistent, and thus these patterns are abstracted over time.

The three perspective-taking frames can generate a range of relational networks, including I-Here-Now, You-Here-Now, I-Here-Then, You-Here-Then, I-There-Now, You-There-Now, I-There-Then, and You-There-Then. Many phrases common to our daily discourse are derived from these eight relational networks, for example, "I am here now, but you were here then" or "You were there then, but I am here now." Of course, when used in actual dialogue, these phrases would often include or substitute words coordinated with particular individuals, places, and times, for example, "It is nine o'clock and I [Ian] am at work [Here and Now], but you [Louise] are still at home in bed" [There and Now]. What appears to make perspective-taking frames particularly useful but also complex is that they cannot be defined in terms of particular words. That is, words such as "I," "you," "here," "there," "now," and "then" are merely examples of the relational cues that control the perspective-taking frames, and a range of other words and contextual features may serve the same function. As for all relational frames, what is important is the generalized relational activity, not the topography of particular cues.

Once the deictic frames of I-YOU, HERE-THERE and NOW-THEN are established in a person's behavioral repertoire, they become an inherent property of most verbal events for that person. In this account, when an individual talks to another, it is from the perspective of I located HERE and NOW about events occurring THERE and THEN. Even in the context of the simple greeting "How are you?" for example, I'm asking HERE and NOW about the situation of YOU (the listener) located THERE (a few feet away) and THEN (when you reply). The same analysis applies to situations in which I talk (typically covertly) to myself. If I think to myself "That was stupid," after making a mistake, for example, then I, HERE and NOW am judging myself THERE and THEN (making the error). In summary, deictic frames establish a constant division between the speaker, who is always HERE and NOW, and the spoken about, which is THERE and THEN.

Empirical Support

Evidence supporting the RFT account of perspective taking as deictic relational framing has been accumulating. McHugh, Barnes-Holmes, & Barnes-Holmes (2004) employed a protocol that focused on the three perspective-taking frames (I-YOU, HERE-THERE, and NOW-THEN), in conjunction with three levels of relational complexity (simple, reversed, and double-reversed relations) to provide a developmental profile of the deictic framing skills of individuals across different age groups. Findings indicated a clear developmental trend. Young children (aged 3–5) produced more errors than all of the older age groups (ranging from 6–30). Furthermore, these differences were broadly consistent with the mainstream cognitive-developmental literature that has reported that performances on simple theory of mind tasks generally develop across the ages of four and five years old, and are usually well established by age six.

Further research has examined how deictic relational framing might be involved in a variety of perspective-dependent skills, including false belief understanding and deception. False belief understanding requires the ability to attribute an incorrect belief to another person and to discriminate when he or she is acting on that belief. False belief understanding is seen as an important milestone in cognitive development as well as a prerequisite for understanding deception, which requires the deliberate creation of a false belief in another (e.g., Perner, Leekam, & Wimmer, 1987). McHugh, Barnes-Holmes, Barnes-Holmes, and Stewart (2006) investigated the role of deictic framing in true and false belief understanding, and McHugh, Barnes-Holmes, Barnes-Holmes, Stewart, and Dymond (2007) conducted a relational frame analysis of deception. Both studies showed clear developmental trends in the performances of participants, aged from early childhood to adulthood, that were supported by significant differences in the number of errors between age groups and a decrease in error rates as a function of age.

These studies showed that the relational repertoires required for perspective taking appear to follow a distinct developmental trend. Furthermore, concordant with the pragmatic focus of RFT, a number of more recent studies have used variations on the McHugh et al. (2004) protocol to assess and remediate deficits in perspective-taking framing in young children (e.g., Heagle & Rehfeldt, 2006; Weil, Hayes, & Capurro, 2011). The two studies cited provide evidence not only of the potential for deictic relational frames to be trained but also how training this form of responding might positively affect performance on alternative perspective-taking tasks and in alternative (including real-world) contexts. Heagle and Rehfeldt (2006) taught three typically developing children between the ages of 6 and 11 perspective-taking skills. This study employed a multiple probe design, which is used in low "n" research to demonstrate the efficacy of a particular intervention by showing that improvement is contingent on the introduction of that intervention. Generalization of perspective taking to new stimuli (i.e., in the context of questions referring to novel situations) and real-world conversational topics (i.e., children were asked more ecologically valid conversation type questions) were also tested. All three children were successfully trained on the perspective-taking protocol and performed with high accuracy on the generalization tests. Weil et al. (2011) also used a multiple probe design to train the perspective-taking protocol with three children, aged between 57 and 68 months. Performance on ToM tasks was tested before, during, and after the training of the perspective-taking protocol, and all three children appeared to show improvement.

Another important extension of the RFT approach to perspective-taking is work investigating deficits in deictic framing in clinical populations. Previous research has found that individuals with autistic spectrum disorder (ASD) show deficits on perspective-taking tasks (e.g., Baron-Cohen, Leslie, & Frith, 1985). Hence, Rehfeldt, Dillen, Ziomek, and Kowalchuk (2007) examined deictic relational framing in children with ASD and compared their performance with that of age-matched typically developing counterparts. Findings indicated that the ASD group made more errors on the McHugh et al. protocol, particularly on reversed relation trials. Mainstream research has also demonstrated deficits in perspective taking in individuals with schizophrenia (e.g., Langdon, Coltheart, Ward, & Catts, 2001). Thus, a number of studies have used the McHugh et al. protocol to assess levels of deictic relational responding in this population. For example, Villatte, Monestès, McHugh, Freixa i Baqué, and Loas (2010) showed that schizophrenic patients showed similar performance to controls on simple deictic relations but poorer performance on reversed and double-reversed relations, indicating a specific deficit.

There has also been investigation of deficits in deictic relations in the subclinical condition of social anhedonia. This is a dimension of schizotypy (a measure of normal personality traits linked with schizophrenia) characterized by social disinterest, withdrawal, and lack of pleasure from social contact, which are important predictors of psychosis. For example, Villatte, Monestès, McHugh, Freixa i Baqué, and Loas (2008) compared individuals with high social anhedonia to nonclinical controls on the McHugh protocol. The social anhedonia group were less accurate than controls on the McHugh protocol, specifically on high relational complexity tasks that included an interpersonal perspective (i.e., those including I-YOU and HERE-THERE relations).

Social anhedonia is associated with low levels of interpersonal interaction, and it is possible that this deficit in interpersonal deictic responding is an effect of lack of social interaction. This suggests that the more severe ToM deficits observed in schizophrenia might result from a developmental history predating the start of the diagnosable condition. Other recent RFT-based work has supported this interpretation by providing evidence that social anhedonia scores can be accounted for by deictic framing, empathic concern, and experiential avoidance (Vilardaga, Estévez, Levin, & Hayes, 2012). This work is based on the idea, explored in greater detail further in this chapter, that a number of factors determine social interaction and that these include levels of deictic framing as well as of skills that emerge from the latter including empathy and acceptance. Since RFT suggests how patterns of responding such as this might be changed (i.e., basic deictic framing can be trained and, as will be seen, so too can the more advanced deictic skills required for emotional acceptance), then this work has both indicated important predictors of the clinical condition of schizophrenia and also suggested ways in which this condition might be made less likely.

In summary, results from a number of recent developmental and clinical studies support the RFT account of perspective taking as deictic relational framing. As suggested previously, this account promises useful new insight into perspective taking and related psychological phenomena, including the strengths and virtues that are of interest to positive psychologists. Some of the studies discussed so far that constitute the most direct evidence for this account have already begun to suggest how this promise might be fulfilled. Having reviewed these studies, we will next begin to consider this approach to perspective taking in the context of a slightly more extended theoretical framework that touches on key related psychological phenomena.

Perspective Taking as Deictic Framing: A Three-Level Guide

Vilardaga and Hayes (2009) provide a three-step guide (see Table 1) to fostering the adult clinical psychotherapeutic relationship in terms of deictic relational responding that both constitutes a specific example of the application of the RFT approach to perspective taking in an applied domain and also suggests a more general theoretical model for approaching perspective taking and related phenomena. Step 1 involves basic perspective (deictic relational) training; step 2 involves empathy (transformation of emotional functions via deictic relations) training; and step 3 involves psychological flexibility (self/other as context) training.

Table 1. Three-Level Guide to Perspective Training Perspective Taking as Empathy

Steps	Theory	Example
1. Basic deictic training	Deictic relational frames specify a relation in terms of the perspective of the speaker. The most important frames are I-YOU, HERE-THERE and NOW-THEN. Acquisition of these frames means learning to differentiate my behavior ("I") from that of others ("YOU") and learning that my current responding is always "HERE," not "THERE" and "NOW" not "THEN."	"If I were you, where would I be?" "If I were you and here was there, where would I be?"
2. Empathy training	Empathy involves the transformation of emotional functions via deictic relational frames. In nontechnical terms, we adopt the perspective of others and this allows us to "feel their suffering." This may prompt us to help them; however, if the suffering is too much, we may avoid deictic framing.	"I feel sad. If you were me, how would you feel?"
3. Self/other-as-context	Deictic framing also enables the experience of self/other-as-context, the invariant in all deictic discriminations (i.e., "HERE and NOW"). Self/other-as-context can be thought of as a transcendence of psychological content that allows acceptance of that content. This includes acceptance of painful content produced through empathic responding to the suffering of others, which can support empathic responding.	"I watch thoughts and feelings come and go. Who is it that is watching them?"

Step 1: Basic Deictic Training

Empirical examples of RFT training of perspective taking have been discussed previously. It seems possible that age- or otherwise context-adapted forms of this training in perspective taking might be made available in mainstream educational curricula. In concert with training in other types of relational responding, this would be an important form of general cognitive training. However, training in perspective (deictic) relations would likely have effects that training in other (nondeictic) relations would not, or at least not to the same degree.

For example, we discussed earlier RFT research that has examined true and false belief understanding and the related phenomenon of deception as deictic relational responding. These are important skills for navigation of our social environment. For example, deception, though it has negative connotations, is frequently important in facilitating positive social interaction, for example, lying to protect the feelings of another person. Training the deictic relations underlying these skills might thus increase what positive psychologists might refer to as social intelligence, which in turn is associated with important benefits both to the individual (e.g., having more friends and an improved sense of well-being) and to society (e.g., increasing the likelihood of prosocial behavior and decreasing that of antisocial behavior). Additional basic RFT research will be needed to develop and optimize deictic relational procedures for training those perspective-relevant phenomena already mentioned as well as other more advanced skills such as complex second order perspective taking in which an individual constructs the beliefs that another person has about him/her or a third party (e.g., Perner & Wimmer, 1985). Future applied research might use these procedures to assess and train increasingly advanced deictic relational skills in particular populations and might also track the long-term effects of such training on social functioning.

Training in perspective relations is also relevant with respect to people's ability to manage their own behavior, referred to as self-control. At a basic behavioral level, the "self" involves responding to one's own responding (see, e.g., Skinner, 1974). This concept, which has been empirically modeled in nonhumans (e.g., Lattal, 1975), provides an important foundation for a behavioral approach to the human self but is not enough to capture the complexity of this phenomenon. RFT argues that a critical addition is that the responding to one's responding is verbal—in other words, it involves relational framing and, more specifically, deictic relations (see e.g., Barnes-Holmes, Hayes, and Dymond, 2001). Verbal self-knowledge is potentially important because a verbal description of one's own behavior, and especially the contingencies controlling it, can alter relevant behavioral functions. Self-control, in which an individual ignores immediate urges for self-gratification in order to gain bigger rewards in the longer term, is an obvious example. For instance, in developmental tests of delayed gratification, young children are typically told that they can have one edible reinforcer (e.g., candy) immediately or two if they wait for several minutes. RFT would suggest that a sufficiently verbally advanced child might relationally frame this situation in accordance with IF...THEN frames such that "waiting" is coordinately framed with "more" while "not waiting" is framed with "less." This may make it more likely that they wait. Alternatively, imagine a child who takes the smaller amount anyway. The child's capacity to describe his or her own behavior and to compare it with the alternative (e.g., "I didn't wait and now I have less than I could have gotten") may well make the candy less reinforcing through transformation of function.

This kind of basic self-control probably does not, strictly speaking, require deictic relations. It does require certain relational frames (e.g., coordination, temporality, and comparison), as well as transformation of functions through these, but deictic relations are not essential. Nevertheless, there is evidence that self-control improves with age, and this may be due to improved deictic relational responding. As such deictic relational training focusing in particular on NOW-THEN relations might be particularly relevant for improving this kind of self-control. Research reviewed earlier (e.g., McHugh et al., 2004) suggested that transformation of functions through temporal deictic (NOW-THEN) relations may emerge later than transformation of functions through I-YOU or HERE-THERE relations. One extrapolation from this that might be relevant to the self-control issue is that very young children might not respond to the future "I" or past "I" in the same way they respond to the present "I." This is supported by research indicating that it is only by age four that children begin to develop a concept of self extended into the future. As suggested above it might not be essential for self-control that deictic relational responding be present; however, it might arguably bolster this phenomenon if a child could respond to his or her future self more similarly to the way in which he or she responds to his or her present self so that a choice between less for the present "I" and more for the future "I" might be more likely to result in a self-controlled rather than an impulsive response. Future RFT research might examine the developmental trajectory of temporal deictic relations in more detail and assess the effect of training such relations, particularly with regard to the outcome of self-control.

Step 2: Empathy Training

Step 2 of the Vilardaga and Hayes (2009) guide involves empathy training. Empathy has been defined as the ability to understand and share another person's emotional state (e.g., Hoffmann, 2000). In general, it is thought to promote positive behavior such as helping and to prevent or reduce antisocial behavior, including aggression and delinquency. In addition, empathy is likely an important element in such virtues as kindness, fairness, and forgiveness.

From an RFT point of view, empathy involves the transformation of emotional functions via deictic relational frames. This account suggests a developmental sequence, including several learning processes (e.g., Valdivia-Salas, Luciano, Gutierrez-Martinez, & Visdomine, 2009). Typically developing children learn to discriminate and label emotional states, and they derive label-state coordination relations (e.g., "I am afraid" becomes coordinated with feelings of fear). Perspective-taking relations are also implicated in the development of such understanding; for example, responding is always from the perspective of I-HERE-NOW, while comparisons can be made with experiences in the past (I-THERE-THEN). Learning to verbally discriminate one's own emotions in this way is one key element in the development of empathy. A second is learning to verbally discriminate the emotions of another. One aspect of this is being able to discriminate and label signs of emotion in others. Once the child begins to correctly discriminate emotions in others, then transfer of function via relations of coordination between names of emotions and particular feelings and thoughts will help to support the subsequent development of transformation of function via deictic relations, the core response required. To directly train and strengthen the latter, multiple exemplar training might be provided, as suggested by Vilardaga and Hayes (2009), by using questions such as "If you were in her place, how would you feel?" After the empathic response is established, further work may be needed to support particular patterns of responding beyond the felt emotion. For example, the child might need to be taught how best to help the other person. In addition, he or she might need to be taught to track rules linking helping behavior with relatively delayed consequences (e.g., "If you help your sister then she'll be happier and the whole family will enjoy the day more").

The above sequence constitutes a possible guide for purposes of research and training in applied arenas. One possible area of relevance is bullying. Sutton, Smith, and Swettenham (1999) argue that bullying among children or adolescents often takes place in a complex social context involving jostling for power among members of a bullying gang in which there is a need by the lead bully to maintain social allegiance by members and that in such interactions, advanced perspective-taking skills are needed at least by the leader. In addition, indirect methods of bullying involving social exclusion and rumormongering would also seem to require well-developed perspective taking. Despite the latter, however, bullies show low levels of empathy. In some rare cases (i.e., individuals classified as having "antisocial personality disorder") there may be genetic abnormalities causing extremely low levels of emotional distress that allow little or no transformation of aversive emotional functions through deictic relations. Such individuals may be incapable of sharing the distress of another and thus difficult or impossible to treat, at least with respect to the possibility of instilling empathy. However, most often there are probably other reasons levels of empathy on the part of bullies are relatively low, such as particular patterns of relational framing with respect to self or other by these individuals in the bullying context or more broadly that make the transformation of functions less likely. For example, perhaps the bully feels emotion but deliberately suppresses it to avoid losing others' respect.

Individuals with autistic spectrum and other developmental disorders may also show extreme lack of empathy. In this case, the primary cause is deficits in relational framing, especially deictic relational framing, which may therefore need to be trained using procedures such as those described earlier in this chapter. Once this repertoire is in place further emotion-relevant training will be needed to properly establish the transformation of emotional functions via deictic relations; however, such training will be more similar to that needed for other populations.

As just suggested, when either perspective taking or the capacity for transformation of emotional functions through deictic relations is absent, training these repertoires can improve empathy. However, even where they are present, empathy is not guaranteed. There are a number of possible reasons transformation of emotional functions might be weakened or absent, leading to a failure of empathy; however, at a purely functional level, they all involve similar issues for which the Vilardaga and Hayes (2009) guide recommends a similar type of intervention. The latter is based on RFT and on Acceptance Commitment Therapy (ACT; Hayes, Wilson, & Strosahl, 2011), a form of RFT-congruent psychological therapy. Critical to ACT and to the intervention suggested by Vilardaga and Hayes (2009) are RFT-based conceptions of self and other that develop via deictic relational responding. In the next section, we explain these concepts.

Step 3: Self-Other Transcendence

Step 3 of the Vilardaga and Hayes (2009) guide involves deictic "self-as-context" training regarding one's own private events. This concept, which is central to Acceptance Commitment Therapy, is based on the RFT approach to self. RFT suggests that, in combination with an extended relational repertoire, perspective taking can establish three functionally different types of self. These are self as content, self as process, and self as context (Hayes, 1995).

SELF-AS-CONTENT

Self-as-content (conceptualized self) consists of elaborate descriptive and evaluative relational networks that a person constructs about himself and his history over time (e.g., "I am a husband and father. I'm a bit standoffish. I love baseball and am a big fan of the Atlanta Braves"). Self-evaluations are always made HERE and NOW about our behaviors that occur THERE and THEN. However, we rarely attend to the process of interpreting and evaluating as it happens in the present moment. Difficulties occur when products of relational responding (e.g., thoughts, beliefs, judgments) are treated as objectively true and inherent aspects of the real world, a process referred to within ACT as *cognitive fusion*. This can be problematic when self-evaluations come to appear as historically

121

rooted and unchangeable; our stories may become rigid and ossified and no longer simply describe our past behavior but also guide future behavior in directions that maintain the coherence of the story.

SELF-AS-PROCESS

Self-as-process (knowing self) is the ongoing verbal discrimination of psychological events as they occur (e.g., "I feel sad"). The knowing self feeds the conceptualized self (e.g., If I discriminate that I frequently feel sad then I may describe myself as "a depressed person") and is also necessary to contact the transcendent self since a self-monitoring repertoire is required to observe the observer.

The knowing self is extremely useful in behavioral regulation both for the socioverbal community and for the person him- or herself. It allows others to predict a person's behavior without knowledge of his or her learning history. For example, if someone says that she feels angry then this allows a level of prediction of her behavior. Self-as-process is also critical in the psychological development of the individual. In order to respond effectively to one's own responding, one must first be aware of the response and its impact. For example, understanding and responding to my thoughts and feelings about other people's behavior in a fluid and flexible manner is critical for establishing personal relationships.

Self-as-process may be underdeveloped if there is inadequate training by the verbal community, such as when awareness and expression of emotions, thoughts, and sensation are punished, ignored, denied, or contradicted, as is often observed in the case of child neglect or abuse. Weak self-knowledge may also be the result of experiential avoidance, the tendency to avoid or escape aversive experiences. Chronic experiential avoidance results in the difficulty observing and describing one's thoughts, emotions, and sensations seen in disorders such as depression for example.

SELF-AS-CONTEXT

Self-as-context (transcendent self) is the invariant in all self-discriminations. If someone answers many different questions about himself and his behavior, then the only aspect of his answering that will be consistent across time is the context from which the answer is given, that is, "I, HERE and NOW." Since self-as-context is an abstraction from the content of verbal responding it is "content-less" and thus constant and unchanging from when it first emerges (i.e., without content there is nothing that could change). It is itself a product of verbal responding, yet as a verbal category that applies to everything that a person has ever done it incorporates both the nonverbal self (as behavioral stream resulting from direct psychological processes) as well as the verbal self (as both object and process of knowledge gained through relational framing) and can thus provide the experiential link between nonverbal and verbal self-knowledge.

Self-as-context is often referred to as the transcendent self, because it is difficult to describe or contact verbally, even though it is a product of relational framing. It cannot be experienced as an object because experiencing it would necessitate adopting a perspective on it that was not one's own perspective, which is impossible. Hence, it is not thing-like and thus can be described as limitless, unchanging, and ever present. For these reasons, it is often linked with spiritual and religious concepts and experiences.

The self-as-context has important implications for how humans experience and regulate psychological pain since this sense of self is not threatened by aversive content in the way that the conceptualized or knowing selves can be. It allows a person to confront deep emotional pain and facilitates willingness, compassion, and intimacy. This characteristic makes this concept of central importance from an ACT point of view.

THE VERBAL OTHER

RFT suggests that just as perspective taking can establish three functionally distinct types of self, it can also establish three distinct types of other, namely, other-as-content, other-as-process and other-as-context (Hayes, 1995). Other-as-content is the verbal construction of the listener. For example, we might assume different things about a new acquaintance we knew to be religious than one we knew to be atheist; in other words, we might verbally construct a different listener in each case and approach certain topics differently on that basis. Other-as-process is also a verbal construction but a more fluid one because in this case, we construct the reactions of the other on a moment-by-moment basis. This tends to happen in conversations as we verbally construct how the other person is reacting to us, especially in more personal conversations in which the person is more likely to reveal his or her feelings (e.g., "I'm a little disappointed to hear you say that"). Other-as-context (the transcendent other) is relatively uncommon, occurring when the speaker is psychologically connected to the listener as a purely conscious person. Transcendence is always experienced as "HERE and NOW" and thus at this level speaker and listener are one, since "HERE and NOW" cannot be more than one event by definition. As such, self-as-context is automatically linked with the transcendent other, and thus the term "self-other-as-context" or "transcendent self-other" can be used to describe this perspective.

SELF AND THE FAILURE OF EMPATHY

This RFT analysis of the construction of self and other can be used to understand and suggest remediation for different examples of the failure of transformation of function via deictic relations (i.e., of empathic responding). One example is when there is such strong fusion with a particular conceptualized self that events tend to be universally framed in terms of their relevance to this self (e.g., narcissistic personality disorder) and thus taking the perspective of another is made less likely. In other cases, transformation of function results in such distress that it produces not sympathy for the other but self-concern (see, e.g., Eisenberg, 2000) and thus the result, once again, is the absence of overt empathic responding. This has been offered as an explanation for lack of empathy in some cases of children and adolescents with disruptive behavior disorder. It may also be relevant with respect to professionals dealing with others' distress, who due to avoidance of excessive emotional distress lose empathy for clients and even experience burnout. In addition to these cases in which transformation of emotional functions via deictic relations is reduced due to psychological processes that are relevant for particular individuals more than others, there are also a number of contextual variables that may make empathic responding more or less likely for any individual. These include similarity between observer and observed, familiarity, social dispositions, cooperative versus competitive context, and how much the observer likes the observed.

From an ACT perspective, all the examples just given involve a degree of fusion with private content that makes empathic responding less likely. The first example involves strong fusion with a particular self-conception to the extent that the other is less salient, while the contextual variables listed at the end of the paragraph all pertain to fusion with particular conceptions of self as being in opposition with other. The other case suggests that fusion with rules dictating experiential avoidance is playing a part. It is to counteract fusion with covert responding such as seen in these examples that in the third level of their guide Vilardaga and Hayes (2009) suggest an intervention to train self/other-as-context in which a therapist has to move flexibly between imagining herself as her client and as herself at different times and in different situations. Their suggestion is aimed at psychotherapists but is likely to be helpful for other situations in which there is a lack of empathy (the differences between the various examples given warrant empirical research, but the process targeted by Vilardaga and Hayes is common to all). From this transcendent perspective in which unhelpful transformations of function in accordance with particular rules (e.g., "I need to be perfect" or "I cannot stand this distress" or "I don't like this person") are made less likely, choosing to act in accordance with values so that responding has the quality of compassion for self and/or empathy for the other becomes possible.

Deictic relations and transformation of function through deictic relations represent potentially fruitful approaches to the domains of perspective taking and empathy, respectively. The newly introduced concept of the three senses of self and other, which is rooted in the concept of deictic relations, also provides interesting avenues for research and practical purposes. Regarding the current context, all of the aforementioned constitutes an important foundation for future empirical analysis of key patterns of complex human behavior in which positive psychologists and others concerned to understand the human condition and maximize human potential are interested.

Conclusion

Positive psychology aims to "achieve a scientific understanding and effective interventions to build thriving in individuals, families, and communities" (Seligman & Csikszentmihalyi, 2000, p. 13). Contextual behavioral science, which includes both RFT and ACT, is an empirically based and practically oriented approach to psychology that has begun to provide new insights into the behavioral origins of key categories of behavior in which positive psychologists are interested. Perspective taking is one such category and is particularly important since it is closely linked with several others including open mindedness, kindness, social intelligence, forgiveness, fairness, self-control, and spirituality. In this chapter we presented the contextual behavioral and more specifically RFT approach to perspective taking. This practically oriented, "bottom up" analysis will hopefully help to facilitate the scientific understanding and effective interventions with respect to these phenomena that positive psychologists seek.

References

Barnes-Holmes, D., Hayes, S. C., & Dymond, S. (2001). Self and self-directed rules. In S. C. Hayes, D. Barnes-Holmes, & B. Roche (Eds.), *Relational frame theory: A post-Skinnerian account of human language and cognition* (pp. 119-139). New York: Plenum.

Baron-Cohen, S. (1994). How to build a baby that can read minds: Cognitive mechanisms in mind reading. *Cahiers de Psychologie Cognitive, 13*, 513–552.

Baron-Cohen, S., Leslie, A. M., & Frith, U. (1985). Does the autistic child have a "theory of mind"? *Cognition, 21*, 37-46.

Dymond, S., Roche, B., & De Houwer, J. In press. *Advances in Relational Frame Theory: Research and Application*. Oakland, CA: New Harbinger.

Eisenberg, N. (2000). Empathy and sympathy. In M. Lewis & J. M. Haviland-Jones (Eds.), *Handbook of emotions* (677-691). New York: Guilford Press.

Hayes, S., Barnes-Holmes, D., & Roche, B. (2001). *Relational frame theory: A post-skinnerian account of human language and cognition*. New York: Plenum.

Hayes, S. C. (1995). Knowing selves. *The Behavior Therapist, 18*, 94-96.

Hayes, S. C., Strosahl, K., & Wilson, K. G. (2011). *Acceptance and Commitment Therapy: The process and practice of mindful change* (2nd ed.). New York: Guilford Press.

Heagle, A. I., & Rehfeldt, R. A. (2006). Teaching perspective-taking skills to typically developing children through derived relational responding. *Journal of Early and Intensive Behavior Intervention, 3*(1), 1–34.

Hoffman, M. L. (2000). *Empathy and moral development: Implications for caring and justice*. New York: Cambridge University Press.

Howlin, P., Baron-Cohen, S., & Hadwin, J. (1999). *Teaching children with autism to mind-read: A practical guide*. Chichester: Wiley.

Langdon, R., Coltheart, M., Ward, P., & Catts, S. (2001). Visual and cognitive perspective-taking impairments in schizophrenia: A failure of allocentric simulation? *Cognitive Neuropsychiatry, 6*(4), 241-269.

Lattal, K. A. (1975). Reinforcement contingencies as discriminative stimuli. *Journal of the Experimental Analysis of Behavior, 23*, 241-246.

McHugh, L., Barnes-Holmes, D., Barnes-Holmes, Y., Stewart, I., & Dymond, S. (2007). Deictic relational complexity and the development of deception. *The Psychological Record, 57*, 517-531.

McHugh, L., Barnes-Holmes, Y., & Barnes-Holmes, D. (2004) Perspective-taking as relational responding: A developmental profile. *The Psychological Record, 54*, 115-144.

McHugh, L., Barnes-Holmes, Y., Barnes-Holmes, D., & Stewart, I. (2006). False belief as generalised operant behavior. *The Psychological Record, 56*, 341-364.

Perner, J., Leekam, S., & Wimmer, H. (1987) Three year olds' difficulty with false belief. The case for a conceptual deficit. *British Journal of Developmental Psychology, 5*, 125-137.

Perner J., & Wimmer, H. (1985). "John thinks that Mary thinks that…" Attribution of second-order beliefs by 5- to 10-year-old children. *Journal of Experimental Child Psychology, 39*, 437–471.

Peterson, C., & Seligman, M. E. P. (2004). *Character strengths and virtues: A handbook and classification.* Washington, D.C.: APA Press and Oxford University Press.

Rehfeldt, R., Dillen, J. E., Ziomek, M. M., & Kowalchuck, R. (2007). Assessing relational learning deficits in perspective-taking in children with high-functioning Autism Spectrum Disorder. *The Psychological Record, 57*, 23-47.

Seligman, M. E. P., & Csikszentmihalyi, M. (2000). Positive psychology: An introduction. *American Psychologist, 55*, 5-14.

Skinner, B. F. (1974). *About behaviorism.* New York: Vintage.

Sutton, J., Smith, P. K., Swettenham, J. (1999). Social cognition and bullying: Social inadequacy or skilled manipulation? *British Journal of Developmental Psychology, 17*(3), 435-450.

Valdivia-Salas, S., Luciano, C., Gutierrez-Martinez, O., & Visdomine, C. (2009). Establishing empathy. In R, A. Rehfeldt & Y. Barnes-Holmes. (Eds.), *Derived relational responding applications for learners with autism and other developmental disabilities.* Oakland, CA: New Harbinger.

Vilardaga, R., Estévez, A., Levin, M. E., & Hayes, S. C. (2012). Deictic relational responding, empathy and experiential avoidance as predictors of social anhedonia: Further contributions from relational frame theory. *The Psychological Record, 62*, 409-432.

Vilardaga, R., & Hayes, S. C. (2009). Experiential avoidance and superstition: Considering concepts in context. *Philosophy, Psychiatry, and Psychology, 15* (3), 269-271.

Villatte, M., Monestès, J. L., McHugh, L., Freixa i Baqué, E., & Loas, G. (2008). Assessing perspective taking in schizophrenia using Relational Frame Theory. *The Psychological Record, 60*, 413-424.

Villatte, M., Monestès, J. L., McHugh, L., Freixa i Baqué, E., & Loas, G. (2010). Adopting the perspective of another in belief attribution: Contribution of Relational Frame Theory to the understanding of impairments in schizophrenia. *Journal of Behavior Therapy and Experimental Psychiatry, 41*, 125-134.

Weil, T. M., Hayes, S. C., & Capurro, P. (2011). Establishing a deictic relational repertoire in young children. *The Psychological Record, 61*, 371-390.

CHAPTER 6

Committed Action

Lance M. McCracken, PhD

Health Psychology Section, Psychology Department, Institute of Psychiatry, King's College London

S ometimes the quality of the actions we take renders them unsuccessful. We are able to recognize some of these qualities when they happen, at least some of the time. These are called half-hearted, pig-headed, tentative, oblivious, passive, unmotivated, giving up, and so forth. There are also some qualities of action that may unexpectedly carry risks for failure. These are called perfect, cautious, knowing, and "just do it." This short chapter considers a quality of effective action, a quality emphasized in Acceptance and Commitment Therapy (ACT; Hayes, Strosahl, & Wilson, 2012), a quality called "committed." Within a framework of positive psychology, committed action falls in the "engaged life" domain and part of what might be called "wise deployment of strengths," or even "perseverance" (Duckworth, Steen, & Seligman, 2005), although here this is a particular kind of perseverance, as will be seen. The objective in this chapter is to examine some of the qualities actions can have, clarify action that is committed from action that is not, and briefly discuss methods for shaping committed action. Chronic pain is used as an example condition here, as it presents some classic threats to effective action that can be neutralized by shaping a flexible committed quality.

ACT and the broader positive psychology approach sometimes differ in how they conceptualize and frame the focus of assessment and study. In ACT it might be more common to say that behavior has certain qualities or functions, while in positive psychology it might be more common to speak of traits or qualities of the person. At the same time it has been argued that it is not enough to simply focus on positive traits and personal characteristics, that traits are not inherently positive or negative, and that it is important to understand the conditions under which different traits enhance or reduce well-being (McNulty & Fincham, 2011). Certainly when positive psychology approaches are more sensitive to context they are also more consistent with ACT. In any case, it is just to say that these approaches are both different in some ways and at the same time compatible. Here committed action will be presented not as a quality of a person, although it is a capacity that a person can enhance. It will be defined as a quality of action that is contextually determined both in its committed quality and in its effectiveness for the goals at hand.

The Problem with Pacing

"Pacing" is a traditional treatment method in rehabilitation and chronic pain management since at least the 1970s. Pacing is also a quality of action, as being discussed here. The problem with pacing is that, despite its immediate appeal and its long history, there seems to be little evidence that it is helpful for chronic pain or for other conditions such as chronic fatigue (see White et al., 2011). In fact, in a recent review of pacing the authors concluded that as a treatment method for chronic pain it "lacks consensus of definition and a demonstrable evidence base" (Gill & Brown, 2009). In this chapter "pacing" will be looked at as an approach to behavior change and improved functioning that is common sense, and even sensible, yet limited. Committed action is proposed here as a better approach.

Pacing has great surface appeal. "Just right" sits between too hot and too cold. People are often drawn away from extremes to the middle, the medium, or the balanced. No doubt this springs in part from success we can achieve from aiming toward the middle some of the time. Our culture is filled with slogans and phrases that reinforce this experience of the "happy medium" or the "middle of the road," or "work-life balance," for instance. Indeed food is better if it is neither too hot nor too cold. Experience and ideas like these are, likely, part of the impetus behind "pacing."

Setting aside that pacing possibly "lacks consensus of definition," let's take just one meaning of the term. According to the ordinary daily use of the term, "pacing" means to set or regulate the rate of an activity, particularly so that an activity can be continued without needing to stop. In chronic pain treatment settings pacing is contrasted with "avoidance" and what is variously called "overactivity cycling," "overactivity-underactivity cycling," "boom and bust," and so forth. Once again, pacing is trying to be somewhere between doing too little, almost all of the time, and doing too much, at least intermittently. Pacing methods teach patients to break up activities into pieces, to use rest breaks, to slow down, to use switching of tasks, and to do what is called the "3 Ps," "prioritize, plan, and pace." It all sounds reasonable, but when these patterns of activity are studied it is typically found that they are associated more with patterns of avoidance, distress, and disability than with patterns of healthy engagement and positive well-being (McCracken & Samuel, 2007). In some studies such patterns seem simply to bear no relation to daily functioning (Karsdorp & Vlaeyen, 2009), which of course should not be the case if they are meant to serve the improvement of daily functioning. Here the "happy medium" in activity seems not to be the answer, but how does that happen?

One of the problems with pacing is that it derives mainly from common sense and not from a deep understanding of how behavior is actually coordinated. As a method based in common sense, training in pacing probably does not typically appreciate the complexity of the behavior change challenge it is trying to tackle. In a sense common sense is not enough. One problem not appreciated is the strength and durability of influences on behavior that coordinate avoidance. For example, if people suffering chronic pain are fearful and avoidant, instructions and reassurance are unlikely to change that in many cases (Linton, McCracken, & Vlaeyen, 2008). More potent and precise methods are needed. Attempting to alter surface features of behavior, however it is structured, such as in rate and pattern over time, may do nothing to undermine the influence of feelings of pain, fear, and anxiety, and the content of thoughts. And, in people who are seeking treatment for chronic pain and pain-related disability it is virtually assured that their thoughts harbor avoidant influences. To say it another way, attempts to impose a new structure of behavior on top of a pattern designed to reduce pain and fear may fail unless there is a focus in treatment on first disintegrating the existing pattern of behavior and its coordinating situations. That means going to the root of what is supporting the existing behavior with effective treatments, such as exposure-based methods in the case of fear and avoidance. It also means using methods to decrease the dominating influences carried in thought content and, essentially, the "stories" we live in, stories about pain, pain management, and ourselves. In ACT terms these processes require methods designed to enhance acceptance or openness, and cognitive defusion, the ability to contact experience outside of our own thoughts about these experiences.

Anyone who has set a goal, sought the goal, and then screwed up, what we can call the "three Ss," already has the direct experience that tinkering with surface features of behavior patterns, even if done with great conviction, does not create success all of the time. Other ongoing influences on behavior, and particularly durable and potentially overwhelming influences, such as those based in cognitive content, remain in control.

Another problem with pacing is that it makes a distinction in behavior that may not in all cases be a psychologically relevant one. In the conceptual frame of pacing there is a distinction made between avoidance and "overdoing it." It seems reasonable to do this because they seem in some ways to be opposites. However this may obscure important similarities. If you notice how patterns of overdoing it unfold, you see that these patterns have more in common with avoidance than it at first appears. If a pattern of high rate of activity leading to subsequent pain increase and then disrupted functioning happens consistently, there is probably some refusal or avoidance of feelings happening before the point that feelings of pain overwhelm other possible influences. Perhaps there is an ignoring of limits or an unwillingness to experience an activity in a way that needs to be modified to accommodate the pain. Perhaps if there was greater awareness and openness to this pain, that could allow more effective functioning and guide a behavior pattern with more flexible persistence. If I develop an ache in my Achilles tendon as I run, I can ignore it, and it may eventually ache more. I can also pay closer attention to it, shorten my stride, and experience that it is possible to keep running as the ache eases, or I may slow down or stop.

Certainly whenever a person with chronic pain consistently repeats a course of action that leads inevitably to the same unwanted result, such as with a high rate of activity that leads to isolation and inactivity, then this pattern reflects psychological inflexibility by definition. So in the context of pain, both overdoing it and avoidance can function as avoidance and can reflect psychological inflexibility. Both can lack openness, have qualities of disconnection with direct experience, and may not serve goals and values.

Open and Aware: Helpful and Not Enough

ACT is a broadly applicable approach to helping people change. It includes some highly effective and now increasingly well-known methods for helping people to open up to their experiences, get out of their thinking, and connect with the present and their values (Hayes, Strohsal, & Wilson, 2012). Its apparently best known process, acceptance, is such an appealing and obviously applicable process for chronic pain that, of all the processes from ACT, it has prompted the most study and integrated itself the most into clinical service developments. Based on its immediate appeal, there were published data on acceptance of pain as early as the 1990s (McCracken, 1998). It was eight years later before studies broadened their focus and finally yielded published data on another one of the ACT processes, values (McCracken & Yang, 2006). Only in recent years have studies finally addressed such processes as "contact with the present moment," and cognitive defusion in chronic pain (McCracken, Gutiérrez-Martínez, & Smyth, 2012), processes which, along with acceptance, constitute the mindfulness-based processes within ACT.

The part of the ACT model that seems most neglected, certainly in chronic pain research, is the part called "committed action." Possibly naively, it seems that most research groups have failed to focus much treatment development work on the *action* component of ACT. We instead pursued a focus on helping people open up to their experiences, get out of their thoughts and beliefs, and connect to their present experience and values. In retrospect, the implicit assumption in all of this was that healthy behavior would emerge from there. If one pursues this route, in training or in providing treatment, there is an interesting result that can happen. You see that it is possible to create the capacity for openness, defusion, and connection with values, without a great deal of action. A piece is missing. In a sense we were taking a focus on mindfulness but without enough of a focus on action.

As far as we know there are no standardized measures of "committed action" as such. Yet, in order to further study committed action and to clarify its role with the wider process of psychological flexibility, means for measuring and tracking committed action are needed.

Commitment Is Not a Mental Act

In everyday usage "commitment" seems to imply a pledge, a state of mental conviction, or a devotion toward a particular goal or even something more abstract, such as a principle or belief. In fact this everyday sense of the term includes a trap, one that can block us from actually doing committed action. In the everyday sense of the word, doing or following a commitment seems to require a strength of mental devotion—hence, no mental devotion = no doing.

In ACT, committed action is "a values-based action that occurs at a particular moment in time and that is deliberately linked to creating a pattern of action that serves the value" (Hayes et al., 2012, p. 328). Hence, three important features of committed action within ACT are that it is situated in the here and now, not in the future; it is linked specifically to values; and it is action. So in contrast with pacing that focuses on future planning of features of action like rate, duration, and scheduling of breaks, the use of rest, and so forth, with pain as a guiding experience, committed action explicitly focuses on the present moment with values as a guiding experience.

In an attempt to reverse the absence of any focus in research into the process of committed action our research group recently began to develop an instrument to measure it. We have done this within a clinical setting of chronic pain management. Once again the purpose here is to one day show that committed action may be a better way than pacing to consider the activation side of chronic pain treatment. Taking the definition of committed action from ACT as the starting point, we created a pool of items intended to reflect committed action and to form the basis for a measure. Translating the items into a measure would next require that we obtain data with them and submit the items to scale analyses and validation. Table 1 includes examples of the items we created. What may be useful about these items in the context of this chapter is that they are at least a preliminary attempt to discriminate committed action from patterns that are not committed. They are exemplars of these classes, and they also give some insight into how one might begin a process of creating a new measure in an area where there is currently no such measure.

Table 1: Sample items from a preliminary instrument to assess committed action.

Positively Keyed Committed Action Items

- I am able to persist with a course of action after experiencing difficulties.
- When I fail in reaching a goal, I can change how I approach it.
- When a goal is difficult to reach, I am able to take small steps to reach it.
- I prefer to change how I approach a goal rather than quit.
- I am able to follow my long-term plans including times when progress is slow.
- When I make commitments, I can both stick to them and change them.
- I am able to pursue my goals both when this feels easy and when it feels difficult.
- I am able to persist in what I am doing or to change what I am doing depending on what helps me reach my goals.
- I am able to let go of goals that I repeatedly experience as unreachable.
- I am able to incorporate discouraging experiences into the process of pursuing my long-term plans.
- I am able to accept failure as part of the experience of doing what is important in my life.
- I can accept my limitations and adjust what I do accordingly.

Negatively Keyed Committed Action Items

- If I experience pain from something I do, I will avoid it no matter what it costs me.

- I act impulsively when I feel under pressure.

- When I fail to achieve what I want to do, I make a point to never do that again.

- I approach goals in an "all-or-nothing" fashion.

- I get stuck doing the same thing over and over even if I am not successful.

- I find it difficult to carry on with an activity unless I experience that it is successful.

- I am more likely to be guided by what I feel than by my goals.

- If I make a commitment and later fail to reach it, I then drop the commitment.

- If I feel distressed or discouraged, I let my commitments slide.

- I get so wrapped up in what I am thinking or feeling that I cannot do the things that matter to me.

- If I cannot do something my way, I will not do it at all.

Goal-Setting and Committed Action

One of the most straightforward and familiar methods for creating patterns of committed action is within the context of goal setting. If goal setting is done in a way designed to organize the participant's actions so they are practical, present-focused, values-directed, and part of an extended pattern of behavior integrated into daily functioning, then it entails committed action. Within ACT, goal setting and committed action methods are connected to values, as already mentioned. Importantly, these methods are also supplemented with methods to increase acceptance and cognitive defusion. This is needed, as potential barriers, in the form of thoughts and feelings, are essentially inevitable in any pattern of values-based action. Table 2 briefly summarizes an approach to committed action through goal setting based on Luoma, Hayes, and Walser (2007).

Table 2: Steps for Enhancing Committed Action

The following outline is a brief guide for how to enhance committed action in the context of goal setting and using methods from Acceptance and Commitment Therapy.

1. Identify relevant high-priority values domains and develop an action plan.

2. Help the patient commit to and take action.

3. Attend to and meet barriers to action with willingness, defusion, contact with the present, and self-as-observer skills.

4. Generalize to larger patterns of action and to wider situations over time.

Goal setting can sometimes feel like a mechanical or didactic process. One way to enhance it is to incorporate experiential components. For example, mental imagery and eyes-closed exercises can be done to investigate and manipulate some of the psychological experiences that play a part in reaching or blocking goals. A specific example follows:

Exercise

First, do appropriate preparations, provide some guidance on characteristics of useful goals (i.e., specific, measurable, attainable, relevant, and time limited), and then have participants sit with eyes closed and focus on your instructions. Next ask them to imagine a goal they have, to picture what it would be like to achieve it, and then ask them to notice what happens as they do that, pausing appropriately. Typically, participants say it feels good to do this—whatever they say is okay at this point. If there is some discussion, it might focus on how in modern Western cultures in particular a strategy of visualizing our goal is often believed to enhance our ability to reach our goals. In fact, when this is studied, it seems that all it does is help us feel better without moving us significantly closer to reaching our goals.

The next phase of the exercise begins with the same visualization task, but then ask the participants to do two additional tasks, first to identify a concrete action they could take in the next two days to pursue their goal, and, when that is done, to watch what happens in their experience when it is said that they have to DO this action, that it is now required. Typically at this point, participants will have any number of thoughts or feelings that essentially "say" this is not possible or that seem to present barriers. They are simply asked at this point to notice and identify their barriers for further examination later.

Discussion following the focus on the experience of both thinking about a goal and doing an action can examine whether participants notice that this seems to be how it works: fantasizing feels good, but getting closer to needing to do something automatically creates apparent barriers. Further discussion might focus on how evidence shows that goals are more likely to be reached if specific actions are planned, potential barriers identified, and methods for dealing with those barriers planned and practiced. Acceptance, defusion, or self-as-observer exercises could be practiced directly with any psychological content that may have emerged during the "now it's time to do it" part of the exercise.

A next phase of this exercise could include identifying a specific goal and asking for a public commitment to be done to support it. This public commitment capitalizes on a final empirically supported goal-setting method, and also provides an additional opportunity to catch, identify, and deal skillfully with potential barriers.

Of course in the end the purpose of committed action methods is to create patterns of committed action that are inherently reinforcing, integrate into daily life, and generalize into different domains of daily functioning. In a sense a verbal statement out loud is itself a kind of committed action as are the actions of making a plan for following, and yet these fall short of the whole pattern of action as it might be specified in a goal.

The final phase of committed action work, if there ever is such a phase, is when patterns of action that are values based and goals reaching are being done persistently and flexibly as ongoing actions. This inevitably means that patients engage in these between sessions and the therapist and patient either observe that these qualities are being achieved or continue to address the stumbling blocks that happen until they are.

Summary

Committed action is action that is present focused, linked to values, and part of a pattern of larger activity that similarly serves one's values. It is sometimes referred to as choosing and choosing again. It is not primarily a kind of pledge for the future. It is a way to create flexible persistence where the behavior pattern might otherwise have the quality of choose, experience an unwanted result, and give up. As it is values based and action oriented it is akin to the domain of "the engaged life" in current conceptual frameworks of positive psychology (Duckworth et al., 2005).

Committed action toward goals that we care about inevitably leads to potential barriers in the form of feelings and thoughts, and this is when methods in ACT that enhance acceptance and cognitive defusion can be very useful. In an overall pattern of successful committed action, thought and feelings, experience of failure, and so forth are not things to be avoided; they are things to be incorporated as part and parcel of the whole pattern of action.

An example was chosen for analysis here; this is the method of training in pacing that is done almost universally in pain management centers that employ psychological methods. Accepting that there can be different meanings of the word *pacing* and a range of methods focused on the same, there is nonetheless a lesson to learn from the approach of pacing. Pacing is an amazingly commonsense approach. It also has been around for more than 30 years—and it has essentially no evidence. Pacing attempts to create a behavior pattern that includes persistent engagement, the capacity to pursue an activity without the need to stop. One of the lessons from pacing seems to be that pacing is too weak as a behavior change method in relation to the strength of the behavior pattern it attempts to replace. That behavior pattern is persistent disengagement, or avoidance. Brute force activation, a quality of "just do it," or activity patterns that are attempts to carry a preordained "just right" structure are not always successful. Rather, it is suggested that effective patterns of activity are contextually sensitive. That means they include openness to experiences that happen during the activity, connection to goals and values and the present situation, and flexible choosing to engage and then choosing that again.

References

Duckworth, A.L., Steen, T.A., & Seligman, M.E.P. (2005). Positive psychology in clinical practice. *Annual Review of Clinical Psychology, 1,* 629-651.

Gill, J. R., & Brown, C. A. (2009). A structured review of the evidence for pacing as a chronic pain intervention. *European Journal of Pain, 13,* 214-216.

Hayes, S. C., Strosahl, K. D., & Wilson, K. G. (2012). *Acceptance and Commitment Therapy: The process and practice of mindful change.* New York: Guilford Press.

Karsdorp, P. A., & Vlaeyen, J. W. S. (2009). Active avoidance but not activity pacing is associated with disability in fibromyalgia. *Pain, 147,* 29-35.

Linton, S. J., McCracken, L. M., & Vlaeyen J. W. S. (2008). Reassurance: Help or hinder in the treatment of pain. *Pain, 134,* 5-8.

Luoma, J. B., Hayes, S. C., Walser, R. D. (2007). *Learning ACT: An acceptance & commitment skills training manual for therapists.* Oakland, CA: New Harbinger.

McCracken, L. M. (1998). Learning to live with the pain: Acceptance of pain predicts adjustment in persons with chronic pain. *Pain, 74,* 21-27.

McCracken, L. M., Gutiérrez-Martínez, O., & Smyth, C. (2012). "Decentering" reflects psychological flexibility in people with chronic pain and correlates with their quality of functioning. *Health Psychology.* Advance online publication. doi:10.1037/a0028093

McCracken, L. M., & Samuel, V. M. (2007). The role of avoidance, pacing, and other activity patterns in chronic pain. *Pain, 130,* 119-125.

McCracken, L. M., & Yang, S-Y. (2006). The role of values in a contextual cognitive-behavioral approach to chronic pain. *Pain, 123,* 137-145.

McNulty, J. K., & Fincham, F. D. (2011). Beyond positive psychology? Toward a contextual view of psychological processes and well-being. *American Psychologist.* doi: 10.1037/a0024572

White, P. D., Goldsmith, K. A., Johnson, A. L., Potts, L., Walwyn, R., J. C. DeCesare, ... Sharpe M. (2011). Comparison of adaptive pacing therapy, cognitive behaviour therapy, graded exercise therapy, and specialist medical care for chronic fatigue syndrome (PACE): A randomised trial. *Lancet, 377,* 823-836.

CHAPTER 7

Positive Interventions: Past, Present, and Future

Acacia C. Parks

Hiram College

Robert Biswas-Diener

Portland State University

Positive Acorn

Positive Interventions: Past, Present, and Future

As positive intervention researchers, we are often approached by proponents of ACT, and the ensuing conversation is frequently the same. The questioners say, "I have always wondered what the difference is between a positive intervention and ACT." Obscured within this polite statement are the questions they *really* want to ask: Is there anything new about positive interventions, or are we "selling old wine in a new bottle"? What do positive interventions bring to the table that other interventions do not? These are, we think, reasonable questions, and ones that researchers in our field too rarely take the time to answer. Equally pressing is a concern that we hear more rarely but are fairly certain lurks in the back of our questioners' minds with some regularity: Isn't it irresponsible to ignore a person's problems? Isn't there a risk that such an approach can do harm to clients?

One central goal of this chapter is to explore the ways in which positive intervention research has and has not been thoughtful about exactly these issues. First, we address the question of what, exactly, a positive intervention *is*. We follow with a review of the different areas of positive intervention, including descriptions of prototypical activities, evidence of their effectiveness, and important considerations for their application. Lastly, we discuss several future directions for positive intervention research; most notable of these is investigation of the possibility that positive interventions, in certain contexts, may be ineffective, or even cause harm. Each of these sections constitutes a step toward our final goal of discussing what distinguishes positive interventions from other approaches in general and from acceptance-based approaches in particular.

What Is a Positive Intervention?

One legitimate criticism of positive intervention research is that it is difficult to determine what actually counts as a "positive intervention." Indeed, there is no definitive definition of a "positive intervention" and no clear set of guidelines for classifying interventions as "positive." However, this is a problem that researchers have attempted to tackle. Our efforts at synthesis led us to three broad conceptualizations of positive interventions: 1) interventions that focus on positive topics, 2) interventions that operate by a positive mechanism or that target a positive outcome variable, and 3) interventions that are designed to promote wellness rather than to fix weakness.

First, "positive" interventions can be defined as those that focus on topics that are positive; in other words, they contain little or no mention of problems, instead emphasizing the positive aspects of peoples' lives. The "positive content" approach is consistent with the positive psychotherapy (PPT) interventions proposed by Seligman, Rashid, and Parks (2006): "The goal [of PPT] is to keep the positive aspects of the clients' lives in the forefront of their minds ... and to strengthen already existing positive aspects." (p. 780). We think that this definition is much too broad; it encompasses any intervention in which individuals do not attend to their problems or do something pleasant. By this definition, procrastinating by playing video games until 4 am constitutes a positive intervention; so does drinking oneself into oblivion to mask anxiety. In other words, while a content-level definition does describe all positive interventions, it also describes a variety of other behaviors that are not positive interventions, and so it is not sufficient.

An intervention can also be defined as "positive" if the mechanism or target outcome is a positive variable such as positive emotion, meaning, and so on (see below for an extensive overview of such variables). The definition used by Sin & Lyubomirsky (2009) in their meta-analysis is a good example of this approach; they define a positive intervention as one that is "aimed at cultivating positive feelings, positive behaviors, or positive cognitions" (p. 1). This definition is better than the last in that it is less inclusive, requiring some level of theoretical development (there must be some positive variable being targeted, so avoidance doesn't fit). However, the definition does not include any requirement that the intervention defines its target variable, nor that the target variable has an empirical basis, nor that the intervention actually *changes* that target variable; "positivity," for example, would be sufficient, even though we have no idea what "positivity" means, nor do we know how to measure or change it. Thus, the variable-level definition encompasses anything with the tag line "be positive" or "think positive"—including, we shudder to say, *The Secret*, and other myriad crackpot self-help approaches.[1]

Lastly, an intervention can be "positive" if the goal of the intervention is to improve rather than to remediate; in other words, the target population is nondistressed, and so the intervention is self-help rather than therapy. The goal of the intervention, then, is to bring individuals from acceptable levels of functioning to "good" or "great." This definition is consistent with the rhetoric that came from Seligman and colleagues during the first few years after positive psychology's inception. For example, when speaking about the general goals of the positive psychology movement, Seligman, Parks, and Steen (2005) stated: "We know very little about how to improve the lives of the people whose days are largely free of overt mental dysfunction" (p. 1379). A positive intervention, by this definition, is one designed for the subset of the population

---

1   We don't have space or license here to do justice to all of the things that are wrong with *The Secret*, nor to sufficiently express how icky it makes us feel when people think *The Secret* is part of positive psychology.

not suffering from a mental disorder. While this definition is more selective than the previous two, it excludes one prominent positive intervention—positive psychotherapy (PPT)—which has been applied in major depression (Seligman, Rashid & Parks, 2006), schizophrenia (Meyer et al., in press), and nicotine dependence (Kahler et al., 2011).

While each of these definitions seems reasonable at first glance, each is uniquely problematic when used as a stand-alone method for classifying interventions as "positive" or not. We believe this is because the goal of creating a single definition may be impractical. Research on positive interventions was well under way before anyone attempted to infuse it with theory, and so the research follows no common theoretical thread. Any definition we create, then, is going to be a post hoc rationalization of the research that has been done so far rather than a theory-driven attempt to classify. It will not be simple because it is an attempt to bring together a broad body of work that was not a cohesive effort. Thus, rather than creating a single definition, we propose a set of criteria derived by integrating and refining the above definitions:

- The primary goal of the intervention is to build some "positive" variable or variables (e.g., subjective well-being, positive emotion, meaning). This criterion eliminates self-indulgent or avoidant behaviors with no real function toward self-improvement.

- Empirical evidence exists that the intervention successfully manipulates the above target variable(s). This criterion eliminates the myriad existing self-help approaches that have no research basis.

- Empirical evidence exists that improving the target variable will lead to positive outcomes for the population in which it is administered. This criterion requires that the target variable has an empirical basis.[2] It allows for special cases in which positive

---

2   We acknowledge that requiring an "empirical basis" is a slippery slope without any formal criteria for what constitutes an empirical basis. We also acknowledge that previous efforts to do this in other arenas have proven fruitful (e.g., the guidelines for what constitutes an "Empirically Supported Therapy" set forth by the APA Task Force on Promotion and Dissemination of Psychological Procedures in 1995). While creating such criteria is beyond the scope of this chapter, we are enthusiastic about doing so in other venues.

interventions are responsibly applied in a clinical population (for example, Kahler et al. [2011] use a positive intervention in smoking cessation because positive affect is a predictor of treatment success). It also excludes interventions that target positive variables in clients for whom this approach would be inappropriate; we would assert, for example, that a gratitude intervention for recent trauma victims would be unlikely to produce positive outcomes, and thus would not be a positive intervention.

We believe that this set of criteria is the right balance of inclusive and exclusive—it encompasses all existing positive interventions but excludes none that we know of.

What Do We Know about the Benefits of Positive Interventions?

Modern positive intervention research began as the study of individual techniques that target specific happiness-related constructs (see below for a comprehensive review). In these seminal studies, many of which are discussed in greater detail below, participants are randomly assigned to practice one of several potential activities—some designed to serve as "controls" and others designed to increase some aspect of well-being. They complete a battery of pre-intervention questionnaires, practice the activity for some predefined time period ranging from one to six weeks, and then complete postintervention questionnaires. In some cases, participants may complete one or more long-term follow-up questionnaires as well.

Other chapters (including at least one written by the first author) have attempted to organize existing positive interventions according to one theoretical framework or another. However, just as there is no common definition of a "positive intervention," neither does there exist any single, empirically based theoretical framework that unifies positive interventions. Unlike many areas of psychology, where theory drives the research, in positive interventions, the opposite is true; data showing that an activity is effective came first, with questions of "how" and "why" tabled for a later date. Thus, the series of summaries below—while, to our knowledge, comprehensive—comes in no particular order. For each area of intervention we discuss, we endeavor not only to describe the most common techniques and the evidence for their effectiveness but also to take a critical approach, highlighting caveats and special considerations as appropriate.

Strengths—Different conceptualizations of strengths exist, with some focusing more on character (VIA-IS; Peterson & Seligman, 2004) and others focusing more on talent (Clifton StrengthsFinder; The Gallup Organization, 1999). Broadly speaking, however, strengths are positive personality traits, and strengths interventions are activities that involve the identification, use, and/or development of one's strengths. The general paradigm for all strengths interventions is the same: an individual takes a strengths test,[3] receives feedback on his strengths, and then changes his behavior in order to use his strengths more often.

Although Gallup has been using a strengths-based model in practice for many years (Hodges & Clifton, 2004) this approach was also popular during the advent of the modern positive psychology movement. Seligman, Steen, Park and Peterson (2005), for example, found that the process of identifying and using one's strengths resulted in increases in happiness and decreases in depressive symptoms, and that these benefits lasted through six-month follow-up among those individuals who continued to practice it. The actual use of one's strengths, above and beyond learning what one's strengths *are*, is an essential ingredient of this activity; participants in an "assessment-only" condition (where they learned their strengths but were not asked to use that information in any way) were indistinguishable from those who practiced a placebo activity (Seligman, Steen et al., 2005).

Recently, researchers have begun to examine potential pitfalls of the "identify and use" approach used by Seligman, Steen et al. (2005). Of particular concern are the implications of treating strengths as stable traits. Pointing to work by Dweck and colleagues, Biswas-Diener, Kashdan, and Minhas (2011) warned that an "identify and use" approach may encourage individuals to think of strengths as permanent and unchangeable, which may in turn lower the individual's motivation to improve. Work by Louis (2011) lends initial support to this view;

---

3 Whereas Gallup's survey is pay only, the VIA strengths inventory is available for free online. This difference, in part, explains why the VIA model is so strongly represented in the literature.

participants randomly assigned to "identify" their strengths reported increases in the belief that strengths are fixed/stable, while those assigned to "develop" their strengths did not experience such an increase. While this study did not evaluate whether more fixed beliefs about the nature of strengths translates into decreased motivation to work on one's strengths, extensive research from Dweck's lab suggests that this phenomenon occurs in other domains (Grant & Dweck, 2003).

Another important issue is the relative importance of working on strengths versus weaknesses—specifically, how do we know that individuals should be further developing their most developed traits (i.e. strengths) rather than attempting to remediate their least developed traits (i.e., weaknesses)? In an informal paper based on data from his students, Haidt (2002) reports that students benefited from both approaches; however, students reported *liking* a strengths-focused approach more. This is consistent with preliminary data from Seligman, Rashid, and Parks (2006), in which participants in positive psychotherapy were noticeably (though not significantly) less likely to drop out than were participants in a standard (remediation-focused) psychotherapy.

In summary, there appears to be evidence that it is worthwhile to identify and promote the *development* of strengths and that these benefits are both psychological and motivational—that is, developing strengths feels intrinsically rewarding to people, and so they are more driven to engage in a strengths-development process. However, we argue that strengths research would benefit from the inclusion of nuance; in line with Schwartz and Hill's (2006) call for "practical wisdom," one should aim not only to use one's strengths more often but to use those strengths *well* and *appropriately*. Humor, for example, can be an invaluable tool for building relationships and for coping with stress if used appropriately; however, humor can also be insensitive or hurtful.

Furthermore, in the authors' various experiences teaching others to develop their strengths, both of us have encountered a common dilemma: it is not always easy to generate concrete ideas of how to use one's strengths. This represents, in our view, an important barrier for practitioners hoping to teach strengths to clients and for individuals hoping to apply positive interventions independently. A person cannot develop her strengths if she has no idea how to go about it, and in the absence of guidelines for advising people in this process, a practitioner is forced to rely on intuition or trial and error. Haidt (2002) provides a list of ideas, compiled by his positive psychology undergraduates, for situations in which each of the 24 VIA strengths can be applied. This list, however, is only the beginning of what needs to be a comprehensive resource to practitioners and clients hoping to promote strengths development.

Gratitude—Some of the earliest positive interventions targeted gratitude, which Wood, Froh, and Geraghty (2010) define as a general habit of noticing and being appreciative of whatever is good in one's life. In their seminal paper, Emmons and McCullough (2003) randomly assigned participants to keep a weekly gratitude journal. In this journal, the participants wrote down up to five things they were grateful for. Compared to participants who kept track of either hassles or neutral events, participants in the gratitude condition scored better on a range of emotional and physical health outcomes. Lyubomirsky, Sheldon, and Schkade (2005) both replicated this finding and found evidence that the "dosage" used by Emmons and McCullough (2003), once per week, may be the ideal frequency for a gratitude journal; participants in a condition that kept a more frequent gratitude journal (3 times per week instead of once) did not experience the same improvements as the once-per-week group, instead reporting that the activity felt stale and overdone (Lyubomirsky, Sheldon, & Schkade, 2005).

Seligman, Steen, Park and Peterson (2005) proposed and tested a related activity, titled the Three Good Things journal. They asked participants to keep a nightly journal of positive events that took place during the day that just ended;[4] this activity resulted in increased happiness and decreased depressive symptoms by 1-month follow-up, with gains continuing to increase over 3-month and 6-month follow-ups. While this finding may at first seem to conflict with Lyubomirsky, Sheldon, and Schkade's (2005) finding that gratitude can be "overdone," there is an important difference between the gratitude journal and Three Good Things: they operate at completely different levels of analysis. Whereas a gratitude journal can and often does revolve around ongoing

---

4   It is debatable whether Three Good Things belongs under the umbrella of "gratitude." This uncertainty is an excellent example of the general lack of theory underlying many existing positive interventions. Three Good Things was designed to make people happier without any specific underlying theory. Only after the exercise appeared to be effective did researchers begin to speculate as to how it works.

areas of gratitude (e.g., family, friends, a good job), Three Good Things requires the individual to focus on events that took place during the current day. Thus, while a gratitude journal might get repetitive if practiced too often, as the content doesn't vary much, a Three Good Things journal has different content every day.

Seligman, Steen, Park and Peterson (2005) report findings on a second gratitude activity, in which participants compose a detailed thank-you letter to someone in their life and deliver the letter in person ("The Gratitude Visit"). In contrast with the previous exercise, The Gratitude Visit led to large initial boosts in happiness—substantially larger than the placebo conditions—but these changes were transient, having faded substantially by 1-month follow-up and entirely by 3 months. While some researchers have presented ideas about how to prolong these effects—for example, a client might keep a daily log of the things her spouse does that she appreciates, then use that log to create "gratitude reports" once per month on an ongoing basis—nobody has tested an "improved" gratitude visit design to date. However, Lyubomirsky, Dickerhoof, Boehm, and Sheldon (2011) did find that writing a gratitude letter, without the added step of delivering the letter to its target, did lead to well-being improvements in their sample. Whereas delivering a glowing letter of thanks to someone may be very powerful the first time, one can imagine that repeated instances could become stale or awkward; by removing the "delivery" step of writing a gratitude letter and the awkwardness that may come along with it, it becomes more plausible that a person might practice this exercise repeatedly.

While the existing literature presents a relatively compelling case that gratitude is a worthwhile practice, gratitude is also one of the few areas in which deleterious effects have been observed.[5] For example, Sin, Della Porta, and Lyubomirksy (2011) report that writing gratitude letters *reduced* immediate well-being for individuals with mild-moderate

---

5   To be clear, gratitude is also one of the only areas in which anyone has looked at moderators of outcome to begin with, and so if deleterious effects do occur in other activities (as, we imagine, they must for some subset of people), these effects are unlikely to have been detected. We discuss these findings not to suggest that gratitude interventions are bad but rather to encourage researchers to do *more* of this type of research on other types of interventions. This type of nuance can only help us apply positive interventions more effectively and with better precision.

depressive symptoms; those participants who believed the activity would work, and thus continued to use it for three weeks despite the initial deleterious effect, did experience eventual improvement, but those who had no such expectation continued to report worsened symptoms as a result of the activity. Sergeant and Mongrain (2011) examined this issue looking at different "types" of depressed individuals and found that individuals whose depressive symptoms were more interpersonally oriented ("needy" rather than "self-critical") experienced no benefits or, in some cases, worsened when doing a gratitude activity. The more self-critical people, by contrast, benefited *more* than average from doing the activity.

It is important, then, to use caution when recommending gratitude activities to people with depressive symptoms. Some data provide direct evidence that gratitude can be useful in mild-moderate depression (Seligman, Steen, Park, and Peterson, 2005), and other data provide more indirect evidence, finding that gratitude interventions can be well-received by people in the mild-moderate symptom range (Seligman, Rashid, & Parks, 2006) or that they are generally efficacious, on average, among people reporting depressive symptoms (Sin & Lyubomirsky, 2009). However, there appears to be some subset of depressed individuals to whom this generalization does not apply, and we are only beginning to understand who they are and how to identify them.

Another factor that we have noticed comes into play with gratitude is culture. The first author has noticed, for example, that activities that involve *expressing* gratitude (e.g., The Gratitude Visit) have sometimes backfired when used by Asian-American students; expressing gratitude can make individuals very uncomfortable, particularly if their cultural norm is to avoid attracting attention. The situation can be further complicated when the target of the letter is an Asian-American parent. In one student's case, her parents viewed her letter as an insult—an acknowledgment of the possibility that they might ever have chosen *not* to give their child appropriate care. We have also noted cases of suspicion on the part of recipients, which can undermine the success of the activity. One student of the first author, for example, reported that her father was suspicious upon receipt of his gratitude letter; he thought that the student was, perhaps, trying to manipulate him into giving her something.

How, then, does one decide to whom one would recommend gratitude activities? Sin, Della Porta, and Lyubomirsky (2011) report that perceived fit is an important predictor of outcome—that is, participants who looked at the gratitude activity and thought it would be helpful for them generally found it helpful. This highlights the importance of choosing positive intervention collaboratively with clients and perhaps even suggests that the "buffet" approach—trying all activities, then selecting those that work best for an individual—may not be optimal for all clients.

Forgiveness—In common parlance, forgiveness is often associated with reconciliation. However, in the forgiveness intervention literature, forgiveness is conceptualized as a primarily internal process. An individual who has experienced a transgression lets go of the negative feelings associated with the transgression and the transgressor, and this change may or may not result in any sort of behavioral change in relation to the transgressor. The emphasis in the literature on emotional forgiveness is largely due to the fact that the emotional aspects of forgiveness appear to play the largest role in the robust link between forgiveness and physical health (Worthington, Witvliet, Pietrini, & Miller, 2007).

The majority of forgiveness interventions follow process-based models, which allow for gradual, stage-like progress toward the decision to forgive (Baskin & Enright, 2004). The "REACH" model is an example of a process-based approach to forgiveness: individuals *recall* the transgression; develop *empathy* for the transgressor, which is an *altruistic* act; *commit* to forgive; then work to *hold* on to that forgiveness. Worthington (2006) provides an example of a 6-session group intervention following the REACH model. A recent meta-analysis focusing only on process-based forgiveness interventions found an average effect size of .82 on forgiveness outcomes, .81 on positive affect, and .54 on negative affect, suggesting that forgiveness interventions can reliably promote forgiveness and improve the emotional damage that grudges can cause (Lundahl, Taylor, Stevenson, & Roberts, 2008).

Smaller scale interventions that target forgiveness also exist. McCullough, Root, and Cohen (2006), for example, tested a writing intervention in which participants spent 20 minutes writing about personal benefits that arose as the result of a transgression they had experienced. Compared to control groups focusing on an unpleasant aspect of the transgression or on a topic not related to the transgression, participants in the benefit-finding condition reported more forgiveness.

Hook, Worthington and Utsey (2009) argue that while forgiveness is valued by both individualistic and collectivistic cultures, collectivistic cultures are distinct in their definition of what constitutes forgiveness. More individualistic cultures tend to consider the emotional aspects of forgiveness to be central; in other words, if an individual has let go of her anger, she has forgiven, even if she does not change her behavior toward the transgressor at all. Collectivistic cultures, on the other hand, prioritize behavioral change, and so forgiveness has not occurred until social harmony is restored (in other words, until the two individuals are able to interact civilly). While no research to date has examined whether forgiveness interventions differentially affect members of individualistic or collectivistic cultures, this question is well worth asking given the apparent cultural differences in how emotional and decisional forgiveness is valued.

It may go without saying that forgiveness may be problematic in certain cases—forgiving a spouse who is regularly physically abusive, for example, would likely lead to continued physical abuse. However, recent work by McNulty (2011) suggests that in the context of romantic relationships, habitual forgiveness can lead to the maintenance and potential worsening of psychological aggression as well. Thus, it is careful to consider whether forgiveness is an appropriate recommendation for a given individual in a given situation. In particular, practitioners should consider whether there is the potential for forgiveness to prolong a negative behavior. It is less likely, for example, that forgiving someone for a single long-past transgression can backfire in this way; adopting a general policy of forgiveness in a relationship, however, has the potential to cause interpersonal problems.

Social Connections—Two branches of research aim to strengthen social connections through positive processes. The first involves acts of kindness (i.e. engaging in altruistic behaviors toward others). Dunn, Aknin, and Norton (2008) report that spending money on others leads to boosts in happiness, and this effect holds up when studied cross-sectionally, longitudinally, and in an experimental manipulation. More recent evidence even suggests that this finding extends across data from 136 different countries (Aknin et al., in press). Lyubomirsky, Sheldon, and Schkade (2005) demonstrated that engaging in deliberate acts of kindness leads to increased well-being, with one caveat: it must be done in such a way that exceeds the individual's normal propensity to be kind. Specifically, engaging in an act of kindness per day for a week does not lead to well-being benefits, but engaging in five acts of kindness in a single day does (Lyubomirsky, Sheldon, & Schkade, 2005). Interestingly, it appears that one can benefit from paying extra attention to the kind acts one has committed without any deliberate efforts to engage in *more* kind acts (Otake et al., 2006). However, these two strategies have not been compared directly, so it is unclear what percentage of the effectiveness of an "acts of kindness" intervention is due to shifts in attention (i.e., *awareness* of one's kind acts) versus shifts in behavior. Furthermore, there has been little effort to standardize acts of kindness interventions or to systematically examine the impact of key variables such as the target of the intervention (a stranger vs. an acquaintance vs. a close other) or whether the act is credited or anonymous. The extent to which these variables matter for "acts of kindness" interventions remains to be seen.

A second branch of research is based on two studies demonstrating that close relationships are more satisfying and long-lived if couples are able to jointly revel in good news (Gable, Reis, Impett, & Asher, 2004). Specifically, they found that the most successful couples were those who responded both actively (with interest and engagement) and constructively (encouraging celebration, responding supportively) to good news when it is shared. For example, in response to one's significant other's receiving a promotion, one might say, concerned for the relationship, "Well, with your busier schedule I guess I'm going to see even less of you now." This would be an active-destructive response, and this type of response is predictive of poor outcomes in relationships. Instead, however, one might focus on the spouse's visible excitement and mirror that excitement, highlighting the way the spouse worked hard to earn the promotion, sharing the news with friends and family members, and so on. Couples that respond to each other in this way report higher relationship satisfaction and are more likely to stay together over time.

Seligman, Rashid, and Parks's (2006) Group PPT intervention included an activity based on this research finding; clients attempted to respond more actively and constructively to people in their lives. While anecdotal responses suggest that this was a helpful activity for some, because Group PPT is a series of activities, it is difficult to isolate the relative contribution of any one exercise to efficacy. Unfortunately, no published studies to date have looked at this activity on its own. However, informal data analyses and anecdotal observations from the first author suggest that active-constructive responding may be subject to what Parks, Della Porta, Pierce, Zilca, & Lyubomirsky (in press) refer to as "degradation." In other words, active-constructive responding may be too complex to teach via simple written instructions (as many positive interventions are), and as a result, it may lose its potency when it is implemented in the real world. Further research should examine the efficacy of active-constructive responding as a sole activity and should disentangle the relative importance of hands-on instruction (as opposed to brief written instructions) for its efficacy.

Meaning—Prevailing theories suggest that people derive a sense of meaning by forming a coherent narrative about their lives (Pennebaker & Seagal, 1999). Thus, it makes sense that the majority of meaning interventions involve writing. Seminal studies on meaning making involve personal narratives of traumatic or stressful life events, but more recently, research has begun to examine the formation of narratives around positive life events and, in particular, events that one expects to occur in the future. King (2001) instructed people to write about their "best possible self"—a future version of themselves who has turned out according to their highest hopes and aspirations—for 20 minutes a day over the course of 4 days. Seligman, Rashid, and Parks (2006) used a similar activity, which they call the "Life Summary," wherein participants write a 1-2 page essay describing their life as they hope to have lived it; as part of the activity, participants are also instructed to consider the ways that they are and are not actively progressing toward the long-term goals described in the essay. Subsequent work by Sheldon and Lyubomirsky (2006) suggests that the benefits of imagining one's positive future are not limited to writing. They asked participants to *think* about their best possible selves at least twice a week and found that doing so was also beneficial.

It is worth mentioning, however, that the first author has encountered a handful of cases where writing about a positive future for oneself has been unpleasant for participants; in particular, relatively anxious students have sometimes reported that trying to imagine their future made them *more* anxious (keep in mind, though, that these are college students, whose futures are quite uncertain; it may be that anxious responses are an artifact of the age group the activity has been tested in). We have also found that more depressed students can find the activity depressing—one student said, in a debriefing with me: "None of this is ever going to happen. What's the point in writing about it?" Anecdotal evidence suggests, then, that meaning-oriented activities may be a better fit for relatively high-functioning clients or for clients who have been in therapy for some time; in clinical populations, one should approach the process of building a life narrative of one's future with caution.

Interestingly, whereas speaking and writing analytically about past negative life events leads to improvements in physical health and well-being, the opposite may be true for positive life events. Lyubomirsky, Sousa, and Dickerhoof (2006) found that participants who wrote about a past positive event reported *lower* satisfaction with life when compared to a control group. Their findings suggest that, when it comes to life's high points, it's best not to overthink things.

Savoring—Savoring is characterized by the deliberate act of deriving pleasure from an experience. In savoring activities, one attends fully to an experience, without preoccupation or distraction ("absorption"), and focuses on the positive aspects of that experience. Typically, savoring activities are brief—just a few minutes at a time—but are nevertheless quite potent sources of positive emotion. Indeed, a consistent practice of savoring experiences is predictive of optimism, life satisfaction, and fewer depressive symptoms (Bryant, 2003).

The prototypical example of a savoring experience involves food— for example, Kabat-Zinn's famous raisin-savoring exercise (2003), wherein the individual focuses on each individual feature of the raisin in turn. This technique is called "sharpening perceptions" and can be combined with absorption to savor any sensory experience: gustatory (e.g., food), visual (e.g., art or a beautiful sunset), tactile (e.g., a massage or a hot bath), olfactory (e.g., the smell of a complex wine), auditory (e.g., music), or any combination of these (Bryant & Veroff, 2007). When the first author directed a group of students through a savoring activity, for example, she used cups of hot chocolate with whipped cream, chocolate shavings, and a wafer from a nearby gourmet chocolatier. Students smelled the hot chocolate, felt the warmth in their hands, then tried each component in turn—the whipped cream, the chocolate shavings, the wafer, and the hot chocolate. They let each sit in their mouths, exploring the texture and the taste, before chewing (as appropriate), then swallowing. They then began experimenting with different combinations of the components, eventually building to a combination of all four.

Having tried each component separately, they were able to fully experience the hot chocolate, tasting each individual aspect and enjoying the interplay between them. The entire process took only a few minutes, but as a group, we (the first author and the students) found it to be a very potent experience—one that was amplified by the fact that we shared it together.

Savoring can be applied to nonsensory experiences as well. One can savor a present moment via "memory building"—taking photographs, for example. These types of activities bring one's attention to the transience of a present experience and lead to better savoring of that experience (Kurtz & Lyubomirsky, in press). Memory building also paves the way for "reminiscence," which is savoring one's memory of a past experience (Bryant, Smart, & King, 2005). Whereas memory building is a technique for promoting enjoyment in the moment, reminiscence is a more cognitive activity, characterized by the use of imagery as one remembers a valued past experience in as much detail as possible. Several published studies have found that deliberately reminiscing more often leads to improvements in depressive and anxious symptoms, as well as increasing positive affect and life satisfaction, particularly among older populations (Bryant, Smart, & King, 2005).

Perspective Taking—Perspective taking has not received much attention from positive psychology proper, but it is, we believe, an important construct, with several successful interventions designed to increase it. Perspective taking is important because it drives people to embrace and help others. By reducing the perceived "distance" between you and your neighbor[6] ("self-other overlap"), your sense of empathic concern makes you feel like your neighbor's problems are your problems, too (Davis, Conklin, Smith, & Luce, 1996). This makes you more likely to help your neighbor and also makes you more interested in helping other people you might group together with your neighbor (Batson, Chang, Orr, & Rowland, 2002).

While perspective taking is often a component of forgiveness interventions (see above), we focus in this section on interventions designed to cultivate perspective taking directly. Perspective-taking interventions have successfully been applied in a variety of contexts, ranging from loved ones (romantic partners, parents and children) to the people one

---

6 Or whomever.

encounters in day-to-day life (patients, for example, if one is a doctor), to members of an outgroup (other race, socioeconomic status, religion, etc.) (see Hodges, Clark, and Myers [2011] for an up-to-date review). In all cases, these interventions have the same basic objective: to increase an individual's ability to go beyond his or her own biases to become aware and appreciative of the perspective of another person.

Myers and Hodges (in press) present a model activity for inducing individuals to take the perspective of someone else—in this case, a member of an outgroup. Participants read a paragraph about a 24-year-old homeless man and are instructed to "imagine what the person thinks and feels about what has happened to him and how it has affected his life." In short, they are asked to focus on imagining the emotional experiences of the other person. It is worth noting that the prompt explicitly asks people to imagine the experience of the other; it does *not* ask them to imagine how they would feel if they were in the same situation. While not found in all studies (Davis et al., 1996), there is some evidence that attempting to put oneself in the shoes of another person (as opposed to imagining their plight from a distance) can evoke anxiety and that anxiety can reduce the likelihood that empathy will result in prosocial behavior (Hodges, Clark, & Myers, 2011).

"Packaged" Positive Interventions. Thus far, we have emphasized research wherein participants use a single activity. This type of study, while ideal from an experimental design standpoint, is not representative of how such activities are actually used by individuals and by practitioners. Parks et al. (in press), for example, found that happiness seekers pursuing happiness on their own (i.e., without being instructed by an experimenter to do anything in particular) report practicing 7-8 activities at a time. Furthermore, they found that when happiness seekers are offered a variety of activities to choose from, those who practiced a wider variety of activities experienced the largest mood benefits. In short, there is no evidence that anyone in the real world picks a single activity and practices it in isolation, and there is also no evidence that doing so is "optimal" in terms of effectiveness. Research examining "packages" of activities, then, is also worthy of attention.

Some of the earliest positive intervention research used a "packaged" intervention design. Fordyce (1977), for example, gave young adults a set of 14 happiness techniques and asked them to practice as many of these activities as possible every day for two weeks. He found that, a year later, these participants were significantly happier than a control group (Fordyce, 1983). This study contains one of the most realistic happiness interventions ever tested, and it was one of the first to demonstrate that happiness can be increased in a way that is not fleeting. More recently, Parks et al. (in press) used a similar "free choice" design with two modifications: the activities used were empirically derived, and the activities were administered using smartphone technology. Because of their broad-stroke nature, it is difficult to draw conclusions from either study beyond the general sentiment that the activities lead to increased happiness. However, given that both studies mimic real-world practice, that is certainly a worthwhile finding.

An alternative "packaged" happiness intervention design requires participants to try each activity for a week, one activity at a time, and *then* select which activities to keep using (Seligman, Rashid, & Parks, 2006; Schueller & Parks, 2012). While this design does have pitfalls—if all participants use every activity in a set, it is difficult to tell which activities are responsible for change—there are other ways in which the design is ideal. For example, while it is difficult to ask questions of person-activity fit at the level of the individual activity using a "package" design, other questions of fit (i.e., whether preference for Activity A predicts preference for Activity B vs. Activity C) can only be answered using a design where the same people practice multiple activities (Schueller, 2010).

Research on "packaged" interventions, then, isn't a *replacement* for single-activity designs—but a worthy complement.

Future Directions

Thus far, we have provided an overview of existing positive interventions. We turn, now, to some important issues that we hope to see the field tackle in the coming years.

Alternative outcomes. One of the preliminary steps in establishing positive psychology as an empirically based endeavor was to include prominent scholars with scientific acumen and well-regarded reputations (Seligman & Csikszentimihaly, 2000). Among these early "recruits" were pioneering members of the positive psychology steering committee, including Mihalyi Csikszentimihaly and Ed Diener. Although certainly unintended, one consequence of aligning so heavily with well-being researchers is the fact that happiness-related constructs became the de facto outcome measures for positive psychology (Biswas-Diener, 2011). In fact, early steering committee discussions explicitly addressed the extent to which happiness can be viewed as the "ultimate outcome measure" (Seligman, 2000, personal communication). While personal well-being is a worthy goal for both policy and intervention, we argue that it is disproportionately valued in positive psychological research over other worthwhile outcome measures. For example, Biswas-Diener, Kashdan, & Minhas (2011) argue that happiness is an individualistic concern and that researchers who confine their attention to happiness as an outcome overlook more group-level outcomes such as trust, friendship, and feelings of connectedness. While those scholars most associated with happiness research advocate a similarly broad understanding of positive psychology outcomes (e.g. Diener & Diener, 2011), it is rare to see measures that are not explicitly focused on the individual represented in positive intervention research.

More nuanced research designs. As we have alluded to earlier, positive interventions, as they are studied in the laboratory, arguably bear little resemblance to those used by people in the real world. Most research studies ask participants to practice a single activity in the exact same way over the course of some time period at the exclusion of other activities (Sin & Lyubomirsky, 2009). However, in practice, happiness seekers practice multiple activities simultaneously, and they intentionally vary the ways in which they practice each activity in order to prevent boredom (Parks et al., in press). Worse, in limiting participants to one activity at a time, it is possible that researchers are actually undermining the effectiveness of that activity; Parks et al. (in press) report that practicing a variety of activities predicts better outcomes than using a single activity, even if level of overall effort is roughly equal. These differences from real-world practice are a problem, then, not only from a conceptual standpoint but from a practical one as well; by using the same activity repeatedly without variation (adapting to it) and by using only one activity at a time (missing out on the benefits of variety), participants may actually be prevented from benefiting fully.

Standards for implementation: Doing harm? One of the strengths of the definition of positive interventions we are proposing is that it demands some sort of evidence, theoretical or otherwise, that an activity will be beneficial to the individual to whom it is being offered. This is, to our knowledge, the first proposal of its kind, but it's an essential one, in our view. In our experience talking with both researchers and practitioners in positive psychology, we have found that the prevailing sentiment is that positive interventions are very unlikely to cause harm, particularly when used in normative, rather than clinical ("more high-risk"), populations. However, recent research is beginning to show that this is an unrealistic viewpoint. Now that the field is beginning to build a substantial repertoire of interventions that we believe to be effective, we must turn to the question of how these interventions can be implemented responsibly.

Evidence already exists that certain activities work better than others for a given individual (Schueller, 2010). Happiness seekers are not homogeneous in terms of their initial levels of happiness and depressive symptoms (Parks et al., in press), nor in terms of their motivation and interest in becoming happier (Lyubomirsky et al., 2011), and so it is inappropriate to assume that a particular activity can be "universally" effective. Individual differences matter, not only for outcome (Sergeant & Mongrain, 2011), but for the likelihood that an individual will use activities in the first place (Sheldon & Lyubomirsky, 2006). In addition to the handful of published studies discussed above, the first author participated in a recent discussion on the FRIENDS-OF-PP listserv in which several members told stories of positive interventions "backfiring" with certain clients. It happens—we just don't know the full extent of when, and for whom, it happens.

On a broader scale, we propose that caution is necessary in how we approach efforts to increase happiness in general. Recent work by Mauss et al. (2011) suggests that holding happiness as a goal makes it more difficult to achieve that goal—by telling oneself that one "should" be happy, one is more easily disappointed by one's own emotional experiences. Work by Louis (2011), mentioned above, highlights the importance of how *the exact same activity*—in this case, taking a strengths assessment and using that assessment to modify one's behavior—is presented to and interpreted by clients. Something as simple as the wording of an activity's prompt can make all the difference between the activity being helpful or harmful.

In short, while the evidence seems clear that individual differences matter, we do not have a great sense of how to use this information in practice. It is our hope that the recent wave of positive intervention research tackling these questions is a trend that will maintain its momentum.

How Are Positive Interventions Distinct from Acceptance-Based Approaches?

In this chapter, we have proposed a new, integrative definition of positive interventions. We have also provided a broad review of existing positive interventions. It is our hope that in doing so, we have clarified what a positive intervention is (and is not). However, we have not yet addressed the question with which we began the chapter: How are positive interventions distinct from acceptance-based approaches? As we see it, there are three key distinctions. First, whereas acceptance-based approaches revolve around engaging in every experience, positive or negative, with the goal of achieving a balanced experience, positive interventions almost exclusively emphasize positive experiences with the assumption that positive experiences are often overshadowed by negative experiences (Baumeister, Bratslavsky, Finkenauer, & Vohs, 2001). We base our approach on work suggesting that individuals function best when the number of positive interactions they experience outweighs the number of negative interactions (Driver & Gottman, 2004; Fredrickson & Losada, 2005).

Second, whereas acceptance-based approaches posit that individuals should not try to change their experiences, but rather accept their experience without judgment, positive interventions revolve around the identification and amplification of positive experiences and sometimes even the creation of new positive experiences. In other words, a positive intervention aims to *replace* negative experiences with positive ones, while an acceptance-based approach makes no attempt to change a client's experience. Third, whereas acceptance-based approaches assume that problems must be engaged with, positive interventions operate under the assumption that positive factors make negative factors less salient, urgent, and important to individuals (Seligman, Rashid, & Parks, 2006).

This is not to say that there are no commonalities between acceptance-based approaches and positive interventions. In fact, we would argue that Acceptance and Commitment Therapy (ACT) and positive interventions have an important conceptual commonality: self-determination theory (Ryan & Deci, 2000). Both approaches acknowledge that both positive and negative emotions play important roles in psychological functioning; despite its reputation as "happyology," positive psychology regularly acknowledges that unfettered positive emotion without negative emotion as an anchor can be quite problematic (i.e., mania). Both approaches aim to help clients pursue their goals in a way that is authentic and self-driven; the techniques differ, but the goals are the same. Nevertheless, we think it is safe to say that positive interventions are, indeed, an approach to improving peoples' lives that is distinct from acceptance-based approaches—both theoretically and practically.

Conclusions

In this chapter, we provided a new definition of a positive intervention: an activity that successfully increases some positive variable and that can be reasonably and ethically applied in whatever context it is being used. We presented evidence that positive interventions targeting a variety of construct exist, and each has at least preliminary evidence of effectiveness, broadly construed. We also argued that caution is warranted when putting positive interventions into real-world practice; we know some of these activities can "backfire" but do not yet understand when, how, and for what activities this occurs. Finally, we argue that positive interventions are distinctive from other psychological approaches in general and from ACT in particular

References

Aknin, L., Barrington-Leigh, C., Dunn, E., Helliwell, J., Biswas-Diener, R., Kemeza, I., Nyende, P., Ashton-James, C., Norton, M. (in press). Prosocial spending and well-being: Cross-cultural evidence for a psychological universal. *Journal of Personality and Social Psychology*.

Baskin, T., & Enright, R. D. (2004). Intervention studies on forgiveness: A meta-analysis. *Journal of Counseling and Development, 82,* 79-90.

Batson, C. D., Chang, J., Orr, R., & Rowland, J. (2002). Empathy, attitudes, and action: Can feeling for a member of a stigmatized group motivate one to help the group? *Personality and Social Psychology Bulletin, 28,* 1656-1666.

Baumeister, R. F., Bratslavsky, E., Finkenauer, C., & Vohs, K. D. (2001). Bad is stronger than good. *Review of General Psychology, 5,* 323-370.

Biswas-Diener, R., Kashdan, T. B., & Minhas, G. (2011). A dynamic approach to psychological strength development and intervention. *Journal of Positive Psychology, 6,* 106-118.

Bryant, F. B. (2003). Savoring Beliefs Inventory (SBI): A scale for measuring beliefs about savoring. *Journal of Mental Health, 12,* 175-196.

Bryant, F. B., Smart, C. M., & King, S. P. (2005). Using the past to enhance the present: Boosting happiness through positive reminiscence. *Journal of Happiness Studies, 6,* 227-260.

Bryant, F. B., & Veroff, J. (2007). *Savoring: A new model of positive experience.* Mahwah, NJ: Lawrence Erlbaum Associates.

Davis, M. H., Conklin, L., Smith, A., & Luce, C. (1996). Effect of perspective taking on the cognitive representation of persons: A merging of self and other. *Journal of Personality and Social Psychology, 70,* 713-726.

Diener, E., & Diener, C. (2011). Monitoring psychosocial prosperity for social change. In R. Biswas-Diener (Ed.), *Positive psychology as social change* (pp. 53-72). Dordrecht, Netherlands: Springer Press.

Driver, J. L., & Gottman, J. M. (2004). Daily marital interactions and positive affect during marital conflict among newlywed couples. *Family Processes, 43,* 301-314.

Dunn, E. W., Aknin, L. B., & Norton, M. I. (2008). Spending money on others promotes happiness. *Science, 319,* 1687-1688.

Emmons, R. A., & McCullough, M. E. (2003). Counting blessings versus burdens: An experimental investigation of gratitude and subjective well-being in daily life. *Journal of Personality and Social Psychology, 84,* 377-389.

Fordyce, M. W. (1977). Development of a program to increase personal happiness. *Journal of Counseling Psychology, 24,* 511-521.

Fordyce, M. W. (1983). A program to increase happiness: Further studies. *Journal of Counseling Psychology, 30,* 483-498.

Fredrickson, B. L., & Losada, M. F. (2005). Positive affect and the complex dynamics of human flourishing. *American Psychologist, 60,* 678-686.

Gable, S. L., Reis, H. T., Impett, E. A., & Asher, E. R. (2004). What do you do when things go right? The intrapersonal and interpersonal benefits of sharing positive events. *Journal of Personality and Social Psychology, 87,* 228-245.

The Gallup Organization. (1999). *Clifton StrengthsFinder.* Washington, DC: Author.

Grant, H., & Dweck, C. S. (2003). Clarifying achievement goals and their impact. *Journal of Personality and Social Psychology, 85,* 541–553.

Haidt, J. (2002). It's more fun to work on strengths than weaknesses (but it may not be better for you). Manuscript retrieved from http://people.virginia.edu/~jdh6n/strengths_analysis.doc

Hodges, S. D., Clark, B., & Myers, M. W. (2011). Better living through perspective taking. In R. Biswas-Diener (Ed.), *Positive psychology as a mechanism for social change* (pp. 193-218). Dordrecht, Netherlands: Springer Press.

Hodges, T. D., & Clifton, D. O. (2004). Strengths-based development in practice. In A. Linley & S. Joseph (Eds.), *Handbook of positive psychology in practice*. Hoboken, New Jersey: John Wiley and Sons, Inc.

Hook, J. N., Worthington, E. L., Jr., & Utsey, S. O. (2009). Collectivism, forgiveness, and social harmony. *The Counseling Psychologist, 37,* 786-820.

Kabat-Zinn, J. (2003). Mindfulness-based stress reduction (MBSR). *Constructivism in the Human Sciences, 8,* 73-107.

Kahler, C. W., Spillane, N. S., Clerkin, E., Brown, R. A., & Parks, A. (2011, July). *Development of positive psychotherapy for smoking cessation.* Paper presented at the Second World Congress on Positive Psychology, Philadelphia, PA.

King, L. A. (2001). The health benefits of writing about life goals. *Personality and Social Psychology Bulletin, 27,* 798-807.

Kurtz, J. L., & Lyubomirsky, S. (in press). Using mindful photography to increase positive emotion and appreciation. In J. J. Froh & A. C. Parks (Eds.), *Activities for teaching positive psychology: A guide for instructors.* Washington, DC: American Psychological Association Press.

Louis, M. (2011). Strengths interventions in higher education: Effects on implicit self-theory. *Journal of Positive Psychology, 6,* 204-215.

Lundahl, B. W., Taylor, M. J., Stevenson, R., & Roberts, K. D. (2008). Process-based forgiveness interventions: A meta-analysis. *Research on Social Work Practice, 18,* 465-478.

Lyubomirsky, S., Dickerhoof, R., Boehm, J. K., & Sheldon, K. M. (2011). Becoming happier takes both a will and a proper way: An experimental longitudinal intervention to boost well-being. *Emotion, 11,* 391-402.

Lyubomirsky, S., Sheldon, K. M., & Schkade, D. (2005). Pursuing happiness: The architecture of sustainable change. *Review of General Psychology, 9,* 111-131.

Lyubomirsky, S., Sousa, L., & Dickerhoof, R. (2006). The costs and benefits of writing, talking, and thinking about life's triumphs and defeats. *Journal of Personality and Social Psychology, 90,* 692-708.

Mauss, I. B., Tamir, M., Anderson, C. L., & Savino, N. (2011). Can seeking happiness make people unhappy? Paradoxical effects of valuing happiness. *Emotion, 11,* 767.

McCullough, M. E., Root, L. M., & Cohen, A. D. (2006). Writing about the benefits of an interpersonal transgression facilitates forgiveness. *Journal of Consulting and Clinical Psychology, 74,* 887-897.

McNulty, J. K. (2011). The dark side of forgiveness: The tendency to forgive predicts continued psychological and physical aggression in marriage. *Personality and Social Psychology Bulletin, 37,* 770-783.

Meyer, P., Johnson, D., Parks, A. C., Iwanski, C., & Penn, D. L. (in press). Positive living: A pilot study of group positive psychotherapy for people with severe mental illness. *Journal of Positive Psychology.*

Myers, M. M., & Hodges, S. D. (in press). Perspective taking and pro-social behavior: Caring for others like we care for the self. In J. J. Froh & A. C. Parks (Eds.),

Activities for teaching positive psychology: A practical guide for instructors. Washington, DC: American Psychological Association Press.

Otake, K., Shimai, S., Tanaka-Matsumi, J., Otsui, K., & Fredrickson, B. L. (2006). Happy people become happier through kindness: A counting kindnesses intervention. *Journal of Happiness Studies, 7,* 361-375.

Parks, A. C., Della Porta, M. D., Pierce, R. S., Zilca, R., & Lyubomirsky, S. (in press). Pursuing happiness in everyday life: A naturalistic investigation of online happiness seekers. *Emotion.*

Pennebaker, J. W., & Seagal, J. D. (1999). Forming a story: The health benefits of narrative. *Journal of Clinical Psychology, 55,* 1243-1254.

Peterson, C., & Seligman, M. E. P. (2004). *Character strengths and virtues: A handbook and classification.* New York: Oxford University Press.

Ryan, R. M., & Deci, E. L. (2001). On happiness and human potentials: A review of research on hedonic and eudaimonic well-being. *Annual Review Psychology, 52,* 141-166.

Schueller, S. M. (2010). Preferences for positive psychology exercises. *The Journal of Positive Psychology, 5,* 192-203.

Schueller, S. M., & Parks, A. C. (2012). Disseminating self-help: Positive psychology exercises in an online trial. To appear in the *Journal of Medical Internet Research.*

Schwartz, B., & Hill, K. E. (2006). Practical wisdom: Aristotle meets positive psychology. *Journal of Happiness Studies, 7,* 377–395.

Seligman, M. E. P. (2000, July). Personal communication during the 2000 annual positive psychology steering committee meeting in Oahu, HI. In attendance, Robert Biswas-Diener, Mihalyi Csikszentimihaly, Ed Diener, Martin Seligman, and George Vaillant.

Seligman, M. E. P., & Csikszentmihalyi, M. (2000). Positive psychology: An introduction. *American Psychologist, 55,* 5-14.

Seligman, M. E. P., Parks, A. C., & Steen, T. (2005). A balanced psychology and a full life. In F. Huppert, N. Baylis, & B. Keverne (Eds.), *The science of well-being* (pp. 275-283). New York: Oxford University Press.

Seligman, M. E. P., Rashid, T., & Parks, A. C. (2006). Positive psychotherapy, *American Psychologist, 61,* 774-788.

Seligman, M. E. P., Steen, T. A., Park, N., & Peterson, C. (2005). Positive psychology progress: Empirical validation of interventions. *American Psychologist, 60,* 410-421.

Sheldon, K. M., & Lyubomirsky, S. (2006). How to increase and sustain positive emotion: The effects of expressing gratitude and visualizing best possible selves. *Journal of Positive Psychology, 1,* 73-82.

Sergeant, S., and Mongrain, M. (2011). Are positive psychology exercises helpful for people with depressive personality styles? *The Journal of Positive Psychology, 6*(4), 260-272.

Sin, N. L., Della Porta, M. D., & Lyubomirsky, S. (2011). Tailoring positive psychology interventions to treat depressed individuals. In S. I. Donaldson, M.

Csikszentmihalyi, & J. Nakamura (Eds.), *Applied positive psychology: Improving everyday life, health, schools, work, and society* (pp. 79-96). New York: Routledge.

Sin, N. L., & Lyubomirsky, S. (2009). Enhancing well-being and alleviating depressive symptoms with positive psychology interventions: A practice-friendly meta-analysis. *Journal of Clinical Psychology: In Session, 65,* 467-487.

Wood, A. M., Froh, J. J, & Geraghty, A. W. A. (2010). Gratitude and well-being: A review and theoretical integration. *Clinical Psychology Review, 30,* 890-905.

Worthington, E. L., Jr. (2006). *The path to forgiveness: Six practical sessions for becoming a more forgiving person.* Unpublished manual. Available online at http://www.people.vcu.edu/~eworth/

Worthington, E. L. Jr., Witvliet, C. V. O., Pietrini, P., & Miller, A. J. (2007). Forgiveness, health, and well-being: A review of evidence for emotional versus decisional forgiveness, dispositional forgivingness, and reduced unforgiveness. *Journal of Behavioral Medicine, 30,* 291-302.

CHAPTER 8

On Making People More Positive and Rational: The Potential Downsides of Positive Psychology Interventions

Mairéad Foody

Yvonne Barnes-Holmes

Dermot Barnes-Holmes

National University of Ireland, Maynooth

Having a sense of self is essential for achieving your values (i.e., because they are "your" values). And so, it is not surprising that common forms of mental distress, such as anxiety, have been associated with problems of the self (e.g., Ingram, 1990). Although clinical practitioners and researchers across the domain of psychology have long recognized the importance of a sense of self in almost everything we do, there is no coherent account of what it is or how it works.

The Role of Self in Positive Psychology

As a discipline, positive psychology attempts to investigate and promote optimum human functioning, including positive and prosocial behavior (Duckworth, Steen, & Seligman, 2005; Gable & Haidt, 2005), and a range of strategies are employed toward this aim (Seligman, Steen, Park, & Peterson, 2005). The most commonly recommended include savoring peak positive moments; identifying talents and strengths of character and finding new opportunities to use them; and building a regular practice of contemplating and expressing gratitude to people (Seligman et al., 2005).

An obvious thread across these practices is an emphasis on the self and promoting commitment to your personal projects and values (often referred to as *flourishing*). Indeed, positive psychologists employ numerous self-related concepts. These include hypo-egoic self-regulation (Leary, Adams, & Tate, 2006); self-compassion (Neff, 2003); self-esteem (Baumeister, Smart, & Boden, 1999); self-efficacy (Bandura, 1999); and self-worth (Crocker & Park, 2004).

Consistent with this array of self-based concepts, numerous positive psychology interventions focus specifically on the self. For example, positive attribution interventions explore the extent to which you attribute positive events to yourself and attribute negative events to external sources (Fredrickson & Joiner, 2002). Hope interventions attempt to increase the extent to which you perceive yourself as effective at achieving your goals (Ciarrochi, Heaven, & Davies, 2007). Optimism interventions attempt to explore your perceived ideal self (Lyubomirsky, Dickerhoof, Boehm, & Sheldon, 2011). And self-compassion interventions seek to enhance self-acceptance (Neff, 2003).

In spite of this emphasis on self, both conceptually and technically, the field of positive psychology has not yet proposed a *complete* account of self, nor of its role in the promotion of positive behavior. In short, different theorists and researchers have focused on specific aspects of self, but these have not yet been collected together into a complete and coherent working definition.

A modern behavioral and functional account of human language and cognition, known as relational frame theory (RFT), has proposed what appears to be a technical account of the self (Hayes,

Barnes-Holmes, & Roche, 2001). The theory proposes that all aspects of human language and cognition, including self-perceptions and perspective taking, are complex "verbal acts" that are generated by individual histories. As we will explain shortly, this approach facilitates an understanding of the self, while accommodating the fact that our histories make us unique. A greater understanding of the self has obvious and broad applicability to the way in which human suffering is perceived and treated, at the level of both individuals and communities.

Chapter Aims

The primary aim of the current chapter is to suggest the applicability, and explore potential sources of overlap, between RFT's technical account of the self and interventions employed by positive psychologists. Self plays a pivotal role in both traditions, and it is often a useful exercise to explore how different approaches interpret common ground. Our key question is whether a functional behavioral account of self can speak directly to the understanding and pursuit of human flourishing, as articulated by positive psychology. In our attempt to build this conceptual bridge, the chapter is divided into two parts. Part one provides a brief summary of the RFT account of self, technical in parts, but necessary for understanding the theory's specific account of self. Readers are referred directly to chapter 1 for a summary of RFT's basic processes. Part two then describes two key exercises promoted by positive psychology that are explicitly focused on the self and involve attempts to manipulate one's sense of self in the service of better psychological health. These include writing about life's positive events and triumphs and expressing gratitude. In the context of each exercise, we offer an RFT interpretation of what appear to be the key underlying psychological processes and the potential pitfalls.

The RFT Approach to Self: Perspective-Taking Relations

For RFT, perspective taking comprises three types of derived stimulus relations, known as I vs. YOU, HERE vs. THERE, and NOW vs. THEN.

Put simply, these describe the three core aspects of your perspective. First, you see the world as I, not as YOU or as someone else (hence, we say, I *versus* YOU). Second, when you see the world as I, you always see it from HERE, not from THERE, or anywhere that is not HERE (hence, we say, HERE *versus* THERE). Third, when you see the world as I, you always see it from NOW, not from THEN, or some other point in time that is not NOW (hence, we say, NOW *versus* THEN). In summary, I always see my world from HERE and NOW and from my perspective, and I always see YOU from THERE and THEN.

I versus YOU. When we operate from the perspective of I, we distinguish, compare, and contrast ourselves to others across a myriad of dimensions. As children, we learn to do this initially through physical attributes (e.g., Mommy is taller than me, but Daddy is taller than her). Harmless as these may seem, the fact that we can already compare and contrast ourselves with others means that we can also evaluate these comparisons. Consider, for example, Ann, who has always felt inferior to her more attractive sister Mary. In relational terms, Ann's perspective holds that Mary is more physically attractive than Ann, more attractive equals better, hence Mary is also better than Ann. Although the initial comparison between the sisters may have been based on a single physical attribute (which may not even have been observed directly by others), Ann's comparative relations have allowed her to contrast this physical superiority, and her coordination relations have allowed her to coordinate this superiority with being better *generally*. Of course, the latter would also quickly have become coordinated with Ann feeling bad about herself. So, it is easy to see how even simple relations and the fact that they involve feelings, can lead us early in our lives toward a path of low self-esteem.

The above example also illustrates how perspective-taking behavior becomes increasingly arbitrary and thus, at one level, moves further and further away from physical attributes. Indeed, as verbally sophisticated adults, most of our comparisons with others are *not* based on physical attributes. For example, I might be consumed by jealousy because, from my perspective, my neighbor appears to be richer than I am, and yet I have no way of knowing how much money my neighbor actually has.

In fact, who we come to know ourselves to be across time emerges on the basis of our perspective on others, such that it seems unlikely that there would be an I without a YOU. What makes perspective taking distinct from other types of relational activity is the paradox that I vs. YOU relations become a constant reference point for our perceptions, even when many aspects of our lives are constantly changing. For example, if I suddenly learn that my "rich" neighbor has lost his job, I may now believe that we are equal in wealth, but we are still different people. That is, aspects of who you are may change constantly, but your perspective from which these changes are observed does not. In short, you always see the world from your own perspective.

HERE versus THERE. There is a long literature on the importance of a sense of place in human development, and, for RFT, this is captured by the spatial relations of HERE and THERE. In conjunction with our I vs. YOU relational development, we learn to distinguish between HERE (i.e., not THERE) and THERE (i.e., not HERE). For example, when Daddy comes home, a child might say, "I am watching TV (HERE), but Mommy is in the kitchen (THERE)." Similar to I-YOU relations, spatial relations become increasingly less based on physical locations and become increasingly arbitrary. For instance, if I say "I am here" at this moment in time, I am in my office, but if I say, "I am here" one hour from now, I will be in my kitchen. In other words, the word "HERE" coordinates with where I am at that point in time, hence it is constantly changing. Paradoxically, much of the language that we use refers to physical space, but in a metaphorical way. Consider Sarah who describes her feelings of depression as "bearing down on her" or as a sense of "carrying the weight of the world on her shoulders."

It is clear from the examples above that I-YOU relations are implicit in HERE-THERE relations because it would be impossible to specify a perspective from a particular location if there was no perspective from which to operate. As a result, Sarah is talking about *her* feelings, which are part of the way she sees herself at that time. As such, the spatial relations are a critical feature of one's perspective because I is always coordinated with HERE (and distinct from THERE) and YOU is always coordinated with THERE (and distinct from HERE).

NOW versus THEN. Temporal relations are another core feature of perspective taking, and RFT refers to these as NOW vs. THEN relations. As the name implies, temporal relations refer to time and are naturally implicit in most everyday sentences. For example, "At two o'clock I was working but by three, I was at home." Again, we learn temporal relations using physical features, especially when we first learn to tell time. Once that skill is acquired, these relations then become largely arbitrary because you can make reference to time without knowing what time it actually is and because temporal relations can be extended across, days, weeks, months, and even years. Consider an athlete who breaks her leg and is unable to participate in any more competitions. She may become fixated on what she was last year and lose sight of her life in the present (e.g., last year (THEN), I was a winner, but this year (NOW) I am a loser). Again, I-YOU relations are implicit in temporal relations because one's perspective is always from NOW and distinct to THEN. Of course, it is important to remember that even if you are referring to how you felt in the past (THEN), the temporal relation from your current perspective is always NOW.

The ACT Approach to Self: The Three Selves

Relational frame theory has offered a detailed account of the development of language, which incorporates an understanding of the darker side of the most natural of human abilities. As the examples above demonstrate, once you have comparison relations, you can begin to compare yourself to others and find that you are wanting. And once you do this, even on only one dimension, you can coordinate this with many other dimensions, even if this is not based on reality. As a result, you can readily come to a place in which you perceive yourself to be truly worthless. Taken together therefore, RFT goes some way toward an understanding of the development of suffering.

Acceptance and Commitment Therapy (ACT) is an approach to human suffering and its alleviation that is related on many levels to RFT (Hayes, Strosahl, & Wilson, 1999). For example, both hail from the same functional behavioral tradition. A growing body of research is currently attempting to explore the empirical overlap between RFT's scientific and ACT's therapeutic concepts (e.g., Luciano et al., 2011). For instance, Foody, Barnes-Holmes, and Barnes-Holmes (2012) have articulated the integration of RFT's perspective-taking relations and ACT's three selves.

According to ACT, the self is conceptualized in terms of three selves, known as self as content, self as process, and self as context (Hayes et al.,

1999). Although the concept of multiple selves has been employed by many other theoretical approaches to the self (e.g., Higgins, 1999), a core distinction forms the basis of the ACT approach. That is, ACT distinguishes between two functional aspects of the self "as a doer and as an observer of the doing" (Hayes, 1995, p. 1). In simple terms, the doer is synonymous with your psychological content (i.e., your thoughts, feelings, emotions, etc.), while the observer is your perspective on this content. Three points are worth remembering about this approach. 1. The doer and the observer are always operating simultaneously. 2. The three selves describe the operations of the doer, not the observer. 3. You can only operate according to one of the selves at any one point in time. Each of these points will become clearer as we walk through the section below on the three selves.

Self as content. As the name implies, self as content is a psychological space in which the distinctions between the observer and the doer are at their lowest. In short, who you are does not appear to be distinct from what you think, feel, remember, etc. In ACT, this shared psychological space is also known as fusion, such that who you are (the observer) is fused with what you think, feel, etc. (the doings). Of course, if your psychological content at any particular point in time is painful or negatively evaluated (e.g., if you are having the thought "I am useless"), the fusion between this and the observer would feel overwhelming. You would feel that you, that is *all of you*, is useless (rather than seeing this just as a thought that you are having at that particular moment). In this way, fusion between the observer and the doer when the doer is negative will practically always lead to you feeling bad and feeling threatened.

On balance, one might argue that fusion between the observer and *positive* psychological content is okay, but in ACT, this is not the case. In short, all fusion between you as the observer and your content is a psychologically unhealthy place from which to operate, because you are much more than the sum of your content. Indeed, as you will see from the two remaining selves, the greater the distinction between the observer and the doer, the more space in your life that can be attributed to the observer so that your overt behavior can then be governed by your values, and so on, and not by psychological content that comes and goes. In other words, you cannot live a rich and full values-based life if you are only what your content says you are and the latter is what is always happening in self as content.

Let's look at an example of self as content in the hypothetical case of Martin, a sufferer of chronic pain who goes for therapy. In the first paragraph, we introduce Martin. In the second, we explore the difficulties created for him by operating in self as content with regard to his pain.

Martin struggles with chronic pain and spends much of his time trying to come up with a foolproof strategy that will ideally get the pain to go away, or at least to let him get some control over it. He firmly believes that he has tried everything but that nothing has worked—some aspect of the pain is always there. Indeed, he can hardly tell anymore whether some type of pain is actually present or not. So the only thing that he can do is to keep trying to come up with the *right* strategy, on the assumption that it has simply eluded him thus far. The pain and his efforts to solve it are demanding, and he believes that they make all other aspects of living difficult, if not impossible. He feels like he is trapped in actual pain or in the pain "waiting room," and so he continues to search endlessly and frustratedly for the *perfect* solution. Nothing less would justify all the effort he has invested.

The pain and the struggle with it have gained such dominance over his life that much of who Martin is psychologically is about pain. In other words, Martin has come to know himself first and foremost as a sufferer of chronic pain. Many other aspects of his life have become secondary to this sense of self (not just in terms of his overt behavior). As such, the identification with the problem has become almost the whole person that he resides in, and other aspects (e.g., husband, father, worker) have, behaviorally, fallen away (e.g., "I can no longer play with the kids because my back will get sore"). And Martin (as the observer) sees this on occasion. He often asks himself where the old Martin went and he knows that his wife wonders about this too. He sees that they both long to have him back, but pain always seems to stand in the way of his going back to the person he used to be. He worries that he might be lost forever. In short, his sense of self is largely fused with the struggle regarding pain.

From an ACT perspective, several steps need to happen to allow Martin's life to be opened up because it has, as he recognizes, been sucked into a vacuum that revolves largely around pain at the expense of valued living. This would primarily involve a change in perspective from viewing himself as nothing but his pain, to perceiving himself as distinct and separate from his pain. Put another way, Martin needs to move from operating mostly in self as content, where his content about his pain has "taken over" much of the observer. We often describe this to clients as "BIG content, small observer," when it should ideally be the other way around.

Now let us consider how RFT can account for what is happening, at the level of process, in self as content. Figure 1 (far left-hand side) distinguishes between the observer and the doer, as in ACT. It is important to note that for RFT, hence in relational terms, the observer is always located HERE-NOW. This is your perspective. And this is the case for all three selves. Although the place from which the observer operates (i.e., HERE-NOW) never changes, the psychological space in which the doer operates does change, depending on which self you are in at any point in time. This is presented on the right-hand side of the diagram.

Figure 1. Conceptualization of the three selves as perspective-taking relations.

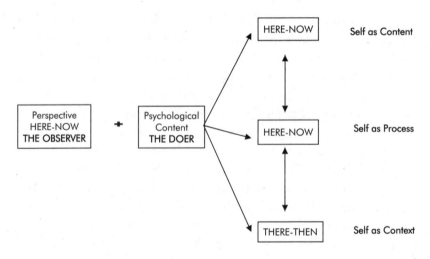

Figure 1 shows that in self as content your psychological content is located HERE and NOW (see figure, top right), as is the observer (the latter is always the case). The coordination between the observer and the doer in this way increases the likelihood that your content will exert control over your behavior. This relationship also accounts for why the sufferer often feels overwhelmed and threatened, because who you know is coordinated with what you think and so on. In essence, *it is the*

relationship between the observer and the doer at any point in time that is captured by the three selves, and in self as content, they are at their most coordinated (or psychologically "equivalent").

Self as process. Self as process is a psychological space in which ongoing activity facilitates continuous distinctions between the observer and the doer. In short, who you are is distinct from what you think, feel, remember, and so on. For ACT, this psychological space does not entail fusion, because the observer can perceive the processes of thinking, feeling, and so on (the doings), and the evaluations that accompany these. Naturally, this distinction has the potential to reduce the previous pain associated with those evaluations (i.e., the observer wouldn't feel as overwhelmed as when in self as content).

The *ongoing awareness* of those content-based processes is a critical feature of self as process. In essence, because you can perceive your content as continuously changing, attachment to it is not facilitated. Consider the example "I feel depressed and am having depressed thoughts, but these are just thoughts and feelings at this moment, and they may be different tomorrow." This ongoing awareness is synonymous with the concept of mindfulness, because you are being mindful of your content as it comes and goes.

Operating in self as process readily permits values-consistent behavior, rather than content-driven behavior, because you have a distinct awareness of your content while remaining open to values. In simple terms, self as process permits both, thereby allowing you greater flexibility with regard to your actions. Hence, you *can* live a rich and full values-based life if you can see your content for what it is. Notice, however, that self as process does not require you to somehow be "content-free" (if that were even possible) but simply offers you a different place from which to observe the ever-changing nature of your content.

On balance, it is also important to recognize that sticky psychological content (with which you have struggled in the past) is likely to create resurgence to self as content. That is, you cannot assume that all you need to do is stay in self as process, because your history will likely dictate that certain powerful content will slide you back into self as content, the minute it shows up. Accordingly, for ACT, there is a very fine line between self as content and self as process, and it is primarily ongoing awareness that keeps you in the latter and away from the grasp of the former. Let us return to our client Martin to illustrate how self as process works.

On a regular basis, Martin feels pain in one part of his body or maybe several at the same time. As soon as this experience occurs, his history of operating in self as content with this experience is almost inevitably brought to bear, and his behavioral flexibility is greatly reduced so that the alleviation of pain is perceived as the only option (i.e., "I must be someone who is pain free"). What this fusion in self as content precludes him from seeing is that even in that instant he does have other options regarding his pain, although they will certainly be difficult. For example, what he cannot see is the logical possibility that the pain can be endured, in the service of values. In short, perhaps, even when pain is present, other valued actions can be conducted. But, none of this can be experienced if pain-related content is not experienced on an ongoing basis, as one pain-related experience after another, and another, and another. Because even before Martin can learn to accept the pain, he must learn to operate from a different place in which the processes of his pain experiences can be observed. This would be self as process.

Now let us consider how RFT can account for what is happening at a relational level in self as process. Look at the right-hand side of Figure 1 again, and you will see that there is no *relational* difference between self as content and self as process, although they are significantly different experientially. In both selves, the doer is located HERE-NOW and, as always, the observer is HERE-NOW also. In self as process, there is a sense of the movement of psychological content from HERE-NOW to THERE-THEN. This means that although psychological content is problematic in self as content because it is HERE-NOW, self as process is different in that your content as HERE-NOW is simply the way we learn to talk about our thoughts, feelings, and behavior, and thus facilitates self-knowledge rather than fusion.

Self as context. Self as context is a psychological space in which there is the strongest distinction between the observer and the doer. For ACT, self as context embodies defusion because who you are is distinct from what you think, feel, remember, and so on. Consider the following example, "I feel depressed and am having depressed thoughts, but I know that who *I* am is more than these negative thoughts and feelings." Naturally, this distinction has the potential to reduce the previous pain associated with content and its evaluations (i.e., the observer wouldn't feel as overwhelmed as when in self as content). To illustrate the ACT approach with regard to facilitating self as context, let us return to Martin.

At the outset of therapy, Martin's experience of his pain, when he discriminates its presence, is always fused with self-knowledge as a sufferer of pain. This dominates his sense of self, such that in the here and now when there is pain, there is little else. Training in self as context would permit Martin to experience a sense of self that is distinct from the pain, as well as highlighting the fact that other experiences can coexist with pain. When Martin learns to make more contact with this sense of self, it also increases his access to values, as a dominant source of behavior, and a greater sense of self as context will allow him to consistently keep his behavior going in that valued direction. Self as context will also foster greater acceptance by him because it opens up a safe place in which pain can be experienced as not completely overwhelming or dominant. It is a part of who he is, but not all that he is.

At a relational level, RFT suggests that in self as context the doer is located THERE-THEN, rather than in HERE-NOW, as was the case with the other two selves (see Figure 1, bottom right). This strong relational distinction between observer and doer renders this the safest place from which to view your thoughts, feelings, and so on, and likely facilitates the greatest distinction between content and overt behavior. In other words, when psychological content is not located in the same place as the observer, the content has no intrinsic power to control behavior. Thus you can live your life in a values-consistent manner without influence from psychological content.

From an ACT perspective, self as context facilitates maximum defusion (or least fusion) because it provides the largest distinction between the observer and the doer. However, there are two important points that should be remembered. First, it might seem that the ideal place from which to operate is self as context, such that you should operate in this mode all the time. But this is neither feasible nor essential, because self as process should suffice for much content and historically sticky content will likely draw you back to self as content anyway. As a result, self as process is perhaps the best mode of operating for most of the time, while self as context is safest when sticky content has a history of sucking you into self as content.

Indeed, a primary goal of ACT is to establish psychological flexibility, which involves the ability to switch among the three selves, as necessary. In short, to minimize fusion, ACT suggests switching from self as content to self as process. But, because self as process is still a relatively dangerous place to be because you can easily get sucked back into self as content, ACT exercises also promote flexibility in switching from self as process to self as context (i.e., to maximize defusion).

Consider again the example of Martin. In the beginning, Martin was operating in self as content with regard to his experiences of pain and became primarily a pain sufferer (i.e., maximum fusion). This fusion then makes it more likely that his behavior will be largely governed by attempts to remove the pain, with thoughts such as "I cannot be who I was until the pain is gone." Teaching Martin to operate with regard to his pain from self as process would allow him to notice on an ongoing basis the nature and frequency of pain experiences and would facilitate some defusion in this regard. For example, his ACT professional might encourage him to notice one pain event after another, and another, and another, like leaves floating down a stream. This self as process exercise would reduce the fusion with some pain events but of course not all, given his history. Hence, at the same time, it would be important to teach Martin how to operate from self as context in which he can come to see that he is much more than his pain experiences (i.e., BIG observer, small doer). In this case, both self as process and self as context can be used to facilitate behavioral flexibility in the service of values because Martin can learn that even when pain shows up, it can be noticed, acknowledged, and yet alternative values-based action can still happen.

In the sections below, we explore the potential overlap between ACT and RFT approaches to self and various exercises from the field of positive psychology. Although each hails from a very different philosophical and psychological tradition, there is much utility in examining potential common ground for both scientific and therapeutic perspectives. In particular, we selected two positive psychology exercises that appeared to have a strong basis in one's sense of self.

An RFT Interpretation of Positive Psychology Exercises

The primary goal of positive psychology is to identify the positive aspects of an individual's personality and to harness these in the service of achieving optimum human functioning. In other words, strategies for promoting well-being lie at the heart of this psychological movement. There are numerous positive psychology strategies that are beneficial in this regard (e.g., Algoe & Haidt, 2009; Cohn & Fredrickson 2010). For example, Sin and Lyubomirsky (2009) conducted a meta-analysis of positive psychology interventions and found that in general they were associated with increases in self-reported well-being and decreases in depressive symptoms. In particular, Seligman et al. (2005) reported that the *gratitude visit, the three good things in life exercise,* and *using signature strengths in a new way* were associated with increased subjective self-reported happiness. There is also mounting evidence to support the use of writing exercises (e.g., Frattaroli, Thomas, & Lyubomirsky, 2011) and gratitude exercises (e.g., Lyubomirsky et al., 2011) in general. In the sections below, we explore RFT interpretations of these two positive psychology interventions.

Writing about life's positive events and triumphs. Positive writing exercises are a well-established tool in positive psychology (Seligman et al., 2005). For example, the *three good things in life* exercise requires you to write down three events that have "gone well" each day for the past week, including the perceived causes of these positive outcomes. Using this intervention, Seligman et al. found increases in self-reported happiness and decreases in depressive symptoms at one-, three-, and six-month follow-ups. In an adaptation of this exercise, King (2001) found that writing down the most positive events that you imagine for your life ahead was also associated with increased subjective well-being at a three-week follow-up. According to King, positive writing exercises facilitate a self-focus on goals, which in turn encourages better behavioral self-regulation.

In contrast, research by Lyubomirsky, Sousa, and Dickerhoof (2006) has reported less positive outcomes for writing analytically about positive life events, relative to simply thinking about these events. Specifically, participants in the former group reported less life satisfaction; personal growth; self-acceptance; and general health. In an attempt to explain these contradictory findings, we will return to this issue later in this section.

The investigation of positive writing is a relatively new endeavor in research and treatment, compared to a traditional focus on the effects of writing about *negative* or traumatic events. Indeed, the literature on what is referred to as *expressive disclosive writing* is simply vast (e.g., Sloan &

Marx, 2004b). In short, this technique requires individuals to write down thoughts and emotions they have about a traumatic life event. Several studies have reported positive outcomes in the use of this technique, including reduced health problems (e.g., Pennebaker & Beall, 1986); faster reemployment after job loss (e.g., Spera, Buhrfeind, & Pennebaker, 1994); better adjustment to college (e.g., Pennebaker, Colder, & Sharp, 1990); and even improved lung functioning for sufferers of asthma (e.g., Smyth, Stone, Hurewitz, & Kaell, 1999). Some researchers have suggested that these outcomes may be mediated by the disclosure of previously inhibited feelings (Pennebaker, 1989) and hence reduced need for emotional avoidance (Sloan & Marx, 2004a).

In between the two approaches above (i.e., writing about positive events and negative events), some therapeutic exercises involve writing down the positive aspects of a negative event. For example, Stanton et al. (2002) demonstrated that women who wrote down their positive thoughts and feelings about their cancer had significantly fewer medical visits, relative to a control group. According to Wing, Schutte, and Byrne (2006), the writing in this case permits deeper cognitive processing through better understanding and assimilation of the emotions associated with these events (Pennebaker & Seagal, 1999).

There may well be benefits associated with writing per se, whether the subject is positive, negative, or somewhere in between. For example, Frattaroli et al. (2011) found that an expressive writing exercise about a forthcoming exam with high school students was associated with significantly higher test scores and lower pre-exam depressive symptoms, relative to controls. Indeed, several authors have suggested that the writing of self-relevant content facilitates greater self-awareness and subsequent self-regulation in terms of one's priorities (King & Miner, 2000). Similarly, Burton and King (2004) proposed that this enhanced self-awareness in turn promotes the integration of one's experiences into the self-concept. In short, writing may serve to facilitate a more clearly articulated sense of self.

There appears to be common ground between positive psychology's promotion of self-writing and the ACT concepts of self as process and defusion. That is, for both accounts, the objective is the ongoing experiencing and describing of thoughts, behaviors, feelings, and so on, which enhance self-regulation in terms of values-consistent behavior (rather than that which is content driven). Indeed for RFT, the writing down of your psychological content is a physical metaphor for defusion, because writing is an act of self as process (i.e., you notice content as you write it). In this way, your content HERE-NOW is simply the manner in which you talk, or indeed write, about your ongoing experiences (Hayes, 1995). In short, they are what you are describing HERE-NOW but not all that you are across time and space.

Consider our previous example of Martin. Imagine his therapist asked him to select a time in which he was experiencing pain or had a sense that pain was imminent. Imagine that she asked him to slowly and systematically write down each pain-related sensation or thought as it emerged, one by one, on sticky notes. She might then ask him to stick each note, one after the other, on his shirt. For ACT and RFT, the physical transfer of the thought, for example, from inside his body to the outside is an act of defusion. The act of writing is self as process as he watches the content emerge continuously in the HERE and NOW. This would differ considerably from what Martin has done to date, in keeping the content tucked away. Notice also that writing in this way is an exercise that is shared with the therapist. Again, this is opposite to what happened previously when pain-related content showed up for Martin and he was unwilling to discuss it with anyone else. Perhaps he even tried to convince himself that it was not actually happening and such experiential avoidance made things worse.

Martin's previous action lacked flexibility at multiple levels. First, self as content was so overwhelming that he could see no alternative but to try to avoid the pain of his content. Second, the more he tried to avoid the content, the more it showed up, and the more likely that he became fused with it, thus reinforcing the view that he was nothing more than his pain. Taken together, these events basically ensured that most of Martin's time and energy were spent in "dealing with" pain, at the cost of any other type of value-based behavior.

From RFT and ACT perspectives, we see one potential limitation in positive psychology's focus on the writing of *positive* experiences, as in the *best possible selves* exercise. For ACT and RFT, there is no functional distinction between positive and negative content; both are types of content that are simply evaluated differently. Indeed, self as content is often problematic, irrespective of the type of content with which you are fused. Similarly, self as process does not concern itself with the experiencing of a particular type of psychological content, but with *all content*.

At an intuitive level, you may be more likely to become fused with your negative content, because it is more painful and more likely to be avoided. So, the harder you fight not to have it, the more of a threat it becomes. This is perhaps less likely to be the case with positive content, which you are less likely to try to avoid. Nonetheless, at a process level, you can become attached to your positive content, and this is indeed what many clients try to do (i.e., "I will be better if I could just have happier thoughts"). But this move would be just as problematic as attachment to negative content, because you are always more than your content (good and bad). In short, neither self as content nor self as process separate out "good" content from "bad"; all content is, by definition, problematic when viewed from self as content and must be observed constantly in self as process. To illustrate this critical difference, consider the example of ACT's metaphor of the chessboard.

> Let us say that the white pieces represent your positive thoughts, while the black pieces represent your negative thoughts. And the different types of thoughts and feelings hang out together in teams. For example, "bad" feelings (like anxiety) hang out with "bad" thoughts (like "I'm useless"). And it's the same with the "good" ones (like feeling happy and thinking that you are in control of your life). So it seems that the way the game is played is that we select which side we want to win. You put the "good" pieces on one side and the bad pieces on the other, and then you get up on the back of the white queen and ride to battle, fighting to win the war against the bad pieces. But from this position, huge portions of yourself are your own enemy. And the more you try to fight the black, the more room you give them to dominate your life. So you have to fight harder and harder and harder. Of course, your hope is that you will knock enough of them off the board so that you will eventually dominate them with white pieces. You feel hopeless, you have a sense that you can't win, and yet you can't stop fighting. If you're on the back of the white horse, fighting is the only choice you have because the black pieces seem life threatening. Yet spending all your time in a war zone is a miserable way to live.

The aim for a client in ACT is to identify with the board as a useful perspective on her content of white and black pieces. The board holds the pieces and they need it, not vice versa. If you are attached to any of the pieces, playing the game is very important and you will be focused on "winning." As the board, you can see all of the pieces, you can hold them, and you can watch the war being played out. You cannot become attached to specific pieces (even white) without abandoning board level. Hayes (2004) captured the essence of operating at board level in the following quote: "ACT clients are encouraged to abandon any interest in the literal truth of their own thoughts or evaluations" (p. 647). As such, no content is to be believed as literally true and/or as saying something about who you are as a person, thereby holding firm to a distinction between the observer and the doer. If you permit attachment to any type of content, even positive, this distinction is sacrificed.

From an RFT/ACT perspective, it seems plausible that positive writing exercises serve one of two functions. The first is that they may facilitate self as content, instead of self as process. This might encourage you to become fused with your positive content if you are seeking to reduce or remove negative content. This type of experiential avoidance is associated with poor mental health outcomes and is not at all consistent with ACT (Hayes, Pankey, & Palm, 2005). The second possibility is that these exercises facilitate defusion and values clarification. For example, you might write "I am a really good parent," if you value sound parenting. The defusion element of this allows you to have distance from any painful experiences you may have of faulty parenting. The values clarification element allows you to see which aspects of parenting you might do better in the future, and this may enhance your motivation for achieving this value. Defusion and values clarification have been critical ACT components since the beginning and there is sound empirical support for their role in positive clinical outcomes (see Hayes, Luoma, Bond, Masuda, & Lillis, 2006).

Therapeutic Suggestions for Expressive Writing Exercises

- Writing exercises should facilitate defusion that allows distance between the writer and the content that is written.

- Writing exercises should facilitate the clarification of values and discourage avoidance of memories of previously nonvalue-based actions.

- Writing exercises should encourage self as process over self as content. Even positive psychological content is problematic when one is attached to it.

An RFT interpretation of "gratitude." Gratitude has been defined by Emmons (2004) as *"a sense of thankfulness and joy in response to a gift, whether the gift be a tangible benefit from a specific other or a moment of peaceful bliss evoked by natural beauty"* (p. 554). Gratitude is an integral part of the positive psychology movement (Bono & McCullough, 2006; McCullough, Kimeldorf, & Cohen, 2008), and numerous interventions based on the experience and development of gratitude have been designed, such as *the gratitude list* (see Wood, Froh, & Geraghty, 2010). Indeed some advocates of positive psychology are so favorable to the concept of gratitude that they have proposed the implementation of its interventions on a national scale (e.g., Bono, Emmons, & McCullough, 2004; Froh, Miller, & Snyder, 2007), as well as in clinical settings (Wood, et al., 2010). In line with this enthusiasm, the available empirical evidence is promising. For example, variations of gratitude exercises have been linked to increases in psychological well-being (Seligman et al., 2005), prosocial behavior (e.g., Tsang, 2006), and general positive emotions (e.g., Emmons & McCullough, 2003).

The "gratitude list" and the "gratitude visit" are two of the most commonly used gratitude-based interventions in positive psychology. The *gratitude list* simply involves writing down the list of people, events, things, attributes, and so on, for which you are most grateful on a daily basis. The benefits of doing so have been demonstrated by a number of studies. For example, Froh, Sefick, and Emmons (2008) reported that adolescents who used the gratitude list over a two-week period showed enhanced optimism and life satisfaction. In addition, Emmons and McCullough (2003) reported that participants who wrote about people or events for whom/which they were grateful made more offers of support to others than participants who wrote about daily hassles.

The *gratitude visit* involves writing and delivering in person a letter of gratitude to someone who has been especially kind to you in the past but whom you have never fully thanked. Seligman et al. (2005) reported that this technique resulted in an increase in happiness and a decrease in depression at one- and three-week follow-ups (although this effect was not maintained at a three-month follow up). However, Lyubomirsky et al. (2011) have reported greater happiness at a six-month follow-up. Furthermore, the amount of effort attributed to the intervention was positively correlated with level of well-being.

Some authors have proposed the concept of *dispositional gratitude* (e.g., Froh, Emmons, Card, Bono, & Wilson, 2011; McCullough, Emmons, & Tsang, 2002). And, others have argued that it is central to generic well-being and prosocial behavior (Kashdan, Uswatte, & Julian, 2006; Tsang, 2006). For example, Wood, Maltby, Gillett, Linley, and Joseph (2008) reported longitudinal findings in which dispositional gratitude appeared to foster social support during a life transition, and to protect from ill effects associated with stress and depression. Other data have also shown that gratitude is an antidote to aggression, in terms of motivating people to express sensitivity and concern toward others (DeWall, Lambert, Pond, Kashdan, & Fincham, 2012). Indeed, some authors have even suggested that dispositional gratitude accounts for as much as 20% of the variance in individual differences in life satisfaction (Wood, Joseph, & Maltby, 2008). There is even evidence demonstrating gender differences between how people perceive and react to gratitude (see Kashdan, Mishra, Breen, & Froh, 2009).

In the language of RFT, gratitude requires complex levels of perspective taking, in terms of recognizing what you value for yourself and how you perceive this should be portrayed to, and appreciated by, others. Consider first the role of the self in gratitude. For me to experience gratitude based on something you did for me, I must be able to recognize that your actions and their outcomes were consistent with something I valued. Without this type of coordination between your action and my values, gratitude as an outcome seems unlikely. At one level, a very deep sense of gratitude suggests a very strong overlap between the actions of others and your values. Consider second the role of others in gratitude. A deep sense of gratitude may involve more than the concurrence of what you do and what I value. In fact, gratitude may also require, at least in the very meaningful instances, a sense that there is overlap or sharing between what you value and what I value. This perhaps accounts for why gratitude connects strongly with prosocial behavior. Furthermore, for this shared value to be appreciated, I must be able to have a perspective on both what I value and what you value. And in turn, you must have a perspective on what I value and what you value.

Consider the following example. As an adult, you realize that your parents had a formative role in your education, which subsequently led to your achieving a professional career that you now highly value. First, consider your *parents'* perspective taking regarding their role in your career. Unbeknownst to you in your youth, your parents were enduring financial hardship to pay your school fees. This is based on the value they placed on your education and the fact that they believed that you would in turn value this in the future. So, they had perspectives on their own values (being good parents, etc.), and their actions and hardships were consistent with these. And, they had a sense of your perspective later in life, and their actions were also consistent with your future values. Now consider *your* perspective taking. At the time, you probably had no perspective on your parents' actions or perspectives, and you perhaps had limited insight into what you valued, even then. You certainly would have been unlikely to have a perspective on what you would value in the future. *Now* you have a perspective on your own values and on your parents', both then and now. As a result of the perspective taking you have on what your parents valued, how they acted on it, and the perspective they had on your future perspective, you have a strong sense of enduring gratitude, because there was coalescence between what they valued and what you now value highly. This complex perspective taking may be illustrated in the following quotation by DeWall et al. (2012): "When experiencing gratitude, a person is sensitive to the emotion, thoughts, and actions that underlie the positive contributions of others … which reflect a shift away from self-interests to mirroring and understanding another person" (p. 2).

As well as demonstrating the complex perspective taking and values-based action involved in gratitude, the example above illustrates how temporal and causal relations, especially IF-THENs, are important. Consider the example again. Your parents' perspective on your future may be described as "*If* we pay for her college fees now and she then gets a career, she will benefit from our efforts *then* because she will value then what we value now." And if you didn't value your career now, you wouldn't feel gratitude for this. However, if you do value your career, your perspective will go something like this: "I am grateful to my parents now because what I value now, they facilitated *then*, and *if* they had not done so, I would not have achieved what I value." In a nutshell, this latter type of perspective taking typifies gratitude.

Furthermore, interventions in both ACT and positive psychology are most often anchored around behavior change in the service of values (e.g., Hayes et al., 2006; Seligman et al., 2005). In ACT, for example, values are highly personalized, and values clarification is designed to facilitate behavior regulation rather than psychological fusion or avoidance (Fletcher & Hayes, 2005). Similarly, in positive psychology, the gratitude list is a primary example of a technique in which you must clarify what you value before you can flourish.

For illustrative purposes, consider again our previous example of Martin. Imagine his therapist asked him to write down three things in his life for which he was grateful. And Martin selected his children, the relationship with his wife, and his career. For ACT, the list serves as values clarification and as a reliable reference against which his behavior may be examined. For example, the therapist may ask, "Do your actions with your children often demonstrate the extent to which you value them?" In response to this, Martin would likely say, "Yes, when I am pain free, we have great fun, but when I am in pain, things are more constrained." "What if," the therapist then asks "you took some time each day to spend with your children, irrespective of how your pain is at that time?" This would likely differ considerably from what Martin has done to date, because pain has been opposed to playing with the children, that is, he thinks that the value "*cannot*" be acted upon when pain is present.

Now, in terms of his relationship with his wife, imagine that the therapist asks Martin to take her perspective on his suffering. He will begin to see that one of the consequences of his suffering is that she has also suffered. And is her suffering in any way less "legitimate" than his? Again, this is unlikely to be a perspective from which Martin has operated to date. He perhaps sees his own suffering as above all else, including values and the suffering of others in the sense that when pain is present, these other things matter less and require less attention. The clarification of these two values may then be highlighted, and Martin's perspective on his wife's and children's perspectives may be enhanced by a gratitude exercise in which he shares with them his perspective and his perspective on their perspective. In addition to showing gratitude, he may make commitments to them to ensure that future actions are more consistent with shared values. Thus, the gratitude exercise facilitates self as context for Martin because he is moving in a values-consistent manner irrespective of his pain.

The sections above highlight a strong overlap between positive psychology's focus on gratitude and the perspective taking and values clarification of RFT and ACT. However, we can identify two possible differences between these approaches, which may have negative clinical implications.

1. When values have been clarified and are genuine, then gratitude is almost inevitable, and the expression of this gratitude likely serves an important purpose in bonding future behavior to these values. In this sense, gratitude is a likely outcome that follows values clarification. Now, think of this the other way around. What if you were advised to express gratitude but values had not been clarified? This may be problematic because you may not experience a sense of gratitude and you would not be sure why you were doing it in the first place. As a result, gratitude exercises are likely to be most effective only in a context of shared values. Gratitude *without this* may be meaningless or even counterproductive.

2. Similar to the concern noted above in terms of a focus on positive writing, it is important to emphasize that ACT adopts the same view of both positive and negative psychological content, in terms of both having the potential to be problematic. Specifically, gratitude exercises clearly involve the expression of positive feelings toward others, and there is nothing surprising or wrong with that. But there is a risk that the exercises tell you how you *should* feel and/or that these feelings should guide your behavior. Put another way, gratitude is an intimate expression of shared values that goes above and beyond what is felt, and gratitude exercises should focus more on the sharing and values aspects than on the feeling aspect. This, of course, raises the possibility that you may engage in a gratitude exercise in the service of something that is valued, even if you don't feel grateful. And that would be consistent with ACT but perhaps not with positive psychology. For example, you might tell your wife that you love her and that you appreciate her after an argument and in the service of returning the relationship to harmony,

even though you feel anger, rather than love and gratitude, at that point in time. In short, the gratitude that you are expressing reflects the effect that many of her previous actions have had on you and on your relationship across time rather than reflecting current feelings. Again, for ACT the focus is on values and not feelings because acting on the basis of current feelings likely reflects self as content. Acting in the service of what your experience across time tells you and what you value are more indicative of self as process and context.

Therapeutic Suggestions for Gratitude Exercises

- In gratitude exercises, you should articulate your perspective and the perspective of your recipient.

- Gratitude exercises must involve values clarification, preferably for both the participant and recipient, and in terms of the participant's perspective on what this will mean for the recipient.

- Gratitude exercises should avoid a focus on what is felt over what is valued in order to encourage self as process or context over content.

Concluding Comments

The current chapter set out to articulate the putative role of RFT's three selves in two key interventions proposed by positive psychology. The interpretation offers a functional, process-based account of what is happening when these techniques are used and why, we believe, they have the outcomes they do. Furthermore, the chapter described a broader overlap between positive psychology and ACT, with a strong sharing of emphasis on the self, defusion, and values clarification. In summary, there is no right or wrong way to do self-enhancement or therapeutic work, and no right or wrong interpretation of what is happening at the level of process. However, there is considerable overlaps across the various traditions in psychology, and the current chapter is an attempt to describe at least some of these and to offer a brief caution of how to watch out for potential pitfalls.

References

Algoe, S. B., & Haidt, J. (2009). Witnessing excellence in actions: The "other-praising" emotions of elevation, gratitude, and admiration. *The Journal of Positive Psychology, 4*(2), 105-127.

Bandura, A. (1999). Self-efficacy: Toward a unifying theory of behavior change. In R. F. Baumeister (Ed.), *The self in social psychology* (pp. 240-279). New York: Psychology Press.

Baumeister, R. F., Smart, L., & Boden, J. (1999). Relation of threatened egotism to violence and aggression: The dark side of high self-esteem. In R. F. Baumeister (Ed.), *The self in social psychology,* (pp. 240-279). New York: Psychology Press.

Bono, G., Emmons, R. A., & McCullough, M. E. (2004). Gratitude in practice and the practice of gratitude. In P. A. Linley & S. Joseph (Eds.), *Positive psychology in practice* (pp. 464-481). Hoboken, NJ: John Wiley & Sons, Inc.

Bono, G., & McCullough, M. E. (2006). Positive responses to benefit and harm: Bringing forgiveness and gratitude into cognitive psychotherapy. *Journal of Cognitive Psychotherapy, 20,* 147-158.

Burton, C. M., & King, L. A. (2004). The health benefits of writing about intensely positive experiences. *Journal of Research in Personality, 38*(2), 150-163.

Ciarrochi, J., Heaven, P. C., & Davies, F. (2007). The impact of hope, self-esteem, and attributional style on adolescents' school grades and emotional well-being: A longitudinal study. *Journal of Research in Personality, 41,* 1161-1178.

Cohn, M. A., & Fredrickson, B. L. (2010). In search of durable positive psychology interventions: Predictors and consequences of long-term positive behavior change. *The Journal of Positive Psychology, 5*(5), 355-366.

Crocker, J., & Park, L. (2004). The costly pursuit of self-esteem. *Psychological Bulletin, 130*(3), 392-414.

DeWall, C. N., Lambert, N. M., Pond, R. S., Kashdan, T. B., & Fincham, F. D. (2012). A grateful heart is a nonviolent heart: Cross-sectional, experience sampling, longitudinal, and experimental evidence. *Social Psychological and Personality Science, 3*(2), 232-240.

Duckworth, A. L., Steen, A., & Seligman, M. E. P. (2005). Positive psychology in clinical practice. *Annual Review of Clinical Psychology, 1,* 629-651.

Emmons, R. A. (2004). Gratitude. In C. Peterson & M. E. P. Seligman (Eds.), *Character strengths and virtues: A handbook and classification* (pp. 553-568). New York: Oxford University Press.

Emmons, R. A., & McCullough, M. E. (2003). Counting blessings versus burdens: An experimental investigation of gratitude and subjective well-being in daily life. *Journal of Personality and Social Psychology, 84*, 377-389.

Fletcher, L., & Hayes, S. C. (2005). Relational frame theory, Acceptance and Commitment Therapy, and a functional analytic definition of mindfulness. *Journal of Rational-Emotive & Cognitive-Behavior Therapy, 23*(4), 315-336.

Foody, M., Barnes-Holmes, Y., & Barnes-Holmes, D. (2012). The role of self in Acceptance and Commitment Therapy (ACT). In L. McHugh and I. Stewart (Eds.), *The self and perspective taking: Research and applications.* Oakland, CA: New Harbinger.

Frattaroli, J., Thomas, M., & Lyubomirsky, S. (2011). Opening up in the classroom: Effects of expressive writing on graduate school entrance exam performance. *Emotion, 11*(3), 691-696.

Fredrickson, B. L., & Joiner, T. (2002). Positive emotions trigger upward spirals toward emotional well-being. *Psychological Science, 13*(2), 172-175.

Froh, J. J., Emmons, R. A., Card, N. A., Bono, G., & Wilson, J. (2011). Gratitude and the reduced costs of materialism in adolescents. *Journal of Happiness Studies, 12*, 289-302.

Froh, J. J., Miller, D. N., & Snyder, S. (2007). Gratitude in children and adolescents: Development, assessment, and school-based intervention. *School Psychology Forum, 2*, 1-13.

Froh, J. J., Sefick, W. J., & Emmons, R. A. (2008). Counting blessings in early adolescents: An experimental study of gratitude and subjective well-being. *Journal of School Psychology, 48*, 213-233.

Gable, S. L., & Haidt, J. (2005). What (and why) is positive psychology? *Review of General Psychology, 9*(2), 103-110.

Hayes, S. C. (1995). Knowing selves. *The Behaviour Therapist, 18*, 94-96.

Hayes, S. C. (2004). Acceptance and Commitment Therapy, relational frame theory, and the third wave of behavioral and cognitive therapies. *Behavior Therapy, 35*, 639-665.

Hayes, S. C., Barnes-Holmes, D., & Roche, B. (2001). *Relational frame theory: A post-Skinnerian account of human language and cognition.* New York: Kluwer Academic/Plenum.

Hayes, S. C., Luoma, J. B., Bond, F. W., Masuda, A., & Lillis, J. (2006). Acceptance and Commitment Therapy: Model, processes and outcomes. *Behaviour Research and Therapy, 44*, 1-25.

Hayes, S. C., Pankey, J., & Palm, K. (2005). The pull of avoidance. In S. C. Hayes & S. Smith (Eds.), *Get out of your mind and into your life: The new Acceptance and Commitment Therapy.* Oakland, CA: New Harbinger.

Hayes, S. C., Strosahl, K. D., & Wilson, K. G. (1999). *Acceptance and Commitment Therapy: An experiential approach to behavior change.* New York: Guilford Press.

Higgins, E. T. (1999). Self-discrepancy: A theory relating self and affect. In R. F. Baumeister (Ed.), *The self in social psychology* (pp. 240-279). New York: Psychology Press.

Ingram, R. E. (1990). Self-focused attention in clinical disorders: Review and a conceptual model. *Psychological Bulletin, 107*(2), 156-176.

Kashdan, T. B., Mishra, M., Breen, W. E., & Froh, J. J. (2009). Gender differences in gratitude: Examining appraisals, narratives, the willingness to express emotions, and changes in psychological needs. *Journal of Personality, 77*(3), 691-730.

Kashdan, T. B., Uswatte, G., & Julian, T. (2006). Gratitude and hedonic and eudaimonic well-being in Vietnam war veterans. *Behaviour Research and Therapy, 44,* 177-199.

King, L. (2001). The health benefits of writing about life goals. *Personality and Social Psychology Bulletin, 27*(7), 798-807.

King, L. A., & Miner, K. N. (2000). Writing about the perceived benefits of traumatic events: Implications for physical health. *Personality and Social Psychology Bulletin, 26,* 220-230.

Leary, M. R., Adams, C. E., & Tate, E. B. (2006). Hypo-egoic self-regulation: Exercising self-control by diminishing the influence of the self. *Journal of Personality, 74*(6), 1803-1832.

Luciano, C., Ruiz, F. J., Vizcaíno Torres, R. M., Sánchez Martín, V., Gutiérrez Martínez, O., & López López, J. C. (2011). A relational frame analysis of defusion in Acceptance and Commitment Therapy: A preliminary and quasi-experimental study with at-risk adolescents. *International Journal of Psychology and Psychological Therapy, 11*(2), 165-182.

Lyubomirsky, S., Dickerhoof, R., Boehm, J. K., & Sheldon, K. M. (2011). Becoming happier takes both a will and a proper way: An experimental longitudinal intervention to boost well-being. *Emotion, 11,* 391-402.

Lyubomirsky, S., Sousa, L., & Dickerhoof, R. (2006). The costs and benefits of writing, talking, and thinking about life's triumphs and defeats. *Journal of Personality and Social Psychology, 90*(4), 692-708.

McCullough, M. E., Emmons, R. A., & Tsang, J-A. (2002). The grateful disposition: A conceptual and empirical topography. *Journal of Personality and Social Psychology, 82*(1), 112-127.

McCullough, M. E., Kimeldorf, M. B., & Cohen, A. D. (2008). An adaptation of altruism? The social causes, social effects and social evolution of gratitude. *Current Directions in Psychological Science, 17,* 281-284.

Neff, K. (2003). Self-compassion: An alternative conceptualization of a healthy attitude toward oneself. *Self and Identity, 2*(2), 85-101.

Pennebaker, J. W. (1989). Cognition, inhibition, and disease. In L. Berkowitz (Ed.), *Advances in experimental social psychology* (Vol. 22, pp. 211-244). New York: Academic Press.

Pennebaker, J. W., & Beall, S. K. (1986). Confronting a traumatic event: Toward an understanding of inhibition and disease. *Journal of Abnormal Psychology, 95,* 274-281.

Pennebaker, J. W., Colder, M., & Sharp, L. K. (1990). Accelerating the coping process. *Journal of Personality and Social Psychology, 58,* 528-537.

Pennebaker, J. W., & Seagal, J. D. (1999). Forming a story: The health benefits of narrative. *Journal of Clinical Psychology, 55*, 1243-1254.

Seligman, M. E. P., Steen, T. A., Park, N., & Peterson, C. (2005). Positive psychology progress: Empirical validation of interventions. *American Psychologist, 60*(5), 410-421.

Sin, N. L., & Lyubomirsky, S. (2009). Enhancing well-being and alleviating depressive symptoms with positive psychology interventions: A practice-friendly meta-analysis. *Journal of Clinical Psychology, 65*(5), 467-487.

Sloan, D. M., & Marx, B. P. (2004a). A closer examination of the written disclosure paradigm. *Journal of Consulting and Clinical Psychology, 72*, 165-175.

Sloan, D. M., & Marx, B. P. (2004b). Taking pen to hand: Evaluating theories underlying the written disclosure paradigm. *Clinical Psychology: Science and Practice, 11*, 121-137.

Smyth, J. M., Stone, A. A., Hurewitz, A., & Kaell, A. (1999). Effects of writing about stressful experiences on symptom reduction in patients with asthma or rheumatoid arthritis: A randomized trial. *Journal of the American Medical Association, 281*, 1304-1309.

Spera, S. P., Buhrfeind, E. D., & Pennebaker, J. W. (1994). Expressive writing and coping with job loss. *Academy of Management Journal, 37*, 722-733.

Stanton, A. L., Danoff-Burg, S., Sworowski, L. A., Collins, C. A., Branstetter, A. D., Rodriguez-Hanley, A., Kirk, S. B., & Austenfeld, L. (2002). Randomized, controlled trial of written emotional expression and benefit finding in breast cancer patients. *Journal of Clinical Oncology, 20*(20), 4160-4168.

Tsang, J-A. (2006). Gratitude and prosocial behaviour: An experimental test of gratitude. *Cognition and Emotion, 20*(1), 138-148.

Wing, J. F., Schutte, N. S., & Byrne, B. (2006). The effect of positive writing on emotional intelligence and life satisfaction. *Journal of Clinical Psychology, 62*(10), 1291-1302.

Wood, A. M., Froh, J. J., & Geraghty, A. W. A. (2010). Gratitude and well-being: A review and theoretical integration. *Clinical Psychology Review, 30*, 890, 905.

Wood, A. M., Joseph, S., & Maltby, J. (2008). Gratitude uniquely predicts satisfaction with life: Incremental validity above the domains and facets of the five factor model. *Personality and Individual Differences, 45*, 49-54.

Wood, A. M., Maltby, J., Gillett, R., Linley, P. A., & Joseph, S. (2008). The role of gratitude in the development of social support, stress, and depression: Two longitudinal studies. *Journal of Research in Personality, 42*, 854-871.

CHAPTER 9

Microculture as a Contextual Positive Psychology Intervention

Robert Biswas-Diener

Portland State University, Positive Acorn

Nadezhda Lyubchik

Portland State University

These words represent the first sentence in an introductory chapter in an academic book connecting Acceptance and Commitment Therapy (ACT) with the science of positive psychology. You, the reader, bring a variety of personal and cultural assumptions to this paragraph including—but not limited to—your particular interest in the topic of this chapter (microculture and contextual psychology), your understanding of edited academic volumes as an intellectual product, and your unique desires for using the information contained herein. We, the authors, also bring a variety of factors to this narrative including our ability to engage you through clarity of writing, evidence of intellectual authority, and novelty and usefulness of our contribution to the helping professions. We are bound together, as authors and readers, but will—ultimately—stop short of co-creating a culture. To take that next social step we need mechanisms to interact with one another: to give feedback, debate, synthesize opinions, modify ideas, and socially share information or technology. It is especially here, in this last point that culture emerges: we must have a shared set of understandings that we can transfer to each other. This is, we hope, a clear illustration of the difference between simple interaction and the emergence of actual culture.

When thinking about the concept of culture, it is tempting to consider this social phenomenon in classic anthropological terms: kinship groups, cosmological beliefs, customs related to dress, and other "visible" aspects. This is particularly true for professionals working across cultural boundaries. There is a large research and theoretical literature concerning the practice of counseling across cultures (Sue & Sue, 2007) just as there is a burgeoning literature addressing cultural factors in the workplace (Ramarajan & Thomas, 2011). To be effective coaches, we need to be sensitive to how culture might present obstacles to effective work or might affect a working relationship. However, guidelines for cultural sensitivity—both at work and in the clinical setting—have been relatively coarse, frequently conceptualizing culture in only the broadest of terms such as those related to ethnic, linguistic, or societal differences (Hofstede & Hofstede, 2005). Among the aims of this chapter is finer attention to the concept of culture. Larger societal cultures encompass smaller "microcultures" that include, but are not limited to subcultures, countercultures, organizational cultures, and artificially constructed microcultures. Microcultures can be thought of as small groups of people who share common history, goals and values, and verbal and nonverbal communication systems (Neuliep, 2009). Microcultural groups, as opposed to subcultural groups based on ethnicity or similar demographic factors, may be of particular interest to interventionists. Although often temporary in nature, artificially created microcultures represent a contextual framework for effecting positive change with individuals and groups.

In the sections that follow we hope to shift from an understanding of culture that is primarily static and related to identity to an understanding that is dynamic and focused on interpersonal processes. Because microcultures can be relatively easily manufactured, especially when compared to typical cultural change interventions such as antismoking campaigns (Biglan, 1995), they are of particular interest to interventionists. Moreover, because microcultures are, themselves, the context in which narrow interventions are delivered, the microculture serves as a meta-intervention that may act as a mediating influence on the effectiveness of other interventions. In this chapter we hope to make the case that context is an important aspect of intervention work.

A Positive Psychology Argument for More Contextual Intervention

There is a temptation in scientific psychology, and especially in the nascent science of positive psychology, to focus on narrow empirically validated interventions (see Parks & Biswas-Diener, this volume). This "tool-based" approach, while certainly a well-intentioned and necessary first step in the development of applied science, represents a limited approach to understanding intervention. By strongly promoting the effectiveness of positive interventions such as the "three blessings exercise" (e.g., Bono, Emmons, & McCullough, 2004), practitioners have implicitly taken the stance that the products of positive psychology are more important than the very people upon whom they are intended to be used. The truth is what we do not know about these interventions outweighs our certainty regarding their use.

Gratitude interventions provide a case study for the current state of positive psychological intervention. There is research evidence suggestive of the emotional benefits of the three blessings exercise and that the effortful expression of gratitude is associated with greater happiness (e.g., Seligman, Steen, Park, & Peterson, 2005). Many practitioners, in our experience, take this as a metaphorical green light to use gratitude interventions with clients of all backgrounds. Unfortunately, the research literature suggests many possible caveats in the prescription and use of this intervention technique. First, there are studies suggesting that gratitude interventions interact with people's cultural backgrounds. For instance, individualists likely benefit more from gratitude interventions than do their collectivist counterparts (Boehm, Lyubomirsky, & Sheldon, 2011). Similarly, there is research suggesting that an individual's religious orientation can affect the benefits of gratitude exercises such that expressing gratitude toward God (as opposed to a more generalized thankfulness) appears to be more beneficial (Rosmarin et al., 2011). A second group of studies demonstrates the importance of client preferences on gratitude effectiveness. Lyubomirsky and colleagues (2011), for example, have found that gratitude interventions appear to provide more substantial benefits if they are chosen by individuals rather than prescribed. Similarly, Schueller (2011) found that individuals who preferred a given positive psychology intervention, such as expressing gratitude, were more likely to actually follow through and complete the intervention. A third group of studies illuminates the possibility that factors related directly to client psychology also affect the potential benefits conferred by gratitude interventions. For instance, it is possible that adolescents who are high in trait positive affect might reach an emotional ceiling, and, therefore, children with more chronically low affect might derive more benefit from these exercises (Froh, Kashdan, Ozimkowski, & Miller, 2009). Along these same lines— and perhaps most alarming among all the research on gratitude—one study suggests that this exercise is sometimes contra-indicated in that it can actually lower self-esteem among people with preexisting depression (Sergeant & Mongrain, 2011). Thus, the gratitude exercise that has long been a workhorse of positive psychology intervention is likely far more nuanced in its real-world application than many practitioners assume.

Many of these studies have only recently been published, and, therefore, a strong argument can be made for the critical importance of keeping abreast of the research to maintain the highest standards of practice. Coaches, therapists, and consultants who are not staying current with positive psychology research limit the potential effectiveness and benefits of interventions and, in some instances, might actually risk harming their clients. It is here that we offer the caution that positive psychology intervention should be looked at as psychological intervention first and as potentially positive only second and in light of the specific context in which it is used. Admittedly, we here posit a strong opinion on the topic; this stance is not made for the sake of effect but, rather, to point out that many practitioners who are informed by positive psychology may have the tendency to overlook issues of person-intervention fit and other contextual factors in favor of an emphasis on the proposed general effectiveness of the tool (Biswas-Diener, Kashdan, & Minhas, 2011). In all fairness we admit that we are guilty of promoting tool-based intervention approaches ourselves (see, for example, Biswas-Diener & Dean, 2007). Our enthusiasm was based on the promise of these tools and the preliminary research findings suggesting their potential. Years later, however, practitioners should demand higher standards for practice and advocate for the science to back these better practices.

The Importance of Microculture to Practice

As positive psychological science improves in sophistication, it grows more elegant in its approach to intervention. Where early positive psychology research focused on narrow outcome measures—usually happiness related—by which discrete intervention tools were validated, more recent work has become necessarily nuanced. For instance, Sin, Della Porta, and Lyubomirsky (2011) argue that attention should be paid to person factors that might influence the effectiveness of positive interventions and that interventions should be accordingly tailored for better individual fit. Similarly, Seligman (2011) argues that the traditional positive psychology focus on individual intervention needs to be replaced by attention to group-level intervention and well-being. This call has been answered by Biswas-Diener and Patterson (2011), Veenhoven (2011), and others who argue that we need to shift our collective attention away from individual happiness as the ultimate outcome toward other desirable outcomes such as increased social capital, greater interpersonal connection, and collective welfare. In this way positive psychology is seen not so much as the science of pursuing happiness but as a mechanism for social change (Biswas-Diener, 2011).

Attention to cultural factors is an important advance for positive psychology and for practice in general. Of the 194 citations that appear in the PsycInfo database for the flagship publication of positive psychology, *Journal of Positive Psychology*, only three are cross-indexed with the keyword "culture"; thankfully, edited volumes have started to appear that address well-being from a cultural perspective (e.g., Delle Fava, Massimini, & Bassi, 2011). We argue that microculture represents a special case of culture that should be of particular interest to interventionists because it is relatively easier to intervene. We offer three comments on microculture interventions that, we hope, establish its usefulness in affecting change with clients:

1. Microculture can be artificially created. This means that although macrocultural influences will always affect individual thinking and feeling, as well as group behavior, it is also possible to use microculture to sidestep *cultural impasses* (impediments

related to feelings toward positive psychology within a given culture). Specifically, artificially constructed microcultures can provide a new context that liberates individuals from cultural constrictions that might otherwise limit their willingness, comfort, or ability to engage in interventions. For example:

When conducting professional skills trainings in collectivist cultures, particularly those in Asia, we have often encountered cultural norms for humility that stand as barriers to the ready acceptance of strengths typical in Western cultures. One approach to working in such a context is to avoid singling out individuals and to accept modesty when it occurs. This can happen by having participants talk about the strengths of others, rather than their own strengths, by working in small groups with less potential for loss of face or by having people offer strengths feedback as a "gift" to other participants. Interestingly, it is also possible to accelerate the learning process by creating local microcultural norms in which modesty is not required. This can be as simple as explicitly stating the new normative language, as in "although Singaporean culture influences everyone in this room, we are also a unique culture unto ourselves … one in which, for this one afternoon, we can speak freely about personal strengths without anyone misconstruing this as bragging." We have been impressed with the appetite for which collectivist workshop participants abandon traditional norms and behave in countercultural ways.

Lest the reader fear that we are insensitive to issues of cultural imperialism, we offer two caveats. First, the norms created in microcultural interventions are temporary and in no way are intended to permanently replace macrocultural norms. For instance, a consultant interacting with an intact work team can artificially create a new microculture in which traditional roles are skewed such that leaders no longer hold positions of power or in which talkative group members have fewer opportunities to dominate conversation. Because microculture is temporary and lacks mechanisms through which these new norms are reinforced and internalized, they will decay quickly, and group members will revert to their traditional roles and interaction styles. In one course we recently taught, for example, we asked students to shout "Whoo-hoo" anytime they heard mention of researchers Martin Seligman or Ed Diener, with the hopes that this would increase learning and engagement. Although there was initial enthusiasm for this new way of doing things students fell back into their more passive roles within 20 minutes. As a second defense against possible charges of cultural imperialism we note that it is just as possible to create new collectivist norms among individualists as it is to create individualistic norms among collectivists. For example, we have created university classroom environments in the United States wherein students are expected to work on all projects together and to be responsible for one another's learning (see Biswas-Diener & Patterson, 2011).

2. Microcultures can be used to sidestep *interpersonal impasses* (impediments related to interactions between people of different cultural backgrounds). Positive psychology, for instance, has sometimes been criticized for being an overly Western—indeed, overly American, discipline (Lazarus, 2003). Wierzbika (2008) argues that much of the language that is central to positive psychology—motivation, well-being, self-interest, quality of life—are not readily translatable to other languages. Wierzbika suggests that the very notion of the "good life" is Anglocentric in nature and rests upon a notion (the good life itself) that translates neither semantically nor culturally to non-Western groups. Further evidence for this criticism of positive psychological concepts comes from Scollon and King (2010), who argue that collectivists such as South Koreans define the "good life" in ways distinct from the individualistic understanding of this concept.

    Rather than allowing broad cultural divides to act as insurmountable barriers to individual connection, it may be that creating new "neutral ground" microcultures can act as a temporary meeting place for people of different backgrounds. A clear example of this can be seen in organizational trainings, such as the type that many psychologists, coaches, and consultants deliver. There are differences in cultural norms around public participation such that people from North America, Africa, and South America are more likely to be vocal and offer personal opinions in a public forum than their counterparts from Asia or the Middle East. When placed in a mixed cultural group those with Western, individualist backgrounds tend to speak up relatively more frequently than do others, and this might actually act as a barrier to participation for non-Westerners. By forming a microculture that emphasizes shared goals or makes shared elements of identity salient, trainers can—to a limited extent—encourage participants to temporarily shed their native culture for the sake of the current learning.

This point is especially germane to positive psychology wherein concepts such as happiness, agency, and self-esteem are, in part, the products of culturally specific thought. Despite arguments against Western biases, researchers and theorists in positive psychology have been largely from the United States and other Western cultures. This can be seen in the published attention given to concepts that are certainly Western in nature, such as the body of literature on Aristotelian notions of well-being based on the fulfillment of individual potential, commonly known as "eudaimonic happiness" (Waterman, Schwartz, & Conti, 2008). Similarly, we should guard against the notion that people from non-Western cultures are capable of appreciating only non-Western positive psychology concepts such as the notion that true happiness is the balance of inevitable negative experiences along with positive ones, where inherent contradictions such as "acceptance" and "change" can coexist (Ho, 2010).

An Introduction to Microculture

Microculture is simply the distinctive culture—the agreed upon ways of temporarily behaving, thinking, or feeling—of a small group of people within a limited geographic area or a small organization such as a school or business. There are, for instance, separate microcultures for riding on an airplane rather than riding on a public bus regardless of geographic location. Riding on a plane, specifically, lends itself to a higher incidence of protracted and—indeed—meaningful interactions between strangers, perhaps because of the longer travel time. Within psychological science there is a long, but not well-known, history of attention to microcultural processes as a research methodology (Whiten & Flynn, 2010). Studies from decades ago employ social learning paradigms to examine the transfer of technology and information from one "generation" to the next. This method has been employed extensively with nonhuman primates (Hannah & McGrew, 1987) and with children (McCrone, 2005). Because a core element in the establishment of all culture, including microculture, is behavioral traditions and rituals, the topic of microculture is particularly relevant to clinical and therapeutic concerns that employ a behavioral methodology. Although Moreno (Fox, 1987), the founder of "psychodrama," was among the earliest to pioneer a therapeutic technique ensconced in a behavioral technique—theater in this instance—modern psychotherapy is replete with therapies that rely on behavioral contexts. These include, but are not limited to, Lego therapy (LeGoff, 2004), which uses the popular children's building toy as an experiential intervention; wilderness therapy (Harper, 2009), which harnesses the natural environment and its physical conditions to build self-confidence; expressive arts therapies (Kossak, 2008), such as the use of painting to encourage cathartic expression; and culture-specific therapies such as *cuento* therapy (Costantino, Magady, & Rogler, 1986), in which local story-telling traditions are harnessed to help clients shift to a healthy narrative of their own life and capacities. The popularity of these therapeutic modalities might reflect an increasing understanding that behavioral contexts are important to therapeutic success.

Design Elements of Microculture

This preliminary chapter is intended not only to argue for the importance of microcultures as meta-interventions but also to offer practical guidance regarding the actual creation of microcultures. We offer recommendations concerning four areas that are important to the creation of microcultures: rituals, role induction, contrasting, and shared experience. We discuss them as individual entities with the understanding that they each impact the others. We have chosen these specific areas because of their conceptual importance to microcultures and the existence of preliminary empirical research into these topics.

1. Rituals/Traditions

Whether it is a Yanomamo ritual in which men strike one another on the chest (Chagnon, 1996) or patriots standing for the national anthem at the onset of a sporting event, rituals and traditions provide a shared sense of purpose and identity. It may even be that engaging in rituals that are closely associated with a cultural identity prime that identity and make certain features of it salient. These habitual behaviors are often engaged in without reflection.

This is particularly important in the psychotherapy context. Clinical delivery has seen a number of innovations since its Freudian heyday of couches and dream analysis. The advent of various technologies has impacted clinical delivery such as the use of physiological monitoring to provide neurofeedback (Masterpasqua & Healey, 2003) and the use of telephonic technologies to allow therapy to be delivered across geographic distances (Jerome et al., 2000). In recent years there has also been a groundswell of popularity in therapeutic techniques related to mindfulness (Vujanovic et al., 2011) and well-being enhancement (e.g., Frisch, 2006). Despite these trends there has been surprisingly little innovation in talk therapy itself as a delivery mechanism for change. Despite variability in therapy duration and theoretical orientations, the basic format of talk therapy follows the same conversational format. Therapists and clients sit in chairs in a private office and discuss problems. One noteworthy exception to this format is the addition of experiential exercises typical to the expressive therapies such as art therapy (Kossak, 2008) and drama therapy (Fox, 1987).

It is surprising how little deviation there is in the format of typical talk therapies until one considers the powerful but subtle influences of cultural norms. Most, if not all, practicing therapists are socialized in graduate school regarding the norms of therapy. This commonly includes discussions of accepting gifts from clients, professional dress codes, and other issues that are not, in themselves, directly therapeutic but which still reflect widespread professional norms. It is curious that therapists have not overtly questioned—in a systematic rather than individual way—whether sitting and talking in a private office is the optimal format. To some degree coaching offers a nice example of strategic experimentation with such issues. Driver (2011), for instance, recommends the use of pacing, walking, or changing positions as a means of pulling back from problems and gaining a fresh perspective (also see Whitworth, Kimsey-House, & Sandhal, 1998). One notable example of incorporating less traditional techniques can be seen in Dialectical Behavioral Therapy (DBT; Linehan, 2006). In many DBT programs clients have access to round-the-clock telephone coaching and participate in mindfulness meditation exercises, often accompanied by chimes, gongs, or similar Eastern cultural artifacts.

Herein lies the power of creating microcultural norms in the consulting room. Therapists have the ability to give permission to clients for a wider range of therapy room behaviors than normally occurs. Discussing the possibility of eating food, writing on a whiteboard, or pacing the room—just to offer three simple examples of deviations from the norm—may enhance client learning or expression. This is an interesting and not inconsequential point: one of the advances in psychotherapy is psychoeducation, including teaching of emotional regulation, mindfulness, and other psychological skills. The focus of these in-session trainings is often on the skills themselves with little attention paid to client learning preferences that might help or hinder this process. The informal presentation of case studies to clients, cooperative learning strategies, modeling, problem-based learning, and other experiential techniques, for example, might be powerful mechanisms for client learning and made more powerful by matching specific strategies to individual client learning styles (Akella, 2010). To effectively pursue this specific route of thinking, clinicians would be called upon to expand the scope of their reading and training to content in education and learning. For example, it might be useful to read research on learning styles and how these might affect the effectiveness of psychoeducation with specific clients.

To be certain, there are some therapists who are already making use of such techniques. Our purpose here is not to criticize the effectiveness of psychotherapy or the clinical wisdom of therapists, or to take aim at therapeutic schools of thought. Indeed, much of this commentary is just as relevant to professional coaching and educational situations. It is our intention to highlight the importance of reflecting on the influence of professional cultural norms in which virtually all therapists are socialized during their education. This process of questioning norms and creating new norms specific to each client reflects the very process of flexible responding at the core of ACT (Luoma, Hayes, & Walser, 2007).

2. Role Induction

Role induction is the use of social influence to assign expectations of specific roles. People, especially those in "power positions," often acculterate new or lower ranking members of a group to how role expectancies will be filled through didactic instruction and/or subtle cues. A business owner, for instance, might indicate to a job applicant where to sit in the office, how formally or informally to behave, or when it is appropriate to shift from the initial "chit-chat" phase of the interview to the more serious part. Similarly, therapists often engage in pretherapy role induction processes, such as discussing the importance and limits of confidentiality, setting expectations for treatment compliance, and opening a dialogue about the nature of the therapeutic alliance. Professional coaches who discuss the distinctions between therapy and coaching with their clients are engaging in a form of role induction that establishes clear cultural parameters for the relationship. In our own introductory coaching sessions we explain to clients that—unlike therapy as it is portrayed in popular media—we, the coaches, will interrupt frequently. We explain that this is done strategically in an effort to move the action forward rather than rehashing past events. Childress and Gillis (1977) suggest that pretherapy role induction is an important predictor of later therapy success because, in part, it clarifies expectations and raises the chances for client compliance.

When thinking about the creation of microcultures, bear in mind that role induction can occur at the level of conscious awareness or as the result of nonverbal *paracommunication*, such as when instructors implicitly reward students at the front of the classroom by being more likely to include them in discussion and call on them when their hands are raised. Similarly, when an executive sits behind a large desk or a workshop leader stands in front of a room full of participants or touches someone on the shoulder, he is using *haptics* (relating to the sense of touch) and *kinesics* (relating to the movement of the body in space) to communicate with others (Beitman & Viamontes, 2007). Facial expression, touch, the strategic use of space, and other nonverbal cues can influence role induction. Seemingly small behaviors such as smiling to reinforce desirable behavior or arranging chairs so that they are angled both toward one another and toward a white board can be subtle but powerful indicators of the role expectancies of both the client and the practitioner.

In a dramatic illustration of role induction, Rose Inza Kim, a therapist working in Seoul, South Korea, limits the number of sessions with clients at the onset to motivate them to seek rapid solutions and expend effort. By addressing limited sessions, Kim explicitly suggests that being resourceful and committed is an essential part of the client role. This may differ from expectations some clients bring to therapy in which they assume therapy is a passive, enduring endeavor.

3. Contrasting

Contrasting is the use of mental comparisons to arrive at a particular emotional, behavioral or attitudinal perspective. Contrasting is a basic part of information processing and everyone engages in cognitive contrasting automatically, as in the case when we use a mental "anchor" point and then adjust our thinking against it (e.g., a charity solicits a donation and requests 50 dollars but allows you to write in any amount—presumably a lesser amount—influenced by this anchor point). Contrasting is occasionally used explicitly for therapeutic outcomes. In a "solutions focus" approach to therapy and coaching, where there is a focus on progress, growth, and possibilities (Jackson & Waldman, 2010), techniques include "scaling" (using numeric or other scales to evaluate progress) and "interviewing for exceptions" (asking clients to identify instances when they have *not* experienced problems or setbacks). Both techniques surprise clients by presenting questions and information that is in stark contrast with client expectations. In solutions focus scaling, for example, a score of a 3 on a 1 to 10 scale assumes that the client automatically attends to the distance between his or her score—a 3—and a presumed perfect outcome of a 10. The solutions focus practitioner transforms this assumption by shifting attention to the distance between the score—a 3—and the presumed worst score of a 1. This perspective change offers clients an opportunity to take stock of progress and resources instead of problems.

There are several reasons contrasting techniques may be useful: they may help clients overcome inhibitions that are influenced by culture (e.g., a Christian client who might be reluctant to engage in mindfulness practices due to spiritual concerns); groups form a sense of shared identity (e.g., human resources experts from a variety of companies view themselves as similar and working toward a common purpose). Contrasting works by highlighting the microculture (its norms, roles, etc.) and making small group membership a salient identity point for clients or training participants. Pointing out the client's culture of origin and explaining the limits of that culture to affect the therapeutic or coaching milieu serves the purpose of re-anchoring them in a new cultural context, albeit temporarily. Macrocultures can influence without dictating microculture thoughts, feelings, and behaviors.

It may be that effectiveness rests on the relative size of the contrast, such that small contrasts are met with more "buy in" than large contrasts that might threaten strongly held beliefs. It is possible, for example, that creating a microculture among Pacific Rim Asians in which personal achievement and interpersonal challenging are the norms would be more difficult than creating one in which it was considered normal to take ownership of one's own strengths to connect with one another.

4. Shared Experience

Shared experience can be a powerful force in the development of a collective identity because it allows individuals a sense of intimacy provided by the perception of increased understanding of one another. People who have been through natural disasters together, for instance, can find a mutual point of connection that can help them make sense of the events. Candau (2010) suggests that shared experiences act as "sociotransmitters" that connect people to one another much in the same fashion that neurotransmitters act as delivery mechanisms for complex connections in the brain. Shared experiences are—perhaps—the aspect of microculture that is the least artificial. Shared experiences, regardless of their specifics, include shared emotions, a common reference point (as in the case of "inside jokes"), and increased self-other overlap (Aron,

Aron, & Smollan, 1992). There is, for example, initial research suggesting that people naturally "sync" with one another by mimicking body language (Vacharkulksemsuk & Fredrickson, 2012) and that mere exposure breeds liking for an object (or person) as well as approach motivation toward that object (or person) (Jones, Young, & Claypool, 2011). Indeed, research suggests that shared experience—especially highly positive experiences—are linked to relationship satisfaction (Reissman, Aron, & Bergen, 1993). These studies point to the importance of shared experience as a relationship and—we would argue here—a microculture building phenomenon at the heart of which is a number of empathic benefits. It should be noted, however, the majority of self-other overlap and shared experience research has been conducted in the context of close or romantic relationships and our understanding of cross-cultural issues or stranger-stranger contact issues is limited.

Case Study

In this penultimate section we offer a brief case to showcase how microcultures can be quickly and intentionally created as well as its effect on people. Rather than make strong pronouncements about specific techniques, we present preliminary observations drawn from real-world experiences. To be clear, we do not believe enough is known about microcultures and their creation to offer clear, strategic advice regarding their construction and use. We leave it, instead, for readers and practitioners to draw their own conclusions about the relative promise and limitations of microculture in the contexts in which they work.

At the biannual conference of the International Positive Psychology Association (IPPA), one of the authors (RBD) gave a 4-hour workshop in which he attempted to create a microculture that would be noticeably distinct from the macroculture in which it existed (American society) and even from the subcultures that might otherwise define it (academia, annual gatherings of professional societies). To gauge the speed of creation, extent of impact, and effectiveness of the microcultural intervention, the author chose to establish a new group norm that would be obviously counter to larger culture norms. In this particular, he decided that no critical questions would be taken from the audience. Critical remarks and clarifying questions have long been assumed to be an integral part of the learning process in general and to the workshop format specifically. While the goal of the IPPA workshop was primarily to teach the application of positive psychology, it was secondarily a demonstration of the power of microcultural norms.

To create a sense of group identity that would support such a strong and arguably disagreeable group norm, the author began by telling a personal story. The specific content of the story is less important than is the acknowledgment that the story was chosen for its emotional value. Contained within the story were moments of high humor and also sobering moments of reflection and self-doubt. This story acted as the anchor point of shared experience for the workshop based on the principles of emotional contagion. The author purposefully included catchphrases and buzz words that he then used throughout the remainder of the workshop to remind participants about their shared experiences and therefore shared identity.

In addition, specific roles were assigned to particular audience members including note-taker, tweeter (actively posting to the Twitter website during the workshop), and photographer. These roles were assigned publicly so that all the participants would understand that the workshop contained specific norms including the use of photography and social media that might differ from other academic experiences. All of the workshop participants also received specific instructions where the microcultural norm was concerned. The author leading the workshop instructed: "Please do not think critically. Critical thinking is negative and can be socially off-putting. Instead, you are encouraged to be curious and explore your sense of wonder about the topics presented. Due to time constraints, however, no broad philosophical questions will be allowed. Only those questions that deal specifically with the clarification of skills and techniques presented here are within the scope of this workshop."

The reaction to this peculiar instruction was a curious phenomenon. There were those in the audience (of approximately 100 people) who naturally wanted to question elements of the workshop with which they disagreed. One man, for instance, questioned the very notion of not questioning. "Isn't this a dangerous group norm to establish," he asked, "as it might lead to group think and interfere with individual thought and creativity?" When the author responded that, although the question appeared to have merit, it was beyond the scope of the training, a number of the other workshop participants actually applauded! We interpret this aspect of the crowd reaction as evidence of the dramatic power of people in leadership positions to establish norms quickly, especially those that appear to serve a useful but temporary purpose. We admit we cannot fully determine the exact mechanisms by which the microculture was established. The role of leader persuasion, the use of humor, the demographic characteristics of the audience, the topic of the workshop, and other factors cannot be ruled out as important facets of microcultural intervention. We do feel confident, however, that local group norms were, in fact, established and learned and reinforced by the members of the group to such an extent that they applauded when an audience member was told he could not ask a legitimate question.

Future Recommendations

Microcultures, as discussed in this chapter, are temporary and artificial cultures that carry unique norms, roles, and rituals. We argue that microcultures can be used as meta-interventions to provide a context through which more traditional interventions can be more effectively delivered. We suggest here that this contextual approach is a necessary step forward for the young science of positive psychology. As an applied science, practitioners have often emphasized the relatively limited number of empirically validated tools that are widely accepted as a core component of the positive psychology cannon. We have argued elsewhere (Biswas-Diener, 2011) that many of these empirically validated tools have been tested on only a narrow range of outcomes and that little is known about the best ways to deliver them, possible contraindications, and client factors that that might affect their effectiveness.

This tool-based emphasis and preference for one's own epistemology is an unavoidable aspect of any intellectual endeavor (Kagan, 2009). As positive psychology matures and explicitly addresses these issues (Schueller, 2011), this nuance and sophistication will better inform other intervention approaches such as coaching and ACT. We believe, in particular, that creating microcultures may represent a means of better understanding the contextual factors of intervention, an approach that converges with the ACT emphasis on context and flexible responding.

Unfortunately, little is known about how to effectively create microcultures or the impact creating such a culture might have on positive psychology intervention. It is likely, in our opinion, that the same social processes implicated in conformity (Asch, 1956), obedience (Milgram, 1963), and de-individuation (Diener, 1980) are implicated—at least in the group setting such as the training example presented above—in the effective establishment of microcultural norms, especially those that might run counter to the norms of the macrocultural context of group members. Although not systematic in our analysis, our training and coaching work in dozens of cultures, including those of African, Asian, and European countries, suggests that even minor attention to the construction of microcultures can have a powerful effect on groups learning and using positive psychology.

References

Akella, D. (2010). Learning together: Kolb's experiential theory and its application. *Journal of Management and Organization, 16*(1), 100-112.

Aron, A., Aron E. N., & Smollan, D. (1992). Inclusion of other in the self scale and the structure of interpersonal closeness. *Journal of Personality and Social Psychology, 63*, 596-612.

Asch, S. (1956). Studies of independence and conformity: I. A minority of one against a unanimous majority. *Psychological Monographs, 70*, 70.

Beitman, B. D., & Viamontes G. L. (2007). Unconscious role induction: Implications for psychotherapy. *Psychiatric Annals, 37*, 259-268.

Biglan, A. (1995). *Changing cultural practices: A contextual framework for intervention research*. Reno: Context Press.

Biswas-Diener, R. (2011). Editor's foreword. In R. Biswas-Diener (Ed.), *Positive psychology as social change* (pp. v-xi). New York: Springer Science + Business Media.

Biswas-Diener, R., & Dean, B. (2007). *Positive psychology coaching*. Hoboken, NJ: John Wiley & Sons.

Biswas-Diener, R., Kashdan, T., & Minhas, G. (2011). A dynamic approach to psychological strengths development and intervention. *Journal of Positive Psychology, 6*, 106-118.

Biswas-Diener, R., & Patterson, L. (2011). Positive psychology and poverty. In R. Biswas-Diener (Ed.), *Positive psychology as social change* (pp. 125-140). Dordrecht: Springer.

Boehm, J., Lyubomirsky, S., & Sheldon, K. (2011). A longitudinal experimental study comparing the effectiveness of happiness-enhancing strategies in Anglo American and Asian Americans. *Cognition & Emotion, 25*(7), 1263-1272.

Bono, G., Emmons, R. A., & McCullough, M. E. (2004). Gratitude in practice and the practice of gratitude. In P. A. Linley & S. Joseph (Eds.), *Positive psychology in practice* (pp. 464-481). New York: Wiley.

Candau, J. (2010). Shared memory, odours and sociotransmitters or: "Save the interaction!" *Outlines: Critical Practice Studies, 12*(2), 29-42.

Chagnon, N. A. (1996). Chronic problems in understanding tribal violence and warfare. In Bock, G. R, Goode, J. A. (Eds.), *Genetics of criminal and antisocial behaviour* (pp. 202-236.) New York: John Wiley & Sons.

Childress, R., & Gillis, J. S. (1977). A study of pretherapy role induction as an influence process. *Journal of Clinical Psychology, 33*, 540-544.

Costantino, G., Magady, R. G., & Rogler, L. H. (1986). Cuento therapy: A culturally sensitive modality for Puerto Rican children. *Journal of Consulting and Clinical Psychology, 54*, 639-645.

Delle Fave, A., Massimini, F., & Bassi, M. (2011). *Psychological selection and optimal experience across cultures: Social empowerment through personal growth.* New York: Springer Science + Business Media.

Diener, E. (1980). Deindividuation: The absence of self-awareness and self-regulation in group members. In P. B. Paulus (Ed.), *Psychology of group influence* (pp. 209-242). Hillsdale, NJ: Lawrence Edbaum.

Driver, M. (2011). *Coaching positively.* Berkshire: Open University Press/McGraw-Hill.

Fox, J. (1987). *The essential Moreno.* New York: Springer Publishing Company.

Frisch, M. (2006). *Quality of life therapy: Applying a satisfaction approach to positive psychology and cognitive therapy.* Hoboken, NJ: John Wiley and Sons, Inc.

Froh, J. J., Kashdan, T. B., Ozimkowski, K. M., & Miller, N. (2009). Who benefits the most from a gratitude intervention in children and adolescents? Examining positive affect as a moderator. *Journal of Positive Psychology, 4*, 408-422.

Hannah, A., & McGrew, W. C. (1987). Chimpanzees using stones to crack open oil palm nuts in Liberia. *Primates, 28*, 31-46.

Harper, N. J. (2009). The relationship of therapeutic alliance to outcome in wilderness treatment. *Journal of Adventure Education and Outdoor Learning, 9*, 45-59.

Ho, S. M. Y. (2010). Universal happiness. In Leo Bormans (Ed.), *The world book of happiness* (pp. 253-255). Belgium: Lannoo.

Hofstede, G., & Hofstede, G. J. (2005). Cultures and organizations: Software of the mind (2nd ed.). New York: McGraw-Hill.

Jackson, P. Z., & Waldman, J. (2010). *Positively speaking.* St. Alban's: The Solutions Focus.

Jerome, L. W., DeLeon, P. H., James, L. C., Folen, R., Earles, J., & Gedney, J. J. (2000). The coming of age of telecommunications in psychological research and practice. *American Psychologist, 55*, 407-421.

Jones, I. F., Young, S. G., & Claypool, H. M. (2011). Approaching the familiar: On the ability of mere exposure to direct approach and avoidance behavior. *Motivation and Emotion, 35*(4), 383-392.

Kagan, J. (2009). *The three cultures: Natural sciences, social sciences and the humanities in the 21st century.* New York: Cambridge University Press.

Kossak, M. S. (2008). Therapeutic attunement: A transpersonal view of expressive arts therapy. *The Arts in Psychotherapy, 36,* 13-18.

Lazarus, R. S. (2003). Does positive psychology movement have legs? *Psychological Inquiry, 14*(2), 93-109.

LeGoff, D. B. (2004). Use of LEGO© as a therapeutic medium for improving social competence. *Journal of Autism and Developmental Disorders, 34*(5), 557-571.

Linehan, M. (2006). *Dialectical behavior therapy with suicidal adolescents.* New York: Guilford.

Luoma, J. B, Hayes, S. C., & Walser, R. D. (2007). *Learning ACT: An Acceptance and Commitment Therapy skills-training manual for therapists.* Oakland, CA: New Harbinger Publications.

Lyubomirsky, S., Dickerhoof, R., Boehm, J. K., & Sheldon, K. M. (2011). Becoming happier takes both a will and a proper way: An experimental longitudinal intervention to boost well-being. *Emotion, 11,* 391-402.

Masterpasqua, F., & Healey, K. N. (2003). Neurofeedback in psychological practice. *Professional Psychology: Research and Practice, 34*(6), 652-656.

McCrone, S. (2005). The development of mathematical discussions: An investigation of a fifth-grade classroom. *Mathematical Thinking and Learning, 7*(2), 111-133.

Milgram, S. (1963). Behavioral study of obedience. *The Journal of Abnormal and Social Psychology, 67*(4), 371-378.

Neulip, J. (2009). *Intercultural communication: A contextual approach.* Thousand Oaks, CA: Sage Publications.

Parks, A., & Biswas-Diener, R. (In press). Positive Interventions: Past, Present, and Future. In T. Kashdan & J. Ciarrochi, Eds., *Mindfulness, acceptance, and positive psychology: The seven foundations of well-being.* Oakland, CA: New Harbinger.

Ramarajan, L., & Thomas, D. (2011). A positive approach to studying diversity in organizations. In K.S. Cameron & G.M. Spreitzer (Eds.), *The Oxford handbook of Positive Organizational Scholarship,* (pp. 552-565). Oxford, UK: Oxford Unviersity Press.

Reissman, C., Aron, A., & Bergen, M. R. (1993). Shared activities and marital satisfaction: Causal direction and self-expansion versus boredom. *Journal of Social and Personal Relationships, 10,* 243-254.

Rosmarin, D. H., Pirutinsky, S., Cohen, A., Galler, Y., & Krumrei, E. J. (2011). Grateful to God or just plain grateful? A study of religious and non-religious gratitude. *Journal of Positive Psychology, 6,* 389-396.

Schueller, S. (2011). To each his own well-being boosting intervention: Using preferences to guide selection. *Journal of Positive Psychology, 6,* 300-313.

Scollon, C. N., & King, L. A. (2010). What people really want in life and why it matters: Contributions from research on folk theories of the good life. In R. Biswas-Diener (Ed.), *Positive Psychology as Social Change* (pp. 1-14). Springer Press.

Searle, R. H., & Skinner, D. (2011). *Trust and human resource management.* Cheltenham: Edward Elgar Publishing, Inc.

Seligman, M. E. P. (2011). *Flourish: A visionary new understanding of happiness and well-being.* New York: Simon and Schuster.

Seligman, M. E. P., Steen, T. A., Park, N., & Peterson, C. (2005). Positive psychology progress: Empirical validation of interventions. *American Psychologist, 60,* 410–421.

Sergeant, S., & Mongrain, M. (2011). Are positive psychology exercises helpful for people with depressive personality styles? *Journal of Positive Psychology, 6,* 260-272.

Sin, N., Della Porta, M., & Lyubomirsky, S. (2011). Tailoring positive psychology interventions to treat depressed individuals. In Donaldson, S., Csikszentmihalyi, M. & Nakamura, J. (Eds.), *Applied positive psychology* (pp. 79-96). New York: Routledge.

Sue, D. W., & Sue, D. (2007). *Counseling the culturally diverse: Theory and practice.* (5th ed.) Hoboken, NJ: John Wiley and Sons, Inc.

Vacharkulksemsuk, T., & Fredrickson, B. L. (2012). Strangers in sync: Achieving embodied rapport through shared movements. *Journal of Experimental Social Psychology, 48*(1), 399-402.

Veenhoven, R. (2011). Greater happiness for a greater number: Is that possible? If so, how? In K. M. Sheldon, T. B. Kashdan, & M. F. Steger (Eds.), *Designing positive psychology: Taking stock and moving forward* (pp. 396-409). New York: Oxford University Press.

Vujanovic, A. A., Niles, B., Pietrefesa, A., Schmertz, S. K., & Potter, C. M. (2011). Mindfulness in the treatment of posttraumatic stress disorder among military veterans. *Professional Psychology: Research and Practice, 42*(1), 24-31.

Waterman, A. S., Schwartz, S. J., & Conti, R. (2008). The implications of two conceptions of happiness (hedonic enjoyment and eudaimonia) for the understanding of intrinsic motivation. *Journal of Happiness Studies, 9,* 41-79.

Wierzbicka, A. (2008). What makes a good life? A cross-linguistic and cross-cultural perspective. *Journal of Positive Psychology, 4*(4), 260-272.

Whiten, A., & Flynn, E. (2010). The transmission and evolution of experimental microcultures in groups of young children. *Developmental Psychology, 46*(6), 1694-1709.

Whitworth, L., Kimsey-House, H., & Sandhal, P. (1998). *Co-active coaching.* Palo Alto: Davies-Black.

CHAPTER 10

Accepting Guilt and Abandoning Shame: A Positive Approach to Addressing Moral Emotions among High-Risk, Multineed Individuals

Elizabeth Malouf

Kerstin Youman

Laura Harty

Karen Schaefer

June P. Tangney
George Mason University

Positive psychology is not the first thing people think about when they think of criminal offenders, nor are values and mindfulness. In our program of research, however, we have found multiple lines of research from positive psychology useful at enhancing inmates' reintegration into the community. In this chapter, we describe three forms of intervention that we have been implementing and evaluating in the context of a larger program of longitudinal research on moral emotions and moral cognitions (Tangney, Mashek, & Stuewig, 2007). We first describe the Impact of Crime (IOC) workshop, an innovative group intervention that draws on a "guilt-inducing, shame-reducing" restorative justice model. Next, we describe our efforts to import components of Acceptance and Commitment Therapy (ACT) into a values-based mindfulness group intervention designed for inmates nearing community reentry. Last, we describe the ways in which we have modified motivational interviewing (MI) procedures to best meet the diverse needs and concerns of "general population" jail inmates.

Across the board, these interventions take a positive approach to cognitive and behavioral change. Inmates are encouraged to take responsibility and commit to their values rather than to simply avoid negative behavior. They are encouraged to take positive action rather than simply avoid further antisocial behavior. Our experience supports the effectiveness of this positive psychology approach in this high-risk population. Moreover, we believe this approach is applicable across many other contexts—at school, in the workplace, anywhere where rules can be violated, harm can be done, and there lurks the possibility of shame.

The Impact of Crime (IOC) Workshop: A Restorative Justice Inspired Group Intervention

The Impact of Crime (IOC) workshop is an innovative group intervention rooted in restorative justice principles. Restorative justice is an alternative to the philosophy of retributive justice (the punishment-focused approach that dominates the criminal justice system in the United States and in many other parts of the world). Rather than focusing on legal processes and punishment of the offender, restorative justice theory emphasizes the harmful effects of crime. Crime is viewed as a violation of the victim and the community rather than a violation of the state. Accountability is defined in terms of taking responsibility for actions and repairing harm caused to the victim and community through restitution, competency development, and community service. In effect, restoration, or making things right, becomes the highest priority of the system rather than the imposition of punishment for its own sake. By taking accountability for their actions, offenders begin to understand the harm they cause to victims and communities, deterring future offenses.

The restorative justice approach aims to initiate significant, lasting change in how offenders *think* about crime, victims, and personal responsibility. The IOC workshop explicitly encourages offenders to reevaluate distorted "criminogenic" beliefs and to shift from a self-centered, egoistic orientation toward a broader appreciation of one's place and role in the community.

The IOC workshop is a voluntary group intervention, providing a cost-effective means of providing a restorative experience to 15-20 offenders at one time. Delivered over the course of 8 weeks, this 16-session workshop is part educational and part experiential. Incarcerated participants have the opportunity to reexamine the ways in which various types of crime (property crime, sexual assault, domestic violence, drug use and distribution, etc.) affect victims, families (of both victims and offenders), and the community as a whole. Participants learn pertinent crime statistics and facts, complete a series of workbook exercises and group discussions about the victim experience, and interact with guest speakers—victims of crime who discuss how specific crimes have affected their lives and those around them. With the aid of a trained facilitator, participants process their reactions to the new information and presentations, drawing connections to their personal experiences. Throughout, the facilitator emphasizes and integrates restorative justice notions of community, personal responsibility, and reparation. An important component of the IOC workshop is the opportunity for offenders to communicate to the community their acceptance of responsibility and their desire to repair the harm done. This is done in powerful discussions with guest speakers and via a joint community service project designed and implemented by each group, over several sessions. A recent IOC group, for example, constructed a calendar with poems, drawings, and messages about the consequences of crime for victims, offenders, and communities. It was distributed to boys' and girls' probation homes with the aim of making a formal apology, actively taking responsibility for their actions, and warning youth about the negative effects of criminal activity. Another group created key chains with a message about the prevalence of drunk driving casualties and gave them to youth at a driving school, encouraging new drivers to consider the impact their behavior has on others.

As inmate participants grapple with issues of responsibility in the IOC workshop, the question of blame inevitably arises.

Upon re-examining the causes of their legal difficulties and revisiting the circumstances surrounding previous offenses and their consequences, many inmates experience new feelings of shame, guilt, or both. Most intriguing to us, restorative justice is essentially a "guilt-inducing, shame-reducing" approach to rehabilitation. Offenders are encouraged to take responsibility for their behavior, acknowledge the negative consequences to others, empathize with the distress of their victims, feel guilt for having *done* the wrong thing, and act on the consequent inclination to repair the harm done. Facilitators model empathy in group (and often one-on-one) discussions about circumstances leading to past offenses and then actively encourage participants to identify ways of repairing the harm they have caused. Using affirmations and highlighting steps offenders have already taken toward reparation shifts the focus from past negative acts to future opportunities for change and restoration. Additionally, group members are encouraged to empathize with and support each other in order to foster openness, collaboration, and sharing of ideas for restoration. Offenders, however, are actively discouraged from feeling shame about *themselves*. In fact, restorative justice approaches eschew messages aimed at condemning and humiliating offenders as "bad people." The emphasis is on bad behaviors that can be changed, negative consequences that can be repaired, and offenders who can be redeemed.

Why is this guilt-inducing, shame-reducing characteristic of the IOC workshop (and restorative justice approaches, in general) so important? Research from our lab, and many others, has shown that shame and guilt are distinct emotions with very different implications for subsequent moral and interpersonal behavior (Tangney, Malouf, Stuewig, & Mashek, 2012; Tangney, Stuewig, & Mashek, 2007). Feelings of shame involve a painful focus on the self—the humiliating sense that "*I* am a bad person." Such shameful feelings are typically accompanied by a sense of shrinking, of being small, by a sense of worthlessness and powerlessness, and by a sense of being exposed. Ironically, research has shown that such painful and debilitating feelings of shame do not motivate constructive changes in behavior. Shamed individuals are no less likely to repeat their transgressions (often more so), and they are no more likely to attempt reparation (often less so) (Tangney, Stuewig, & Hafez, 2011). Instead, because shame is so intolerable, people in the midst of a shame experience often resort to defensive tactics, or what ACT refers to as experiential avoidance. They may seek to hide or escape shameful feelings, denying responsibility. They may seek to shift the blame outside, holding others responsible for their dilemma. And not infrequently, they become irrationally angry with others, sometimes resorting to overtly aggressive and destructive actions. In short, shame serves to escalate the very destructive patterns of behavior we aim to curb.

Contrast this with feelings of guilt, which involve a focus on a specific behavior—the sense that "I did a bad thing" rather than "I am a bad person." Feelings of guilt involve a sense of tension, remorse, and regret over the "bad thing done." Research has shown that this sense of tension and regret typically motivates reparative action (confessing, apologizing, or somehow repairing the damage done) without engendering all the defensive and retaliatory responses that are the hallmark of shame (Leith & Baumeister, 1998; Tangney, Stuewig, & Mashek, 2007; Tangney, Youman, & Stuewig, 2009). Most important, guilt is more likely to foster constructive changes in future behavior because what is at issue is not a bad, defective self but a bad, defective behavior. And, as anyone knows, it is easier to change a bad behavior (drunk driving, theft, substance abuse) than to change a bad, defective self.

Many offenders come in to treatment with a propensity to experience shame rather than guilt. Some are so defensive that they feel little of either emotion. The IOC workshop utilizes cognitive-behavioral techniques to foster a more adaptive capacity for moral emotions by (a) using inductive and educational strategies to foster a capacity for perspective taking and other-oriented empathy; (b) encouraging participants to broaden their vision through a better understanding of the impact of crime and a greater taking of accountability, cutting through minimization and denial of criminal actions; (c) understanding the relationships between victims, offenders, and the community; (d) encouraging appropriate experiences of guilt and emphasizing associated constructive motivations to repair or make amends; and (e) explicitly avoiding language that may be construed as condemning or humiliating inmate participants as "bad people." Instead, the strong message is that redemption is possible.

The IOC curriculum begins with discussions of crime, its consequences, and how to repair the harm caused, in the abstract. Over time, the completion of workbook exercises, group discussions, and interactions with guest speakers prepares participants to look at their own actions honestly and to use their newfound understanding to change their behaviors. Recently, one participant revealed that he was experiencing intense shame about his history of drunk driving. He spoke very little in class but responded thoughtfully to homework exercises and responded well to the facilitator's written and verbal praise of his efforts. As he began to speak up in class to support other participants' attempts to understand and change their behaviors, he likewise received empathic and encouraging responses that allowed him to confront his past actions and identify ways to repair the harm he caused. A turning point occurred for him during the lesson about drunk driving, when the guest speaker, the mother of a girl killed by a drunk driver, explained that the one thing that she would want from the man who killed her daughter would be for him not to drive drunk again. For this participant, the idea that restoration is possible allowed him to view himself as someone who could change and redeem himself. At the end of the workshop, he led the group in a community service project that petitioned Congress for a law to make built-in breathalyzers mandatory in cars in an effort to curb drunk driving casualties. In short, the intervention emphasizes that inmate participants can take steps to repair the fabric of their relationships and the community, and they can make lasting positive changes in their behavior moving forward.

Currently, we are conducting a randomized clinical trial to assess the efficacy of the IOC workshop in reducing postrelease reoffense and in enhancing adjustment in the community. A key hypothesis is that the IOC workshop will reduce recidivism via its impact on moral emotions and cognitions—that is, by enhancing adaptive feelings of guilt, reducing problematic feelings of shame, and restructuring criminogenic beliefs.

The Re-Entry Values and Mindfulness Program (REVAMP)

Research has shown that a majority of jail inmates have significant psychological and behavioral problems. Upwards of 70% of jail inmates in our sample had clinically significant elevations on one or more symptom clusters. For example, 47% scored in the clinical range for drug problems, 26% for alcohol problems, 10% for anxiety, and 19% for depression (Drapalski, Youman, Stuewig, & Tangney, 2009; Youman, Drapalski,

Stuewig, Bagley, & Tangney, 2010). Additionally, a remarkable proportion (31.7%) report clinically significant symptoms of borderline personality features (Conn, Warden, Stuewig, Kim, Harty, Hastings, & Tangney, 2010). Few of these inmates have sought or received traditional mental health treatment in the community, and there are limited resources for mental health treatment in jails (Drapalski et al., 2009; Meyer, Tangney, & Stuewig, under review; Youman et al., 2010). While anecdotal evidence suggests that few inmates perceive themselves as living a rewarding life in accordance with their own values, little empirical research in this population has investigated positive psychological outcomes. It is as if the possibility that inmates might have a sense of meaning, happiness, optimism, or gratitude hasn't been considered.

With an awareness of the need to reduce symptoms and enhance value-based living in this population, we developed a short-term group intervention specifically designed for jail inmates nearing reentry to the community: the Re-Entry Values and Mindfulness Program (REVAMP). This program, derived primarily from Acceptance and Commitment therapy (ACT), empowers the individual and is flexible enough to address the diversity of problems and life experiences encountered in a jail population (Hayes, 2004; Hayes & Smith, 2005). In addition to ACT, REVAMP draws tools from several mindfulness- and acceptance-based interventions, notably mindfulness-based relapse prevention (Bowen, Chawla, & Marlatt, 2011), dialectical behavioral therapy (Linehan, 1993), VA Maryland Health Care System ACT group manual (VAMHCS ACT Therapy Team, 2007), and skills for improving distress intolerance (Bornovalova, 2008).

REVAMP is distinguished from other jail-based programs by its acceptance-based approach to symptom reduction and its focus on values in action. Psychological interventions for inmates generally only focus on reducing symptoms of psychological distress and/or behavior problems. However, REVAMP aims to both reduce symptoms, *and* improve individuals' ability to lead a values-driven, personally meaningful life. These dual aims of reducing symptoms and enhancing valued action are intrinsically linked. Symptoms often serve as barriers between individuals and their values. In turn, values serve to motivate the behavior change necessary to reduce symptoms. Thus, enhancing valued action and reducing suffering represent two major overarching, interconnected themes throughout the REVAMP program. We discuss each in turn, outlining how both reinforce each other and highlighting how each serves to overcome treatment barriers for this challenging population.

Focus on Values-Based Action: Clarifying Values and Setting Goals

The REVAMP program begins with a focus on personal values. By starting with an identification of personal values, defensiveness is decreased and personal investment in the program is heightened. This also appears to be a refreshing change for individuals who are used to being judged and who are accustomed to being told what to do and when to do it by the correctional system. REVAMP facilitators emphasize that there are no "right" or "wrong" answers and encourage participants to say what they really believe rather than what they think we want to hear.

One might wonder what sorts of values inmates generate and if this might be a foolhardy or even dangerous endeavor. Given their often extensive criminal histories, might inmates' values orient them in a direction that would be harmful to the community? For example, inmates might value material wealth attained by any means necessary or risky sexual behavior.

Our experience with multiple groups of inmates over the course of the treatment is that they consistently identify prosocial values. Inmates' values often not only reflected a desire to achieve well-being for themselves but also to positively contribute to others (see Table 1). In fact, across program participants, there were no examples of clearly antisocial values (though a few mentioned different sets of values they had at younger ages that they now see as misdirected).

Table 1: Example of Inmate's Values and Goals

Values	Goals
Be a friend and partner for my spouse	Find activities that we both enjoy and do them

A close family	Talk to my relatives at least once a month
Be a man who protects, provides for, and shelters his wife	Get and keep a good-paying job
Live drug and alcohol free	Sobriety one day at a time
Help uplift my community	Coach a little league team
Be a person who respects other people's thoughts	Listen more to other people
Live my religion	Attend church every Sunday

Once values are generated, REVAMP leaders facilitate a refinement of these values to an appropriate level of specificity. For example, a participant might identify "family" as a personal value. He or she would be encouraged to elaborate—e.g., "providing for my family" or "making my family proud." A helpful values metaphor is to have participants imagine themselves as a bus driver with the value as the direction they want to drive their bus (Hayes & Smith, 2005, p. 153). At the end of the first session, inmates are asked to write their own epitaph. This exercise, which is employed in ACT and other acceptance-based interventions, focuses inmates on defining their intended legacy, what they want their lives to stand for (Hayes & Smith, 2005, p. 170). During the second session, inmates expand this by identifying their specific personal values with a worksheet listing major life domains (e.g., career, family, health) and prompts to identify a value in each domain (Hayes & Smith, 2005, p. 170). They rate the importance of each value to help prioritize the values they would like to begin working toward. Inmates then set goals consistent with their values, or in terms of the bus metaphor, stops they want to make on the journey toward their values.

Barriers to Values: Bridge from Values Enhancement to Reduction of Suffering

Inevitably, these values exercises begin to raise awareness of discrepancies between inmates' values, their recent behavior, and their current situation. In fact, a key aim of Sessions 1 and 2 is to highlight the discrepancies between where inmates are and where they want to be heading. In group, having identified a broad list of values, the perceived barriers (e.g., "yeah, buts…") begin to flow. Participants focus on the genuine difficulties they anticipate facing when they return to the community (e.g., poor economy, stigma related to a criminal record, racism, disappointed family members, logistical requirements of probation that complicate maintaining successful employment).

Inmates may also acknowledge obstacles to their values that involve their own behavior. However, inmates are often ambivalent about their own role in contributing to these difficulties. They may acknowledge partial responsibility, yet often externalize blame to flaws in the legal system, discrimination, or other circumstances beyond their control. Perceptions of unjust treatment associated with their current incarceration may exacerbate inmates' defensiveness, heightening their awareness of external obstacles and increasing reluctance to focus on the role that they have played in their own suffering.

Given that the immediate jail environment can further elicit defensiveness, REVAMP is careful not to imply judgment, while still encouraging a focus on one's own behavior. This is accomplished by openly probing for perceived barriers to valued action and validating the emotional response to these barriers (e.g., frustration). Next, the program provides psychoeducation about the distinction between "external" obstacles (problems in the environment they are returning to) and "internal" obstacles (one's thoughts, emotions, and behavior). Facilitators present the outline of a person and ask participants to classify the obstacles they identified as either internal or external (see Figure 1). When external obstacles are identified (e.g., burdensome probation requirements) they are written outside of the outlined figure, and facilitators probe for related internal obstacles (e.g., frustration, missing meetings), writing these in the interior of the figure. Often, participants spontaneously recognize connections between internal and external obstacles.

(These connections are also incorporated into the figure, providing visual emphasis.) Following the group discussion, participants identify the internal and external obstacles they will face as individuals. Because both values and obstacles are defined by the participant, the perception of judgment or blame is minimized.

Figure 1: Internal and External Barriers

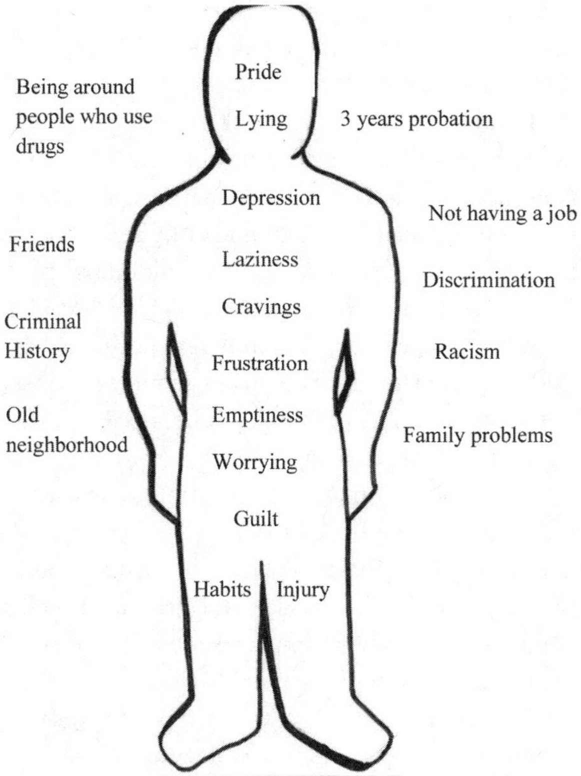

In a collaborative process, REVAMP facilitators acknowledge that participants' ability to achieve a values-driven, meaningful life is hampered by both external and internal barriers, which often are interconnected. However, REVAMP directs attention to that which individuals can directly impact while still incarcerated: the internal barriers.

Reducing Suffering: Confronting and Breaking Barriers to Values

Given that jail inmates are diverse, there is substantial variety in both the internal and external barriers they face. Therefore, a successful reentry program must provide flexible tools to prepare participants to overcome a range of behavior problems and life challenges.

The theoretical underpinning of REVAMP provides such flexibility. REVAMP identifies and focuses on a common factor related to many of the psychological and behavioral problems experienced by inmates: the maladaptive avoidance of emotional pain (Hayes, Wilson, Gifford, Follette, & Strosahl, 1996). Pain is understood as a normal and inevitable part of life. Although many essential aspects of life involve pain, individuals may try to avoid or escape pain. This unwillingness to experience pain can manifest as a variety of problematic avoidance behaviors, such as substance abuse, social isolation, and risky sexual behavior. In turn, problematic avoidance behaviors result in additional pain (e.g., health problems, loneliness, strained relationships). This "extra" pain resulting from one's own attempt to avoid pain is referred to as "suffering." Over time, patterns of problematic avoidance behavior may become habitual and difficult to break (Hayes & Smith, 2005, pp. 1-16).

This conceptualization is applicable to a variety of distinct problem behaviors found among inmates. To illustrate, consider two examples. Inmate A reports that he began to drink heavily soon after the unexpected death of a loved one. He describes his drinking as becoming "out of control," leading him to lose his job and straining his relationship with his surviving family members. Inmate B describes being "addicted" to the power and quick money of selling drugs, which he attributes to his impatience for the slow pace it takes to improve one's status through education and entry-level positions. Following previous incarcerations, he has tried to maintain employment but says he cannot tolerate the mundane routine of the type of job that he can attain given his criminal record. He adds that his daughter has "expensive tastes" and pressures him to provide her with expensive things.

As shown in Table 2, these vignettes illustrate that a common element of two different problematic behaviors (alcohol abuse and illegal activity) can be conceptualized as avoidance behavior. While each inmate faces

Table 2: Pain and Suffering Conceptualization

	Difficult Situation	Pain	Avoidance Behavior	Suffering
Inmate A	Death of a family member	Feelings of loss	Excessive alcohol use	Legal trouble Unemployment Strained relationship with family members
Inmate B	Long history of incarceration and separation from family Daughter asking for money	Feeling of powerlessness, frustration, shame	Selling drugs to make quick money	Legal trouble Separation from daughter and loss of her respect

different situations and experiences different emotional reactions, both attempt to escape their pain through risky avoidance behavior. In REVAMP, one's relationship with pain is a major target of treatment. In this way, the program's focus is on the common element of different problem behaviors. By focusing on one's relationship to affective experience, rather than on specific types of experiences, REVAMP is able to accommodate the diverse group of participants represented in a jail setting.

During session 3, inmates are provided with psychoeducation about the difference between acceptance and avoidance of pain, and the relationship with suffering. Two metaphors often employed in ACT are used to illustrate these concepts: quicksand and Chinese finger traps (Hayes & Smith, 2005, pp. 3-4, p. 37). First, participants are asked to imagine their reaction if they were to find themselves caught in quicksand. Most imagine that they would panic and would try to pull, swim, or run out. In quicksand, the more you struggle the more you sink, so these frantic movements would cause someone to sink deeper and deeper. It is clear that, for most people, acting on the first impulse would serve to make a bad situation worse, which illustrates the concept of suffering. Next, participants are provided with Chinese finger traps—woven straw tubes just large enough to insert an index finger into each end. The tubes are constructed to "trap" the inserted fingers when one quickly attempts to pull out the fingers directly. But by pushing in, the finger trap relaxes allowing the fingers to become freed. Inmates are asked to imagine that the finger trap represents pain. Inmates experience how their first impulse, which usually is to jerk the fingers apart, serves to tighten the trap and restrict their flexibility. The Chinese finger trap allows inmates to experience, in a physical way, the paradox of acceptance. By allowing the fingers to go further into the trap, essentially doing the opposite of one's immediate avoidance impulse, more space and flexibility are created, which ultimately allows escape. While some might be skeptical that criminal offenders would appreciate the abstract nature of metaphors, our experience has been that inmates readily identify with these metaphors. Several have generated additional metaphors to illustrate their own futile struggle with pain (e.g., swimming against a riptide). Both in group and individually, participants reflect on their own experience of suffering resulting from impulsive avoidance behavior. Individually, by completing worksheets, inmates reflect on how acceptance would allow them to lead a life more in line with their values.

After the rationale for pursuing a healthier way to react to pain is established, participants are taught concrete skills to better manage pain. Sessions 4, 5, and 6 cover three major classes of skills: present awareness, short-term distress tolerance, and defusion skills. During session 4, which is devoted to present awareness, participants are taught about the concept of automatic behavior, action without awareness, and automatic pilot mode (Bowen et al., 2011, pp. 32-47). During automatic pilot mode, individuals' behaviors are influenced by their thoughts and feelings without conscious awareness of this process, such that a situation can trigger harmful automatic reactions. Facilitators explain that awareness is necessary in order to respond to internal states with intention and choice, rather than automatically. Participants engage in several exercises to bring awareness to their experience. First they complete a body scan (Bowen et al., 2011, pp. 42-43), which involves focusing on sensations experienced in each part of the body, without reacting to them. Participants then bring awareness to their thoughts by writing what goes through their minds, or their "mental chatter," for 2 minutes (Hayes & Smith, 2005, p. 55). Later, participants further raise nonattached awareness of their thoughts with a mindfulness exercise in which they picture their thoughts as leaves floating down a stream (Bowen et al., 2011, pp. 140-141).

Session 5 focuses on adaptive management of emotional pain. In this session, group leaders acknowledge that bringing acceptance to pain is not an immediate fix. Similar to other acceptance-based interventions, REVAMP takes the stance that sometimes taking healthy action to temporarily reduce the pain can be the best option (Linehan, 1993). The difference between adaptive and maladaptive coping action is explained in reference to the outcome of the behavior; adaptive coping behaviors have positive outcomes, while maladaptive coping behaviors have negative long-term outcomes. Participants brainstorm examples of each type of coping behavior and identify the consequences. In an individual exercise, participants monitor changes in their distress as they practice several coping behaviors (Hayes & Smith, 2005, p. 28). These short-term distress tolerance skills are presented as quick fixes to be used during times of intense pain rather than as permanent solutions. Session 6 presents a long-term strategy to manage distress by transforming the relationship participants have to their own thoughts and feelings. Inmates are provided with psychoeducation on observer perspective and defusion. Group leaders explain that taking a step back from thoughts and emotions and adopting an outside perspective can reduce the automatic impact on behavior. To illustrate this, group leaders present an ACT metaphor of a chessboard (Hayes & Smith, 2005, p. 96). Inmates are instructed to imagine their internal struggle as a chess game with positive and negative thoughts and emotions as two opposing teams of chess pieces. Group leaders then ask the inmates which part of the metaphor represents them (e.g., the pieces, the player, or the board). Participants usually immediately respond that they are the pieces or the player. Group leaders explain that the board represents an observer perspective; it holds the internal content (e.g., thoughts and emotions) but is not a part of the struggle. Inmates then participate in a visualization-based centering exercise referred to as the mountain meditation (Bowen et al., 2011). In this meditation, an image of a mountain is used to represent a grounded, unmoving, nonreactive presence.

The worksheet assigned at the end of session 6 integrates distress-monitoring material from sessions 4-6. Participants are first instructed to identify their own past maladaptive reactions to distress. Then they are asked to reflect on the distress that they will likely experience in the future and describe alternative adaptive reactions. This allows participants to apply the material related to present awareness, short-term adaptive coping, and/or observer perspective to their own anticipated distress (Bornovalova, 2008).

Session Structure

REVAMP is designed to have a consistent structure across sessions to provide a challenging, yet predictable, group experience. Session 1 differs from the other sessions due to the need to orient participants to the program by presenting its purpose and goals, enhancing curiosity and interest in the remainder of the intervention, creating a safe environment to promote personal participation, and introducing centering exercises for the first time. Sessions 2-8 each follow the same pattern:

- Centering exercise

- Review/discussion of previous assignment

- Curriculum beginning with bridge from last class and often including a new or expanded metaphor

- Exercise that illustrates the lesson of the day

- Discussion of the curriculum and exercise

- Assignment of worksheet to be completed prior to the next session to personalize the lesson for each inmate and/or practice putting the lesson into action

- Distribution of a take-home message providing the curriculum in a succinct phrase or two

- Centering exercise

For example, session 7, which focuses on integrating values-based living with distress tolerance skills, begins with the mountain meditation for the centering exercise, followed by a review of the distress-monitoring worksheet assigned at the end of session 6. Next, group facilitators present the curriculum, which focuses on valued action, goal setting, and overcoming barriers. Group facilitators utilize the bus metaphor to reinforce material on values (direction the bus is heading), goals (stops along the way), internal barriers (distracting passengers on the bus), and external barriers (traffic jam). An exercise in which participants set short-term achievable goals is followed by a discussion of overcoming barriers in the community. Participants are then given a worksheet to identify potential barriers and strategies to overcome these barriers. Next, participants are provided with a "take-home message": "Practicing mindfulness and trying new things can help you live the life you want to live." Finally, participants complete a present awareness-based centering exercise.

The final group, session 8, follows the same general structure as sessions 2-7, with a few differences to promote reflection of what has already been presented and how the group experience can help each person when he or she reenters the community. We start with a centering exercise, as usual, but the group chooses one of three previously used exercises. We also review the worksheet assigned during the previous session. Then, instead of introducing a new lesson during the curriculum section, we review: the goals of the program; the theoretical rationale for each goal; and how each goal was promoted in the lessons, exercises, centering techniques, and discussions. Instead of having one discussion section after the curriculum review, we discuss the personal application of each course goal for each individual. We also distribute a compiled list of all of the take-home messages. Finally, the group again selects a final centering exercise from a menu of previous centering exercises.

Acceptability

Outcome data are not yet available from our pilot randomized clinical trial, but evidence suggests that REVAMP is well received by a diverse group of inmates. All participants were given anonymous feedback forms to complete. Overall, feedback has been very positive. Participants provided ratings on a scale of 1-4 of the intervention's quality (M= 3.3), usefulness (M= 3.5), and their overall satisfaction with the program (M= 3.6). Retention throughout the program has been strong for a jail-based program, comparing very favorably with attendance observed in other multiweek programs and interventions offered at this jail.

Applicability

REVAMP was designed to be generally applicable to a broad range of inmate participants that are diverse in terms of age, ethnicity, criminal history, values, and barriers (e.g., mental health concerns, substance abuse problems, etc.). Accordingly, participants in REVAMP were eligible for the study if they met basic requirements meant to ensure the ability to participate in the program (e.g., were assigned to the general population, had remaining sentences long enough to participate in the program, would be released directly to the community). Participation in REVAMP was entirely voluntary. Thus far, participants in this program have ranged in age (from 18 to 81), criminal history, and type of instant offense.

In sum, the 8-session REVAMP treatment has dual aims of reducing distress and enhancing values-based living. REVAMP is specifically tailored to the jail setting, and preliminary feedback suggests that it has been well received by a diverse group of inmates. We are in the process of collecting empirical data on REVAMP's effectiveness.

Motivational Interviewing with "General Population" Inmates

What Is Motivational Interviewing?

Motivational interviewing (MI) is a brief intervention developed by Miller and Rollnick (2002). Often, MI is used as a "pretreatment" intervention, typically delivered in 1-2 individual sessions just prior to the initiation of treatment. In other contexts, it is provided as a stand-alone intervention, in anticipation of treatment or change.

The goal of the motivational interview is to enhance a person's motivation to change. MI is especially useful for "resistant" or "uncommitted" clients—people in need of treatment who are ambivalent about change or who are not committed to change. Using a directive, yet client-centered approach, the MI clinician: (a) probes to make the client's goals and personal values salient; (b) highlights discrepancies by helping the client identify ways in which his or her current behavior and life circumstance are at odds with those values and goals, and (c) helps the client utilize dissonance arising from recognition of such discrepancies as a source of motivation for (and commitment to) positive change. In the MI interview, the clinician works from the client's perspective, expresses empathy, highlights discrepancies in the client's current circumstance and future goals, reframes resistance, and supports the client's sense of self-efficacy. Initially developed for the treatment of alcoholics, MI has evolved into a broadly applicable technique and associated theory, complete with specified mechanisms of action including motivation for change, stages of change, "change talk," and "commitment talk" (Miller & Rollnick, 2002).

Although not explicitly developed within the context of positive psychology, motivational interviewing techniques stem from positive psychology principles. MI techniques to enhance self-efficacy focus on the client's positive individual traits (e.g., "What strengths do you have that will help you make this change?"). Additionally, MI techniques to enhance motivation focus the client on the positive results of enacting a change (e.g., "If you make the change, what would be better about your life?").

Empirically, How Has Motivational Interviewing (MI) Fared in the Community?

Motivational interviewing techniques have been employed in conjunction with many different kinds of treatment aimed at changing behavior in a variety of domains. There is now an impressive body of research documenting MI's effectiveness in increasing treatment motivation and subsequent behavior change. Three meta-analyses, each of somewhat different study samples, converge—MI yields medium effects across diverse samples and in a variety of problem areas, both when evaluated as a stand-alone intervention *and* when assessed as an additive effect in combination with a focal treatment (Burke, Arkowitz, & Menchola, 2003; Hettema, Steele, & Miller, 2005; Rubick, Sandbaek, Lauritzen, & Christensen, 2005).

Why Is MI Especially Relevant to Inmates?

Some limited research with individuals who are incarcerated or on probation has yielded promising results (Ginsburg et al., 2002; Walters et al., 2007). For example, a motivational enhancement intervention with domestic violence offenders increased readiness to change substance use (Easton, Swan, & Sinha, 2000). Among incarcerated adolescents, motivational interviewing reduced the frequency of postrelease drinking and driving, and being a passenger in a car with someone who had been drinking, especially among those with low levels of depression (Stein et al., 2006). In addition, MI appears effective with individuals who are angry or oppositional and with individuals who are not motivated to change (Hettema et al., 2005; O'Leary Tevyaw & Monti, 2004). Moreover, a meta-analysis found that the effects of MI are significantly larger for minority samples than for Caucasian samples (Hettema et al., 2005), especially relevant to a jail setting given that minorities are disproportionately represented in jails and prisons.

Special Challenges in Using MI with Prerelease Jail Inmates

MI is typically employed in contexts where the actual target of change is unambiguous (e.g., among individuals referred specifically for substance abuse treatment, among adolescents with eating disorders, among clients seeking mental health treatment for depression). In most contexts, the ultimate focus of change is clear from the outset—to both client and interviewing clinician.

In contrast, jail inmates nearing community reentry, especially those with comorbid substance dependence and psychiatric disorders, face myriad challenges and a long list of potential targets for change. For some, the primary goal is to obtain employment and find a place to live. For others, abstinence from substance use is paramount. For others, continuation of psychotropic medication (often first prescribed during incarceration) and supportive therapy is at the top of the list. In the absence of MI, inmates typically express a fervent wish to live life differently from their pre-incarceration days, but plans to reach and maintain these goals are underdeveloped or entirely absent. In short, the use of MI procedures with jail inmates, especially those with comorbid substance dependence and psychiatric disorders, is complicated by the need to clearly identify achievable goals (emanating from personal values) and to then move on to the prototypical MI business of enhancing motivation, delineating plans for action, and bolstering self-efficacy for implementation.

Having obtained extensive training in MI procedures and having piloted these procedures with jail inmates nearing reentry into the community, we are convinced that the use of MI in this context is necessarily quite different from its use in more conventional contexts (e.g., substance abuse treatment programs). Conventional approaches must be modified because of the need to identify idiographic targets of change. There is a diversity of potential goals and targets of change among general population offenders (e.g., reducing or eliminating substance use, gaining employment, strengthening family ties, desisting from criminal activities). It is also especially important to minimize the potential for inmates to feel judged, stigmatized, or even shamed by the MI clinician.

Our initial efforts to probe to identify person-specific targets of change appeared to do just that. We tried opening our interviews by saying "Mr. X, you're due to be released from the ADC in XX weeks. Thinking about rejoining the community, what kind of changes would you like to make to avoid being incarcerated in the future?" The interviews fell flat. We met with considerable resistance. A number of inmates bristled at the idea that they needed to make changes to avoid re-incarceration. Many responded with stories about external factors—especially how the system had failed participants. Others stated categorically that they weren't going to return to jail. They'd already made all the changes they needed to make. In effect, we communicated our assumption that participants *needed* to make changes. Our opening question inadvertently implied that inmate participants were deficient in some fundamental way and that we knew they needed to make changes (and likely that we knew best what needed to be changed).

We spent several months piloting a number of strategies, and one approach clearly emerged as more effective than the rest: tapping into inmates' personal values and goals right from the outset. We now begin MI interviews with inmates by thanking them for meeting with us and asking, "So Mr. X, what kind of things are most important to you? What do you value most?" Using this approach, the way opens like magic. As in the REVAMP program, inmates have no difficulty coming up with personal values—values that are, almost without exception, positive prosocial values that most of us share. The interview opens on an upbeat note. Rapport is readily established, as inmate participants feel respected and valued as individuals.

Having identified personal values, it is a short step for the MI clinician to note how a criminal activity and incarceration have interfered with pursuing personally relevant values and associated goals. "Developing discrepancy," a key MI technique, is a natural transition—done in a way that inmate participants experience as not threatening or judgmental but rather as supportive and caring. Targets of change are much more readily identified. Inmate participants readily move through one or more stages of change. And the interview concludes on a positive note, reaffirming the participant's own values and goals and the changes she identified that would pave the way toward reaching these personally relevant goals.

Summary and Conclusion

There is a tremendous need for psychological interventions tailored to the needs of inmates and the constraints of the jail or prison environment. Because of their severity and potential danger to society, a focus on inmates' psychological and behavioral problems may seem more important than a focus on positive outcomes. And in fact, whereas recent years have seen a growth in empirical research on positive psychological interventions in clinical and community settings, little work has focused on translating this research into interventions for inmates.

In this chapter, we described three treatment approaches designed for "general population" jail inmates. Several common threads run through each of these interventions. First, these approaches are shame-reducing in nature. Each intervention takes a slightly different response to the inevitable shame resulting from inmates' reflections. Consider, for example, this inmate's expression of shame: "Now that I am clean and sober in jail I see how my substance use has hurt myself, my family, and my community. I am so stupid for having let this go on for so long." IOC encourages inmates to take responsibility and to develop and carry out a reparative plan. REVAMP encourages acceptance and refocusing on valued action. In MI, therapists express empathy, reframe and affirm clients' strengths and values, and encourage a sense of self-efficacy in order to enhance motivation. While these approaches are not mutually exclusive, they help illustrate ways in which each treatment can address clients' experiences of shame.

Second, these treatment approaches share an emphasis on making positive change for the future. Modifications were necessary for both MI and the ACT-inspired REVAMP. Pilot testing of both led us to anchor the intervention in an initial discussion of personal values and goals.

Our work has emphasized that encouraging "the positive" and curing "the negative" are not necessarily mutually exclusive. Our experience across interventions has shown that inmates' motivation to change is strongest when it is driven by positive motivations (e.g., a valued goal or restoration following an offense) rather than by simple avoidance of shame, further punishment, and re-incarceration. In sum, working to enhance values and reduce symptoms can be complementary and mutually reinforcing in this population. Offender rehabilitation could be substantially enhanced by a greater consideration of constructs and interventions emanating from the field of positive psychology.

References

Bornovalova, M.A. (2008). Distress tolerance treatment for inner-city drug users: A preliminary trial. (Doctoral dissertation). Retrieved from Digital Repository at the University of Maryland. (http://hdl.handle.net/1903/8446)

Bowen, S., Chawla, N., & Marlatt, G. A. (2011). *Mindfulness-based relapse prevention for addictive behaviors: A clinician's guide.* New York: Guilford Press.

Burke, B. L., Arkowitz, H., & Menchola, M. (2003). The efficacy of motivational interviewing: A meta-analysis of controlled clinical trials. *Journal of Consulting and Clinical Psychology, 71,* 843-861.

Conn, C., Warden, R., Stuewig, J., Kim, E. H., Harty, L., Hastings, M., & Tangney, J. P. (2010). Borderline personality disorder among jail inmates: How common, and how distinct? *Corrections Compendium, 4,* 6-13.

Drapalski, A., Youman, K., Stuewig, J., & Tangney, J. P. (2009). Gender differences in jail inmates' symptoms of mental illness, treatment history and treatment seeking. *Criminal Behaviour and Mental Health, 19,* 193-206.

Easton, C., Swan, S., & Sinha, R. (2000). Motivation to change substance use among offenders of domestic violence. *Journal of Substance Abuse Treatment, 19,* 1-5.

Ginsburg, J. L. D., Mann, R. E., Rotgers, F., & Weekes, J. R. (2002). Motivational interviewing with criminal justice populations. In W. R. Miller & S. Rollnick (eds.), *Motivational interviewing: Preparing people for change* (2nd ed.) (pp. 333-346). New York: Guilford Press.

Hayes, S. C. (2004). Acceptance and Commitment Therapy, relational frame theory, and the third wave of behavioral and cognitive therapies. *Behavior Therapy, 35,* 639-665.

Hayes, S. C., & Smith, S. (2005). *Get out of your mind and into your life: The new Acceptance and Commitment Therapy.* Oakland, CA: New Harbinger.

Hayes, S. C., Wilson, K. G., Gifford, E. V., Follette, V. M., & Strosahl, K. (1996). Experiential avoidance and behavioral disorders: A functional dimensional approach to diagnosis and treatment. *Journal of Consulting and Clinical Psychology, 64,* 1152-1168.

Hettema, J., Steele, J., & Miller, W. R. (2005). Motivational interviewing. *Annual Review of Clinical Psychology, 1,* 91-111.

Leith, K. P., & Baumeister, R. F. (1998). Empathy, shame, guilt, and narratives of interpersonal conflicts: Guilt-prone people are better at perspective taking. *Journal of Personality, 66,* 1-37.

Linehan, M. M. (1993). *Cognitive behavioral treatment of borderline personality disorder.* New York: Guilford Press.

Meyer, C. R., Tangney, J. P., & Stuewig, J. (under review). Why do some jail inmates not engage in treatment and services?

Miller, W. R., & Rollnick, S. (2002). *Motivational interviewing: Preparing people for change* (2nd ed.). New York: Guilford Press.

O'Leary Tevyaw, T., & Monti, P. M. (2004). Motivational enhancement and other brief interventions for adolescent substance abuse: Foundations, applications and evaluations. *Addiction, 99,* 63-75.

Rubak, S., Sandbæk, A., Laurizen, T., Christensen, B. (2005). Motivational interviewing: A systematic review and meta-analysis. *British Journal of General Practice, 55,* 305-312.

Stein, L. A. R., Colby, S. M., Barnett, N. P., Monti, P. M., Golembeske, C., & Lebeau-Craven, R. (2006). Effects of motivational interviewing for incarcerated adolescents on driving under the influence after release. *The American Journal on Addictions, 15,* 50-57.

Tangney, J. P., Malouf, E. T., Stuewig, J., & Mashek, D. (2012). Emotions and morality: You don't have to feel really bad to be good. In M. W. Eysenck, M. Fajkowska, & T. Maruszewski (Eds.), *Warsaw lectures on personality and social psychology. Personality, cognition and emotion* (Vol. 2). New York: Eliot Werner.

Tangney, J. P., Mashek, D., & Stuewig, J. (2007). Working at the social-clinical-community-criminology interface: The George Mason University Inmate Study. *Journal of Social and Clinical Psychology, 26,* 1-21.

Tangney, J. P., Stuewig, J., & Hafez, L. (2011). Shame, guilt and remorse: Implications for offender populations. *Journal of Forensic Psychiatry & Psychology, 22*(5), 706-723.

Tangney, J. P., Stuewig, J., & Mashek, D. J. (2007). Moral emotions and moral behavior. *Annual Review of Psychology, 58,* 345-372.

Tangney, J. P., Youman, K., & Stuewig, J. (2009). Proneness to shame and proneness to guilt. In M.R. Leary & R.H. Hoyle (Eds.), *Handbook of individual differences in social behavior* (pp. 192-209). New York: Guilford Press.

VA Maryland Health Care System Acceptance and Commitment Therapy Team. (2007). *Acceptance and Commitment Therapy Group Therapy Protocol: Addictions Intensive Outpatient Program PTSD/Substance Use Dual Diagnosis Program.* Unpublished therapy manual.

Walters, S.T., Clark, M.D., Gingerich, R., & Meltzer, M.L. (2007). *A guide for probation and parole: Motivating offenders to change.* Washington, DC: U.S. Department of Justice, Office of Justice Programs, National Institute of Corrections.

Youman, K., Drapalski, A., Stuewig, J., Bagley, K., & Tangney, J. P. (2010). Race differences in psychopathology and disparities in treatment seeking: Community and jail-based treatment seeking patterns. *Psychological Services, 7,* 11-26.

CHAPTER 11

Using the Science of Meaning to Invigorate Values-Congruent, Purpose-Driven Action

Michael F. Steger

Colorado State University

North-West University, South Africa

Kelly Sheline

Colorado State University

Leslie Merriman

Colorado State University

Todd B. Kashdan

George Mason University

There's an interesting parallel between Acceptance and Commitment Therapy (ACT) and positive psychology. Both strive to help people achieve their best possible futures. But there is a key difference. ACT is based on a theory that integrates the positive and negative with a large set of interventions aimed at reducing barriers that prevent people from striving toward healthy aims, being autonomous when striving, and being able to integrate these strivings into a reasonably coherent life plan. Positive psychology has been defined by diverse research that emphasizes subject matter that has been labeled as good, desirable, or "positive" such as happiness, gratitude, and kindness without sufficient integration among different forms of positivity, much less the rest of the spectrum of human experience. As a contrast, ACT has put people, not surface-level positivity, at the center.

Positive psychology has gained a great deal of ground focusing on the ways in which happy people are alike and creating relatively universal interventions (e.g., expressing gratitude or kindness more regularly to other people). ACT has gained ground by relying on the assumption that a primary source of suffering is common to all people: language. From this starting point, ACT practitioners focus on the dormant aspirations aligned with each person's unique configuration of values.

Perhaps the meeting ground of these two perspectives is each person's unique journey toward a common vision of a well-lived life. In this chapter, we describe some of the ways in which meaning in life takes a step outside the typical terrain of positive psychology to provide this meeting ground. After highlighting the ways in which ACT has already invested in meaning in life, we use a case example to show how meaning in life enhances ACT and provides new insights to help people achieve their best possible futures.

ACT, Positive Psychology, and Meaning in Life

Meaning in life had often been included in models of optimal human functioning that predated the introduction of positive psychology. For example, Ryff's (1989) model of psychological well-being included purpose in life, and many investigations seeking to understand the basic building blocks of well-being included measures of meaning and purpose in life (e.g., DeNeve & Cooper, 1998; Harlow & Newcomb, 1990). However, most of the well-being research completed in the 1970s–1990s focused on personality traits, emotions, and life satisfaction. Perhaps it was to be expected that the positive psychology movement would also focus on personality traits (called character strengths) and positive emotions, and embrace the research that combined emotions and life satisfaction into the notion of subjective well-being. Although calls to focus on other variables were issued (e.g., Ryan & Deci, 2001), few ideas were able to penetrate the fog of enthusiasm about positive emotions.

However, the one or two successfully competitive ideas are highly instructive. First, mindfulness captured enthusiasm in the media and among practitioners. Second, meaning in life began to appear once again on lists of important variables in social psychology, and among the targets of interventions in palliative and oncology nursing. Mindfulness is central to ACT, and one aim of this chapter is to demonstrate that meaning in life as well. Thus, it could be argued that the "second wave" of positive psychology strongly resembles the "third wave" of behavior therapy.

Most often, and unfortunately, business-as-usual positive psychology has seemed overly focused on gratification, success, and enjoyment in the moment. This can be seen in its most common application: simplistic behavioral tallying techniques to draw attention to positive experiences as in "counting blessings" or writing down three good things from the day. These tools might inspire people to pursue positive emotions or urge people to do what comes easily, enjoyably, and naturally. Positive psychology 1.0 (cf. Wong, 2011) is positioned to be delivered as a commodity and to be accumulated by consumers in an almost materialistic manner. This strong focus on positive experiences has created a strange economics of utility—forgive someone, it'll make you feel better; express gratitude, it'll make you feel better.

Positive psychology 1.0 also has focused on relatively static character strengths, although rather than simply basking in appreciation of one's attractive qualities, the spotlight recently has begun to shine on the promising avenues of using strengths, or even developing new strengths (Biswas-Diener, Kashdan, & Minhas, 2011). Other encouraging trends include adaptations of cognitive therapy to promote resilience. Positive psychology can continue to grow by adapting to the complex and dynamic texture of life as it is lived, full of the good, the bad, the ambivalent, and the uncertain. A thoughtfully orchestrated merger between ACT and meaning in life work could help achieve this growth.

Meaning in life research is about going beyond "feel-good" motives to address a more complex landscape of human strivings. Although most would associate a meaningful life with feeling good, people are also adept at finding meaning under awful circumstances. Everyone's life brings some ambiguity, some struggle, and some unique burden. Meaning in life is built from all of those experiences, as well as the happy moments. The birth of a child and the death of a parent are both meaningful, though either could be positive, negative, or a blend. As another example, creating meaning in life can often lead to scapegoating and the creation of enemies. In ambiguous situations where something bad happens, we look to make sense of it all (Sullivan, Landau, & Rothschild, 2010). Threats of meaninglessness increase the likelihood of blaming other people for the unfortunate situation, which temporarily restores a sense of meaning (Sullivan, Landau, & Rothschild, 2010). Thus, when and how the pursuit of meaning is healthy is not a simple question with a single answer.

Meaning in life shifts the emphasis from what feels good for the individual to what is important for the individual, for his/her group, and for the wider universe. Meaning in life also focuses on the journey, rather than the hedonic outcomes of the journey (Steger, Kashdan, & Oishi, 2008), and thereby provides a language and stable framework for sustaining fulfillment even in the face of pain and setbacks. With the right interventions to guide people, the emphasis can be on the greatest psychological benefits and the least costs to detecting and creating meaning in areas that matter the most.

This suggests an immediate resonance with ACT's emphasis on experiential acceptance rather than avoidance. Much of the research literature on avoidance has contrasted the erosive influence of attempting to avoid negative states, thoughts, and experiences with the constructive influence of attempting instead to achieve, or obtain, positive states, thoughts, and experiences (e.g., Elliott & Thrash, 2002). Although the message that "avoiding bad is bad" has generally gotten across in positive psychology, perhaps the message that "seeking good is good" may have been overapplied. At times, the clamor for more happiness seems to have created a warped psychological tourism, with metaphorical busloads of people being driven past a sequence of great positive attributes to acquire.

Character strengths! Positive emotions! Optimism! Gratitude! Curiosity! Meaning in life! The concern that positive psychology would devolve into a singular focus on the acquisition of the good—and only the good—things in life has been with the movement since the beginning (Lazarus, 2003). In this chapter, we emphasize that the best things in life involve both positive and negative experiences.

Each individual is faced with the challenge of making sense of an existence beset by threats, change, confusion, and failure. Despite grave existential issues around the threat of death, the pain of loneliness, and constraints on autonomy, humans cope. Humans continue to find a wide number of sources of meaning in life and show great creativity in comprehending what is happening to carve out a purpose in life (McKnight & Kashdan, 2009). Perhaps this is because among positive psychology constructs, meaning in life is notable for its origins in clinical work. Perhaps it is unsurprising that many people are willing to forego short-term gratification because of the wisdom that meaning grows from hard work, not easy work (e.g., couples craving parenthood, military recruits, graduate school applicants) (King & Napa, 1998; King & Hicks, 2007). Like ACT, the ideas central to meaning and purpose in life evolved in response to the special partnership of client and therapist, facilitator and organization.

Meaning in Life—What Is It and How Does It Connect with ACT?

Clinicians and researchers across the field of psychology have written about the importance of meaning making in cultivating a life worth living (e.g., Baumeister, 1991; Frankl, 1963; Ryff & Singer, 1998; Wong & Fry, 1998). At various times, different psychologists have meant different things by the term "meaning in life." It is often meant to convey the sense that people make in life, capturing the idea that, similar to meaning making in language, meaning in life holds symbolic content. As a sentence conveys information, so then does life. This is the cognitive quality of meaning in life. Steger (2009, 2012; Steger, Frazier, Oishi, & Kaler, 2006) has referred to this aspect of meaning as comprehension. Meaning has also been used to describe the point of life: what people are trying to do, accomplish, and aspire to. This dimension has been nearly universally referred to as purpose (Kashdan & McKnight, 2009; McKnight & Kashdan, 2009; Reker, 2000). Taken together, meaning in life is the degree to which an individual makes sense of and sees significance in their life and believes his or her life to have an overarching purpose (Steger, 2009).

These two dimensions of meaning in life are readily connected to key processes that ACT proposes lead to psychopathology and rigidity. Comprehension links nicely with the dominance of people's ideas about their past and their future, which prevents nondefensive, open contact with what is being experienced in the present. When people become lost in their ideas about the past and future, it blocks self-development and the ability to grow from wanted and unwanted experiences that occur in each moment. Experiential avoidance renders people's comprehension systems inaccurate, fragile, and constantly in need of protection.

Comprehension also can be linked to people's attachment to the self as they conceive of it rather than as they experience it. When the self is viewed through the prism of feelings, thoughts, and ideas about who one is (the content of one's mind; Luoma, Hayes, & Walser, 2007), the potential for personal growth is limited. As with the first pathological process of experiential avoidance, becoming overly attached to particular conceptualizations of ourselves can divide us from knowledge of our true self. The comprehension dimension of meaning in life emphasizes the important role played by our conceptualizations and understandings of ourselves, the world around us, and our interactions with the world. By incorporating the world as the context for personal experience and by calling attention to the ways in which people understand the dynamic interactions of their selves and changing contexts, the comprehension dimension is broader than the two pathological processes identified in ACT. Yet, by addressing people's orientation to past and future events as potential barriers of authentic experience, ACT is broader than meaning in life theory. Whereas ACT often focuses on creating a better life by helping people detach from unhelpful self-concepts (defusion) and maintain an accepting attitude about what is happening in the present moment (mindfulness), meaning in life is about how to elaborate the sense of self in a productive way. That is, by attending to meaning in life, individuals create a better life through the expansion of the self out into the world and into the abstract realm of people's ultimate concerns. Both ACT and meaning in life can be strengthened through collaboration.

A Little More about Meaning in Life

Generally, research has focused on whether people have meaning in life or how much of it they have. Hundreds of studies have linked the presence of meaning in life to desirable characteristics, ranging from character strengths and well-being variables to less distress and even lowered risk of Alzheimer's and death (Shin & Steger, in press; Steger, 2009; Steger et al., 2006). However, research also suggests a distinction between the presence of meaning and the degree to which people search for meaning (Steger et al., 2006; Steger, Kashdan, Sullivan, & Lorentz, 2008). The search for meaning refers to the active pursuit of meaning in life ("I am seeking a purpose or mission for my life") and is related to neuroticism and negative emotions (Steger et al., 2006). Searching for meaning may range from straining to establish a minimal level of meaning to viewing life as a continuous attempt to understand one's purpose in life (Steger, Kashdan, et al., 2008). It appears to matter whether people are searching for meaning from a position of strength—trying to build an already healthy sense of meaning in life—or from a position of desperation—trying to rebuild or simply find some way for life to hold meaning. People who are searching for meaning in the absence of meaning in life are less happy and satisfied than people who are not searching for meaning; yet searching for meaning does not appear to detract from happiness among people who feel their lives are meaningful (e.g., Park, Park, & Peterson, 2010; Steger, Kashdan et al., 2008; Steger, Oishi, Kesebir, 2011).

Helping people find healthy and effective ways of constructing meaning therefore appears important for how well people are able to live their lives (Read, Westerhof, Dittmann-Kohli, 2005). Although the focus of meaning in life research and interventions is on the overarching, encompassing comprehension and purpose people create in their lives as a whole, other research has focused on the way in which people make meaning from specific events (e.g., Davis, Nolen-Hoeksema, & Larson, 1998). King and Hicks (2009) demonstrated that negative events are more likely to be perceived as meaningful. Finding meaning in negative events such as chronic or life-limiting illnesses like cancer and conges-tive heart failure appears to support health (e.g., Cohen, Mount, Tomas, & Mount, 1996).

We have taken a brief look at some of the complexity that meaning in life theory can add to the current landscape of positive psychology. We have also quickly outlined some of the ways in which ACT and meaning in life overlap and can be combined to create new insights. In the next section, we will use a case study to illustrate how we think ACT and meaning in life can be used together to yield interventions.

◆ Understanding Mandy

Mandy is a 34-year-old woman whose divorce was finalized 6 weeks ago. She shares custody of her two daughters with her former husband. If you ask Mandy why she is divorced, she says it's because her husband wanted to "upgrade his wife." In fact, he is already living with someone. Like her ex-husband, her ex's new partner is a middle manager at a large electrical parts man-ufacturing corporation. Mandy has been working for a title company for 12 years, moving up to underwriter during the start of the housing boom. Her income at the peak easily rivaled her ex-husband's and they enjoyed a high standard of living. In the past few years, so few home sales have closed that Mandy's income has plummeted.

Mandy expresses little hope for the future, worries about the bad influence of the new woman in her children's lives, and has recently emerged from a prolonged major depressive episode. She now expresses constant worries about doing a poor job of raising her kids, having something bad happen to them while they are in her ex-husband's custody, and losing her job and her house. She says that her sleep and work performance have suf-fered because of the time she spends worrying and the intensity of her anxiety, particularly over the weekends when her children are in her ex-husband's care. When pressed, Mandy admits that she deeply misses the days when her income was so high that she never worried about money.

Mandy is obviously dealing with tremendous change and stress. One way to work with someone in Mandy's situation is to explore Mandy's self-concept, or in ACT terminology: the "conceptualized self." Many of her worries stem from the seemingly vast divide between how she once saw herself and how she now sees herself. She once lived a life of few worries and many pleasures. As she goes through her days, she dwells on how hard things are now and how great things were before. She also revisits the pain of being left by her ex-husband and the humiliation of learning that he already had replaced her. As the weekends approach, she grows increasingly anxious about the time her children will spend with her husband. By ruminating about the greatness of the past and worrying about the future, Mandy has no idea how to rebuild her life.

From an ACT standpoint, Mandy may be suffering from the dominance of her conceptualizations of the past and the future, as well as from a narrow and unhelpful self-concept. She has poor contact with the present moment.

From a meaning in life standpoint, the core components of Mandy's comprehension of her life are no longer accurate, useful, or nurturing. Instead, they have been broken down by her divorce and all that has resulted from it. Instead of guiding Mandy's actions, cradling her values, and shaping her purpose, her meaning system degrades and demoralizes her. Because Mandy's life has changed so much, she needs to accommodate or alter the defining features of her self-concept (i.e., her meaning systems).

We would suggest two approaches to working with clients to help them revisit, restore, rebuild, or revitalize their basic comprehension of their lives. They are similar to values exploration exercises that are commonly used within ACT, although they may be even more basic.

1. *Givens.* "We hold these truths to be self-evident..." The authors and signatories of the United States Declaration of Independence boldly and clearly stated their given assumptions about the equality of all men. Aside from the fact that many of these signatories had slaves who were treated with anything but equality, this "given" puts the rest of this document in context. How often do we, or out clients, express the fundamental "givens" that put our lives in context? This exercise simply asks clients to take a week to think about the things they assume are true, the things

they believe and never have to question, or the truths that they hold to be self-evident. For example, clients might think about their family life. I will never turn down a hug from my children. Each child will be treated as a unique individual. Whenever possible, the family will eat dinner together. Or, I will never discipline my children like my parents disciplined me. When clients return with this homework, clinicians lead a discussion about the implications and the themes of these givens, helping to illuminate the fundamental assumptions—the most basic comprehensions—people have. These may need to be challenged in order to move forward, so clients should be encouraged and empowered to be completely honest about their givens. In the parenting examples above, despite their laudable nature, "absolute" phrasing often reveals reactive givens—those that are generated because of somewhat unresolved pain. This is most clear in the given about never disciplining like one's parents. This might or might not be a great idea, but the absolute nature of that given likely sets a person up for failure and may even be used to prevent effective and reasonable responses to a child's behavior. Therapists and coaches are a great resource for helping clients discover and reconsider their most basic comprehensions of the world.

2. *Values Work.* The aim of both ACT and a meaning in life standpoint is to assist and inspire people to live in accordance with what they care most deeply about. This is tough to do without exploring one's values; an act done less often than presumed. Here, we draw on Schwartz, Kurtines, & Montgomery (2005) to give clients a concrete way to think about values (for additional activities, see Shin and Steger, 2012).

    Ask your client to identify one or two of the important life choices or dilemmas he or she has faced in the past. Ask the client to describe what made that situation so difficult. For example, many clients face hard choices between dedicating their time and effort to their careers or to their families. Often clients will say that there were no good choices or that whichever decision they made they would let someone down. Make note of the themes that arise, but do not address them yet. These reasons provide powerful clues about your client's values. Next, ask your client to talk about the decision, and in particular how selecting the chosen option made him or her feel. Then, depending on your preferences in working with this client, you have two choices. You can help the client draw links between the feelings that resulted from the decision and the reasons the client gave about why the choice was so tough. A client who chose to focus on family rather than career might say that she favored family because she was raised with the notion that being a parent is the most important job she will ever have. Immediately after choosing to forgo an important career opportunity, our client might have felt great pride but also worries that friends and family would feel she'd made a stupid decision or failed to reach her potential. In this case, you could help her explore how strongly and deeply this client actually valued parenting versus career pursuits, as well as self-direction versus the importance of others' opinions. Alternatively, you can continue to explore with your client why she thinks she felt that way and how she feels about her decision now. To continue our example, our client might now feel smothered by family and feel inadequate in comparison with friends flaunting the milestones of career success. Here, work with this client might focus even more tightly on the importance given to others' expectations, as well as on how large a role those expectations might have played in driving the client's apparent valuation of parenting. Whichever approach seems relevant to you, the idea is to work to help clients see what is important to them because this is what drives both decisions and feelings in their aftermath.

Some clients will lack sufficient insight to identify their values without considerable assistance. They may characterize their givens and decisions in mechanical or concrete terms ("I guess I didn't have a choice, I didn't want to go to jail"). They should be guided to explore their values in similarly concrete terms ("Perhaps that is because you couldn't be there for your family if you were in jail?"). In helping clients explore—and commit to—their values, we should always be aware that we ourselves may have values that conflict with those of our clients. We recommend an exercise developed by Luoma and colleagues (2007) that asks you as a clinician about what you do best, what you most want to give to your clients, and the lasting impact you would most desire to have on clients. Their exercise can provide a language you can use when working with clients to explore their values. This includes those moments when there is conflict between your values and those of clients. Managing conflicts requires tolerance for tension, self-honesty, and candid dialogue with clients about how our values impact the way we interpret what our clients tell us.

Finally, we must face the possibility that some people's values are morally objectionable. As one of the authors (MFS) likes to say "Saints have holy purposes, and assholes have assholey purposes." Based on available research, most people have pretty decent purposes, some have awe-inspiring purposes, and a small portion have horrible purposes. Working with this latter group is difficult, and therapy may need to proceed by showing how it is eventually in the client's selfish interests to figure out how to have reasonably prosocial values and purpose.

• Mandy's Meaning Making

Mandy tells her therapist that she once had great plans for herself. She was a good student in high school and college, and always felt that she was well-liked. When she met her ex-husband, she had already decided to get involved in the real estate business. She initially worked as a real estate agent, but then she had her first child; she agreed to stay home with the baby for the first year. She went to work for the title company part-time, only gaining promotions as her daughters grew older and were in school full-time. Now that the real estate market has gone bust, Mandy says she can't see any way that she'll be successful. Even making a little money these days takes following many dead ends, watching appraisals fall short, banks pull out, and deals fall apart at closing. She can't see herself doing anything else and seems convinced that her next step will be poverty. She says that her daughters would never forgive her for destroying their lives like that and maybe she should just go ahead and give up custody so that they can have a better life with her ex-husband.

Here we begin to see that Mandy's rigid attachment to "how things were" has become despairing paralysis in the face of her new reality. Beyond feeling stuck in her present circumstances, Mandy seems to struggle to figure out who she really is and how her life can "return to normal." Much of the way she frames her situation is in terms of what cannot be done and the failures that seem to await her.

One way of looking at her problem is that her predivorce comprehension system—the network of beliefs about self, world, and self in the world—has been shattered and has failed to adapt to the impact of this difficult event. Elsewhere, we have speculated that when difficult things happen, two kinds of comprehension systems might predict the best outcomes (Steger & Park, 2012). The first is an exceptionally rigid, one-size-fits-all meaning system. In such a system, people have unquestioning confidence that their relatively simple comprehension system can explain all life events. One possible example comes from religious comprehension systems, in which the belief that "it is God's will" can be used to account for everything that happens. Such systems may be able to withstand significant impacts from negative life events without requiring any alteration. However, it seems possible that any event(s) that could shatter such a comprehension system would be devastating, leaving people without much of an intact way of understanding and integrating their experience.

The second comprehension system is one that is flexible, iterative, and dynamically responsive to life events. People adapt their comprehension as they gain feedback from living their lives. These systems may be more resilient in the face of negative life events (Kashdan & Rottenberg, 2010), but it may be that people fall into the tendency to overthink and show a lack of commitment to completing important life projects, like the perfectionist author who can never stop tinkering with a manuscript.

Mandy seems to need to make meaning from her divorce and perhaps reexamine her comprehension system. Cognitive therapy already uses cognitive restructuring to help people work on similar tasks, and narrative therapy has several techniques for helping clients re-author their stories. We consider an additional way of helping people articulate their comprehension system. We are currently researching this approach and are excited about its use in the context of ACT because a large part of what it is about exists entirely apart from language. Although it may be well suited for helping clients chart out their existing values and comprehension systems, we believe it can also be used to revise and clarify a newly emerging comprehension system in the wake of negative life events. We call this intervention "The Photojournalist." We also suggest another way of eliciting growth narratives from clients, which can be used to alter or rebuild comprehension systems.

1. *The Photojournalist.* In the most basic application of this intervention, participants are simply given a digital camera and asked to take 10-12 photos of "what makes your life meaningful." Because not everyone is in close proximity to the things that make life meaningful (a child may have moved out of the house, and not everyone lives in their ideal vacation destination), we tell people they can take photos of mementos or even other photos. When they return the camera, their photos are uploaded to a computer and printed off in a format of one photo per page, with a space provided for writing. When the photos are printed, the client is asked to describe what it is a photo of and how it contributes to life's meaning. In our lab, we also ask people to rank-order photos in terms of centrality to their life's meaning. This allows us to gauge whether there are any discrepancies in what people say about their values or purpose and how they rank photos that seemingly align with those values or their purpose. For making meaning from negative life events, we would suggest altering the instructions to allow clients to choose to take photos of one of the following: what makes life meaningful, what used to make life meaningful, or what someday will make life more meaningful. The eventual point is to lead clients in a discussion of what is different about the photos they took to address each of the three choices. Perhaps a new comprehension system can be built on what is meaningful now, perhaps new versions of what used to make life meaningful can be found or a comprehension system can be built that no longer needs those things, and of course it will be important to help clients find ways to bring into their lives that which they hope will give meaning to their lives someday. Not all clients will be able to see a hopeful, meaningful future, which is why we like providing those three choices.

2. *Growth Narrative.* This intervention would ask a client to reflect on life, beginning in childhood and adolescence, and have her or him identify two areas in which growth has occurred (e.g., where he or she gained a newer, more adaptive and mature self-awareness, insight, or positive self-transformation). The clinician would ask the client to anchor these growth areas with specific life examples. As the clinician asks for details, she or he is also helping the client to identify themes and how the growth that was accomplished aligns with the client's values. Finally, the client is asked to propose a future vignette exemplifying future growth, including in what areas growth would need to occur and what the client's activities, internal experience, and social circumstances would look like.

These interventions should be helpful in assisting clients to explore the landscape of their present and future comprehension systems. However, stopping here might trap clients in an artificial world dominated by their conceptualizations of the "big picture," "what life's really all about," or "the meaning of life." The critical next step is to help clients put their meaning into action. This is done through purpose.

• Mobilizing Mandy

When her therapist asks her about what she wants to accomplish in her life, Mandy is vague. She says she wants her daughter to be happy and that she wants to be successful again, but when pressed for details, she seems to become hopeless and says she'd just be content if her ex-husband would pay for what he did. Mandy says she is a good person at heart and that she still trusts people, but that she feels vulnerable because of this experience and "not like herself." She perseverates about her husband's new life and frets over comparisons between herself and his new wife. She is not sure what she wants to accomplish any more, but she says that the most important thing to her right now is to give her daughters a good role model. Part of this, for Mandy, is showing how to be strong and recover from setbacks.

Mandy is aware of some of her core values. In particular, she is consistent about wanting to bear up for her daughters and give them a good life. Bearing up under strain is a noble aim, but it is inherently a limited one. What does bearing up look like? What purpose does being strong serve? What does it mean to recover from a setback? What comes after the bearing up? Mandy wants to do right by her daughters, but it really is not clear what that looks like, and it appears that thoughts of vengeance and inadequacy slip into the gaps created by that lack of clarity. In the end, our values can come to define us only if we do something to stand up for them and act them out. ACT identifies a lack of clarity and contact with values as a pathological process because in the absence of this knowledge, short-term needs can dominate. Mandy needs to move away from treading water and find something to move toward. We are fond of saying that purpose is the anchor we throw to pull us to our future. Mandy needs help discerning her purpose.

The basic process of discerning a purpose calls for a careful and honest exploration of the comprehension side of meaning in life. This exploration then must lead to a shift from static knowledge to what that knowledge implies about how people should act in the world. At this point, comprehension is used to give people a sense of what they are about and what they are good at doing, what the world needs, and the ways in which people are best at navigating the world around them to accomplish their aims. In Mandy's case, the straightforward question about what she wants to accomplish was not sufficient. She needed a process that is not so overwhelming. We suggest two intervention strategies for helping people discern a purpose.

1. *Mobilizing Values.* A question many clients should have after exploring and clarifying their values is "so what?" In reality, how often are people really called to task for their values? The aim of this intervention is to answer the question "so what?" by showing that one of the "points" of having values is turning them into action. If values work has already been done, such as the activities we suggested above, those that ACT manuals recommend, or others clinicians are comfortable with, then the output of those activities can be used. Otherwise, you can ask clients to tell you about what they stand for, what they believe in, what makes them proud about their own conduct, and so on. Then

you can ask your client how she or he shows the world that these are important values. Essentially, how do other people know what your client stands for without your client verbalizing. This line of questioning may identify behaviors your client has already used to activate values. You can continue this line of questioning by asking your client about what she or he is really good at doing, what people compliment her or him for, and what she or he does that feels most authentic. In other words, you are asking your client about personal strengths. Finally, you can ask your client what it would be like to use his or her strengths to act out their values for the world to see. This line of questioning should continue to push your client to talk about what the end result of all of this would be—ideally, if we used the best of ourselves to act out what we truly valued, we would do so in the service of a natural purpose.

2. *What the World Needs Now.* This intervention strategy starts on the other side of the equation. Rather than beginning with what clients value and do best, it starts with what the world needs. You can ask clients about one or two things they would change about the world, or about news stories they have read recently that have really moved them, or even what part of their experiences they would want most to spare their children and those they care about. This identifies some things that people may want to work toward as part of their purpose. Continued dialogue can help clients find the most magnetic need in the world. When paired with the "mobilizing values" intervention, people can be helped to find a purpose they care about and articulate some rough ideas about how they would like to pursue it.

• Keeping Mandy Moving

Mandy has been struggling to do the things that are necessary to make a title company's work successful in a down market. She doesn't see the point. When the market was good, Mandy loved the excitement and making as much money as her husband. Now, the work seems like pointless drudgery. As Mandy explores her stagnant career with her therapist, she realizes that although she enjoyed it at its peak, being a title officer was a job she backed into rather than chose. Through her work experience, she came to appreciate her talents and came to enjoy some of her work activities. Currently, she cannot see how what she is doing at her present job does anything to support her value of providing a better life for her daughters. As she relinquishes her desire to compete with—and hurt—her ex-husband, she explores her values, talents, and interests. She realizes that she can provide a better world for her daughters in a way that has nothing to do with whether she earns as much as her ex-husband. This will entail making sure that her daughters understand what happened to their family and that, even though she is hurt, Mandy is still strong, raising them with positive values, encouraging their dreams. In her work, she sees that she can use her bookkeeping skills to maintain steady employment while she attends weekend classes in property law at a law school that caters to midcareer professionals. In Mandy's case, her value of a better future for her daughters mingled with the craving for stability and permanence that grew from the divorce to prompt a new purpose: working to preserve the landscape for future generations through conservation and agricultural easements.

Among the many values Mandy identified, a few consistently rose to the top. She emphasized her daughters' future, she liked variety and growth in her work, and through the divorce she had come to value things that stood for timelessness, permanence, and the preservation of good things. The main task for Mandy at this point was to commit to some purpose and engage in the activities that would help her pursue it. ACT points to the damaging effects of inaction, impulsivity, and avoidant persistence. When people are gripped by any of these processes, they cease to act in self-determined ways and instead act sporadically or fearfully. Being able to align daily activities with one's purpose is an antidote. But there can be a large difference between discerning and pursuing a purpose. In this section we provide suggestions for helping clients engage with their purpose through planning, goal setting, progress monitoring, and flexible responding to obstacles.

1. *Signs of Progress.* One's purpose can sometimes be frustratingly abstract. "Make the world a better place." "Be a good parent." "Heal suffering." There are a million ways to try to do these things. Clients often need help breaking the large task of pursuing their purpose into small markers of progress. A big part of this is helping clients accept that a purpose is not easily accomplished, and that, at least in some ways, a purpose might be best if it cannot be accomplished at all. That is, purpose is best defined as a central, self-organizing life aim that provides direction rather than a terminal end point to be completed. For instance, the desire to be a loving father (life journey) rather than being dedicated to spending at least one day each weekend with his daughter and helping her get to college (tangible targeted outcomes). Rather than having clients focus on how they will check their purpose off their list, we want to encourage them to see their purpose as an ever-unfolding way of expressing their values and their selves in the world around them. So, encourage your client to work backward. Whatever his/her purpose is, what are some things that could be accomplished over the next 5 years that would show movement toward purpose? Within that 5 year span, what are some specific milestones that can be identified? What are 3-5 goals that add up to the first milestone? What activities need to be done in order to accomplish the first of these goals? How can these activities be implemented this month? This week? Today?

2. *Rerouting.* At the heart of ACT is psychological flexibility, which is the ability to adjust one's behavior and thinking to best pursue valued goals based on an authentic understanding of the moment (Kashdan & Rottenberg, 2010). Flexibility is at the heart of successful, sustained pursuit of purpose. Define purpose as a journey rather than an outcome to accomplish. This sets the stage for clients to view their purpose as being attainable by an infinite number of paths. In this intervention, this theme is reinforced by using metaphors. We like the metaphor of a GPS unit that keeps the destination in mind but is able to update a new course depending on wrong turns, road closures, or side trips. A key skill for clients to learn is to be mindful of how their behavior is

reflecting their purpose. This awareness can help them identify when they have encountered an obstacle to their pursuit of purpose and help them reroute. You can help your clients by using thought experiments about helpful responses to obstacles. The ACT techniques directed at defusion are critical here. There are many roads to one's purpose, and although it may be tempting to judge obstacles on one of them as being disastrous, it is just one obstruction on one road.

In Mandy's case, once she had identified a purpose for her career, it became clear that there was a conflict with another purpose. Mandy could not both attend a traditional law school and be there for her daughters during the week. Rather than giving up and viewing her purpose as unobtainable (and herself as worthless), Mandy found another road. She registered for weekend classes through a nontraditional law school to gain competencies and qualifications to work effectively in her chosen area of land preservation easements. In making this decision, she needed to be creative and relinquish superficial needs for prestige (in the eyes of others). It was a longer road to her career purpose, but she found a way to encounter both life aims along the path she chose.

Additional Collusion between ACT and Meaning and Purpose in Life

Mandy's case helped us discuss suggestions for ways in which the pathological processes identified in ACT could be addressed in ways rooted in meaning in life. These processes are not the only ways in which ACT and meaning in life can be brought together. Two other areas for collusion are mindfulness and suicide.

Mindfulness

Whereas ACT has brought a great deal of attention to mindfulness, meaning in life research and practice has been mostly silent. Maintaining an accepting attitude as each moment unfolds in the present would seem to set the stage for meaning making. One isolated research study has found that a 6-week-long interpersonal mindfulness training program reduced people's tendencies to chronically search for meaning in life among participants. This is an interesting finding because people who are chronically searching for meaning typically report less well-being (Steger, Kashdan et al., 2008). However, with so little research, we explore the theoretical links among mindfulness, ACT, and meaning in life.

Mindfulness has been described as a nonjudgmental way of paying attention to the internal and external qualities of our experiences. Life is what we pay attention to. Therefore, this refinement of attention may give people a key way to live a better life. Indeed, mindfulness may directly contribute to well-being and happiness by adding clarity and vividness to experience (Brown & Ryan, 2003). Yet, despite a history rooted in Eastern meditative practices and new attempts to integrate mindfulness into clinical interventions (Baer, 2003), mindfulness hasn't really caught on as a stand-alone therapeutic tool. In this way, mindfulness is the psychological equivalent of eating more kale: everyone knows it's good for you, but few people really commit to it.

ACT strives to make mindfulness more accessible to clients by breaking it down into distinct processes that can be targeted individually, none of which are implicitly linked to the task of meditation: contact with the present moment, acceptance, defusion, and self-as-context. Mindfulness is not only a route to gaining psychological flexibility but to building existential strength from the wider range of possibilities the self can inhabit, once its content is shed and a broader context is adopted. Redefining one's self has implications for wrestling with life's existential dilemmas, as "one answer to the existential dilemma of death is to transcend one's mortal self" (Steger & Shin, 2010, p. 98).

What then, does meaning in life research have to offer ACT, via the concept of mindfulness? Both perspectives value how mindfulness helps us to understand the reality of the self and foster a more universal identity, apart from the stories and thoughts we narrowly use to define our lives. ACT's clearly stated desirable outcome is to bring behaviors in accordance with values, and mindfulness is embedded in the model as a means to reach that goal. Mindfulness is a tool to live well, not a replacement for living. Mindfulness provides the link for clients to bring their behaviors and activities into accord with their defining values, by paying attention to whether what one is doing is aligned with core, central values.

Of course, aligning action with values and purpose is a central aim of meaning in life theory and practice as well, so those focusing on meaning in life should consider incorporating ACT's approach to mindfulness. At the same time, meaning in life theory makes some place for mindfulness in its emphasis on self-transcendence (Reker, 2000). Although most meaning in life theorists are agnostic about what kinds of meanings are "best," several have argued that as people mature, their meaning in life becomes increasingly directed at a greater good that transcends their momentary, individualistic desires. This notion of self-transcendence is often a descriptor used of people experiencing a mindful mindset (Brown, Ryan, & Creswell, 2007).

But again, we see a divergence in what ACT has often focused on— freeing people from paralyzing conceptualizations of the past and future—and what meaning in life has focused on—freeing people from being engrossed by the fidgety distractions of daily life. We also see an apparent conflict. Whereas ACT encourages people to be open and non-judgmentally aware of their present experience, meaning in life seems to beg people to judge whether their activities in the present are aligned with and are helpful in achieving their purpose at some point in their future. Although ACT encourages people to assess how present actions align with values, those values do not necessarily invoke any particular future state. Meaning in life seems to have the potential to shift people's focus toward the future and the potential fulfillment of their purposes. ACT could provide the pursuit of meaning in life with a healthy dose of present centeredness, and perhaps meaning in life could help people connect their values with their overall aims in life.

The subtext we perceive running through ACT is that with training, people's tendency to automatically frame life in judgmental, avoidant, fearful, rigid language can be rendered less powerful. With mindfulness, people learn to let go of these language processes. You can still have these language processes, but they no longer dominate everyday existence. Within ACT, mindfulness has two aims: (a) loosen the hold of unhelpful language processes (through defusion, self-as-context work) and (b) put people in greater touch with the world of experience beyond mere words (through values clarification and behavioral commitment to these values).

We argue for the benefit of also altering language itself so that greater attention is given to the dimensions of meaning: (a) comprehension and (b) purpose in life. Rather than frantic avoidance, nervous rigidity, or, we would say, ceaseless pursuit of the secret key to the good life, the language and narrative of people's lives should be founded on cherished values, beliefs they have tested, a clear-eyed appraisal of their abilities and shortcomings, and ultimate aspirations for their one shot at existence. If meaning is woven into the language by which people meet the world, then mindfulness does not need to conflict with a desire to live in accordance with one's purpose—it is a way of filling one's present moments with gentle reassurances of what one comprehends in life and navigational nudges toward one's purpose.

A meaning in life approach offers ACT a way to conceptualize those "larger and larger patterns." Meaning in life research directly addresses how behaviors and values, as a holistic unit, bring one's life into harmony by serving a greater purpose. In conjunction with ACT's model, meaning in life offers the people we work with greater cohesion in mindfully instilling the moments of their lives with value and purpose.

Suicide, Meaning, and Early Applications of Acceptance and Commitment Therapy

What happens when people have so little meaning in their life that they can justify killing themselves? Suicide research suggests that people who feel that they are connected to others and personally effective have a stronger will to live (Joiner, 2005). These two dimensions map onto the comprehension and purpose and aspects of meaning in life. An important component of comprehension is the way in which we understand the world around us. Research consistently demonstrates that the most important elements in our environment are other people—that people create the context in which we live (Baumeister & Leary, 1995). Paying attention to the ways in which people comprehend their worlds automatically implicates their sense of belonging and connectedness, and research shows that people who invest in their relationships experience greater meaning in life (Steger, Kashdan, & Oishi, 2008). Our sense of effectiveness, the view that we are not burdens but rather contributors to life, is related to the purpose dimension of meaning in life. Purpose captures the sense that we are useful, functioning, important parts of the world, that we ourselves "have a point." Losing this sense of contribution and usefulness was among the earliest identified causes of suicidal behavior (Durkheim, 1897/1953). Developing an individual's sense of meaning in the context of a therapeutic relationship has promising applications for decreasing suicidal ideations and possibly preventing suicide.

Research indicates that suicide is associated with hopelessness, a negative perception of one's future (Beck, Rush, Shaw, & Emery, 1979), and a lack of meaning in life (e.g., Rothermund & Brandtstädter, 2003). Unfortunately, there are few empirical studies examining meaning-based interventions in suicidal populations. Research by Edwards and Holden (2001) suggests that life meaning acts as a buffer between coping style and suicidal manifestations, and the authors argue for the addition of meaning variables to improve the accuracy of the prediction of suicidality. Having reasons for living and/or leading a meaningful life is incompatible with suicide. This is an idea supported by research in which early retirees who expressed suicidal ideation were enrolled in a personal goals management program (Lapierre, Dubé, Bouffard, & Alain, 2007). Following the program, participants reported increased self-efficacy in reaching their goals and greater psychological well-being. Meaning in life is all about linking goals to a grander life purpose.

Conclusions

As we have argued throughout this chapter, the core processes of ACT—encouraging clients to think about what they really want in life, reflecting on avoidance and control strategies, and focusing on becoming aware of important personal values and making decisions based on those values—are not merely harmonious with, but perfectly suited to take advantage of the additional leverage provided by meaning in life. As a growing body of literature has shown, ACT can achieve medium to large clinical effects among people with depression (e.g., Bohlmeijer, Fledderus, Rokx, & Pieterse, 2011), and research is ever-emerging on its benefits for those with other psychological disorders. We suggest that by combining the applications of ACT with the encompassing perspective of meaning in life, more effective treatment strategies can be developed to help clients live the lives they want. By anchoring clients' personal values in their overall comprehension of their lives, and anchoring their willingness to be flexible in pursuit of valued life aims in their purposes, clients can be drawn toward positive, hopeful, futures of contributing to those around them.

References

Baer, R. A. (2003). Mindfulness training as a clinical intervention: A conceptual and empirical review. *Clinical Psychology: Science and Practice, 10*, 125–143.

Baumeister, R. F. (1991). *Meanings of life.* New York: Guilford Press.

Baumeister, R. F., & Leary, M. R. (1995). The need to belong: Desire for interpersonal attachments as a fundamental human motivation. *Psychological Bulletin, 117*, 497-529.

Beck, A. T., Rush, A. J., Shaw, B. F., & Emery, G. (1979). *Cognitive therapy of depression.* New York: Guilford Press.

Biswas-Diener, R., Kashdan, T. B, & Minhas, G. (2011). A dynamic approach to psychological strength development and intervention. *Journal of Positive Psychology, 6*, 106-118.

Bohlmeijer, E. T., Fledderus, M., Rokx, T. A. J. J., & Pieterse, M. E. (2011). Efficacy of an early intervention based on Acceptance and Commitment Therapy for adults with depressive symptomatology: Evaluation in a randomized controlled trial. *Behaviour Research and Therapy, 49*, 62-67.

Brown, K. W., & Ryan, R. M. (2003). The benefits of being present: Mindfulness and its role in psychological well-being. *Journal of Personality and Social Psychology, 84*, 822-848.

Brown, K. W., Ryan, R. M., & Creswell, J. D. (2007). Mindfulness: Theoretical foundations and evidence for its salutary effects. *Psychological Inquiry, 18*, 211-237.

Cohen, S. R., Mount, B. M., Tomas, J. J. N., & Mount, L. F. (1996). Existential well-being is an important determinant of quality of life. *Cancer, 77*, 576-586.

Davis, C. G., Nolen-Hoeksema, S., & Larson, J. (1998). Making sense of loss and growing from the experience: Two construals of meaning. *Journal of Personality and Social Psychology, 75*, 561-574.

DeNeve, K. M., & Cooper, H. (1998). The happy personality: A meta-analysis of 137 personality traits and subjective well-being. *Psychological Bulletin, 124*, 197-229.

Durkheim, E. (1897, 1953). *Suicide.* New York: Free Press.

Edwards, M. J., & Holden, R. R. (2001). Coping, meaning in life, and suicidal manifestations. *Examining Gender Differences, 57*, 1517-1534.

Elliot, A. J., & Thrash, T. M. (2002). Approach-avoidance motivation in personality: Approach and avoidance temperaments and goals. *Journal of Personality and Social Psychology, 82*, 804-818.

Frankl, V. E. (1963). *Man's search for meaning: An introduction to logotherapy.* New York: Washington Square Press.

Harlow, L., & Newcomb, M. (1990). Towards a general hierarchical model of meaning and satisfaction in life. *Multivariate Behavioral Research, 25,* 387-405.

Joiner, T. E. (2005). *Why people die by suicide.* Cambridge, MA: Harvard University Press.

Kashdan, T. B., & McKnight, P. E. (2009). Origins of purpose in life: Refining our understanding of a life well lived. *Psychological Topics, 18,* 303-316.

Kashdan, T. B., & Rottenberg, J. (2010). Psychological flexibility as a fundamental aspect of health. *Clinical Psychology Review, 30,* 865-878.

King, L. A., & Hicks, J. A. (2007). Whatever happened to "what might have been"? Regret, happiness, and maturity. *American Psychologist, 62,* 625-636.

King, L. A., & Hicks, J. A. (2009). Detecting and constructing meaning in life events. *Journal of Positive Psychology, 4*(5), 317-330.

King, L. A., & Napa, C. K. (1998). What makes a life good? *Journal of Personality and Social Psychology, 75,* 156–165.

Lapierre, S., Dubé, M., Bouffard, L., & Alain, M. (2007). Addressing suicidal ideations through the realization of meaningful personal goals. *Crisis, 28,* 16-25.

Lazarus, R. S. (2003). Does the positive psychology movement have legs? *Psychological Inquiry, 14,* 93-109.

Luoma, J. B., Hayes, S. C., & Walser, R. (2007). *Learning ACT: An Acceptance and Commitment Therapy skills-training manual for therapists.* Oakland, CA: New Harbinger Publications.

McKnight, P. E., & Kashdan, T. B. (2009). Purpose in life as a system that creates and sustains health and well-being: An integrative, testable theory. *Review of General Psychology, 13,* 242-251.

Park, N., Park, M., & Peterson, C. (2010). When is the search for meaning related to life satisfaction? *Applied Psychology: Health and Well-Being, 2,* 1-13.

Read, S., Westerhof, G. J., & Dittmann-Kohli, F. (2005). Challenges to meaning in life: A comparison in four different age groups in Germany. *International Journal of Aging and Human Development, 61,* 85-104.

Reker, G. T. (2000). Theoretical perspective, dimensions, and measurement of existential meaning. In G. T. Reker & K. Chamberlain (Eds.), *Exploring existential meaning: Optimizing human development across the life span* (pp. 39-58). Thousand Oaks, CA: Sage Publications.

Rothermund, K., & Brandtstädter, J. (2003). Depression in later life: Cross-sequential patterns and possible determinants. *Psychology and Aging, 18,* 80-90.

Ryan, R. M., & Deci, E. L. (2001). On happiness and human potentials: A review of research on hedonic and eudaimonic well-being. *Annual Review Psychology, 52,* 141-166.

Ryff, C. D. (1989). Happiness is everything, or is it? Explorations on the meaning of psychological well-being. *Journal of Personality and Social Psychology, 57,* 1069-1081.

Schwartz, S. J., Kurtines, W. M., & Montgomery, M. J. (2005). A comparison of two approaches for facilitating identity exploration processes in emerging adults: An exploratory study. *Journal of Adolescent Research, 20,* 309-345.

Ryff, C. D., & Singer, B. (1998). The contours of positive human health. *Psychological Inquiry, 9,* 1-28.

Shin, J. Y., & Steger, M. F. (in press). Promoting meaning and purpose in life. In A. Parks (Ed.), *Positive psychology interventions.* Chicago, IL: Wiley.

Steger, M. F. (2009). Meaning in life. In S. J. Lopez (Ed.)., *Oxford handbook of positive psychology* (2nd ed.). (pp. 679-687). Oxford, UK: Oxford University Press.

Steger, M. F. (2012). Experiencing meaning in life: Optimal functioning at the nexus of spirituality, psychopathology, and well-being. In P. T. P. Wong & P. S. Fry (Eds.), *The human quest for meaning* (2nd ed). New York: Routledge.

Steger, M. F., Frazier, P., Oishi, S., & Kaler, M. (2006). The Meaning in Life questionnaire: Assessing the presence of and search for meaning in life. *Journal of Counseling Psychology, 53,* 80-93.

Steger, M. F.; Kashdan, T.B.; & Oishi, S. (2008). Being good by doing good: Daily eudaimonic activity and well-being. *Journal of Research in Personality, 42,* 22-42.

Steger, M. F., Kashdan, T. B., Sullivan, B. A., & Lorentz, D. (2008). Understanding the search for meaning in life: Personality, cognitive style, and the dynamic between seeking and experiencing meaning. *Journal of Personality, 76,* 199-228.

Steger, M. F., Oishi, S., & Kesibir, S. (2011). Is a life without meaning satisfying? The moderating role of the search for meaning in satisfaction with life judgments. *Journal of Positive Psychology, 6,* 173-180.

Steger, M. F., & Park, C. L. (2012). The creation of meaning following trauma: Meaning making and trajectories of distress and recovery. In T. Keane, E. Newman, & K. Fogler (Eds.), *Toward an integrated approach to trauma focused therapy: Placing evidence-based interventions in an expanded psychological context.* Washington, DC: APA.

Steger, M. F., & Shin, J. Y. (2010). The relevance of the Meaning in Life questionnaire to therapeutic practice: A look at the initial evidence. *International Forum on Logotherapy, 33,* 95-104.

Sullivan, D., Landau, M. J., & Rothschild, Z. (2010). An existential function of enemyship: Evidence that people attribute influence to personal and political enemies to compensate for threats to control. *Journal of Personality and Social Psychology, 98,* 434-449.

Wong, P. T. P. (2011). Positive psychology 2.0: Towards a balanced interactive model of the good life. *Canadian Psychology/Psychologie canadienne, 52,* 69-81.

Wong, P. T. P., & Fry, P. S. (1998). *The human quest for meaning: A handbook of psychological research and clinical applications.* Mahwah, NJ: Erlbaum.

CHAPTER 12

Nurturing Genius: Using Relational Frame Theory to Address a Foundational Aim of Psychology

Bryan Roche

National University of Ireland, Maynooth

Sarah Cassidy

Smithsfield Clinic, Co. Meath, Ireland

Ian Stewart

National University of Ireland, Galway

Authors' footnote: Visit RaiseYourIQ.com for online relational frame training designed to improve general intellectual ability.

In the current chapter we will outline our vision of how psychologists can, for the first time, embark on an empirically supported program of research and practice to literally "nurture genius" in children. We are not merely referring here to a program of early and intensive educational intervention to ensure that disadvantaged children reach their scholastic potential, or to the use of teaching methods that are more efficient and effective than those already in use. We are talking about new and radical developments in the experimental analysis of human behavior that may be opening the way for the intelligence quotients (IQs) to be raised by degrees previously thought impossible. That is, recent research in the field of relational frame theory (RFT; Hayes, Barnes-Holmes, & Roche, 2001) has suggested that by using what is called a relational frame training intervention, real and profound differences can be made to the intellectual abilities of children. Of course, this RFT intervention did not come out of thin air: it emerged from two decades of research into language and cognition and a concerted effort to understand what it is we mean by intelligence and how we might go about raising it. In effect, our mission has been consistent with one of the original aims of psychology as a profession and one which has recently been revisited by positive psychology, the mission to *nurture genius* (see Seligman & Csikszentmihalyi, 2000).

In this chapter, we will begin with a brief history of the behavior-analytic approach to intellectual development to show how the pathway to the recently developed RFT intervention was carved. We will then go on to consider the concept of intelligence itself, and how it is viewed from the broadly Skinnerian analytic perspective shared by RFT. Finally, we will consider the RFT approach itself and illustrate how it orients us toward the types of environmental histories and current interventions that maximize intellectual capacity.

Intelligence as the Behaviorist Views It

Our modern behavior analytic approach to human intellectual development focuses on the exploration of human potential rather than its limits. From our perspective, IQ tests simply measure the speed and accuracy with which an individual can perform tasks associated with educational attainment (e.g., add numbers, translate metaphors, remember information, deal with objects in 3-D space) in our culture today. Stated this way, the concept of intelligence cannot be used to quantify individuals, but it can be used to index their skill levels in various domains.

As behavior analysts, we concur with the positive psychology position that psychologists require a broadening of our view of intelligence that makes it amenable to intervention (Duckworth, Steen, & Seligman, 2005). Indeed, Sternberg (2003) described the traditional view of intelligence as a form of "negative psychology," one in which IQ tests measure intellectual *limits* rather than potential. According to this traditional view, the measurement of intelligence serves institutions but not individuals. Interestingly, Sternberg also emphasized that positive psychology as a movement sorely requires studies that show real and empirical effects of interventions designed to improve the potential and fulfillment of individuals if it is not to be seen as "soft" by serious scientists. Modern behavior-analytic interventions designed to measurably raise intellectual achievement constitute just such an instance of hard, persuasive science.

Seligman, Ernst, Gilham, Reivich, and Linkins (2009) view educational interventions as key to reaching the goals of the positive psychologist. Seligman and colleagues proposed that school interventions provide an excellent opportunity to reach entire populations and therefore are a powerful way to enhance the lives of whole communities. In particular, they suggest that any interventions that serve to enhance the frequency of positive emotions in one's life will serve to enhance learning. More specifically, positive emotions are associated with broadened cognitive focus (e.g., Basso, Schefft, Ris, & Dember, 1996) and enhanced creativity and insight in learning situations (e.g., Estrada, Isen, & Young, 1994; Isen, Daubman, & Nowiki, 1987). In short, it appears that "more well-being is synergistic with better learning" (Seligman et al., 2009, p. 294), which is the aim of traditional education. It is important to note, however, that while well-being is an end in itself, its potential impact on intellectual ability is also important because intellectual ability roughly predicts educational success (Deary, Strand, Smith, & Fernandes, 2007) and is associated with a range of several positive life outcomes (Schmidt & Hunter, 1998). One study (Frey & Detterman, 2004) found a high correlation of 0.82 between IQ and American Standard Aptitude Test (SAT) scores. The latter are widely used as selection criteria for college places and other training and employment opportunities. Another study (Deary et al., 2007) found a correlation of 0.81 between IQ and British GCSE scores (a measure of scholastic success administered to all high school graduates in the United Kingdom). Taken together, these findings strongly suggest that any enhancement of intellectual skills will broaden educational and employment opportunity for the individual.

The reader may be surprised at this point to hear us speak confidently about the possibility of raising the measurable intelligence quotients of individuals. After all, IQ is supposed by many to index an invariant trait. However, intellectual ability *does* vary across the life span, contrary to the best efforts of psychometricians to correct for these routine variations in the statistical computation of IQ scores. Indeed, it has been known for some time now that any intensive educational program can lead to IQ gains (Ceci, 1991). Moreover, new evidence provided in a recent article published in *Nature* shows that IQ can vary considerably in the teenage years as a function of environmental influences (Ramsden et al., 2011). The specific challenge for the current research, then, is not just to raise IQ but to improve intellectual skills by factors sufficient to raise full-scale IQ scores into new qualitative ranges (e.g., from subnormal to normal) or by more than a standard deviation (typically around 15 points). Before examining how RFT can help us reach this goal, we should first consider some previous attempts to raise intelligence.

Previous Attempts to Raise IQ

There have been numerous claims made in the literature and by online software companies about various interventions that supposedly raise intelligence levels. Most of these are of dubious merit (e.g., the "Mozart effect"; Rauscher, Shaw, & Ky, 1993; but see Chabris, 1999; Lorant-Royer, Spiess, Goncalvez, & Lieury, 2008; McKelvie & Low, 2002; Newman, Rosenbach, Burns, Latimer, Matocha & Vogt, 1995; Steele, Bass, & Crook, 1999). However, some respectable studies have shown that intellectual stimulation in the form of "cognitive training" can help to slow down cognitive decline in the elderly and among those with dementia and Alzheimer's disease (Belleville, Gilbert, Fontaine, Gagnon, Menard, & Gauthier, 2006; de la Fuente-Fernandez, 2006; Spector et al., 2003; Willis et al., 2006; Wilson et al., 2002). Nevertheless, while neurogenesis (the stimulation of nerve brain growth) is a well-established phenomenon, there is no known link between engagement in cognitive exercises and improvements in full scale IQ (i.e., IQ as assessed by a full standardized IQ test), although improvements in one aspect of intelligence known as fluid intelligence[1] have recently been reported (Jaeggi, Buschkuehl, Jonides, & Shah, 2011).

Much of the best support for brain training comes from studies examining its effects on stroke recovery and management of dementia in the elderly (e.g., Smith et al., 2009). The skills improved by such training are generic skills, like memory and attention, which had already been well established at an earlier time. For instance, the *Advanced Cognitive Training for Independent and Vital Elderly* (ACTIVE) clinical trial is the U.S.'s largest study of the effects of cognitive or "brain" training. Ball et al. (2002) found that this program could produce improvements in cognitive ability sufficient to stem age-related cognitive decline. That study also found that weekly regular training, with a range of cognitive tasks for five weeks, led to measurable improvements in memory, reasoning, and information-processing speed. However, the big challenge is to show that such interventions do more than simply improve people's skills at the very tasks at which they practice. What is needed is evidence that training at one task generalizes to real-life situations (e.g., involving problem-solving or remembering) or to other aspects of cognitive functioning.

A promising research program into the generalized effects of cognitive training has been led by Susanne Jäeggi, John Jonides, and colleagues at the University of Michigan. These researchers found that practice on a demanding memory task known as the dual n-back procedure[2] led to gains in fluid intelligence (the ability to reason and to solve new problems independently of previously acquired knowledge, and denoted as Gf; see Jäeggi, Buschkuehl, Jonides, & Perrig, 2008). Fluid intelligence (not full-scale intelligence) was measured using the Raven's Matrices test

---

1 In Cattell's original 1963 formulation, fluid intelligence was hypothesized to "reflect the physiological integrity of the organism useful for adapting to novel situations." (Lohman, 1989, p. 339).

---

2 In an n-back task, a subject is presented with a series of stimuli, such as letters or words or pictures, one by one across separate trials. The object of the task is to indicate when the stimulus on screen is the same one presented a given number of trials previously. For example, in a 3-back task, the subject has to respond whenever he or she sees a stimulus that was also on the screen three trials previously. More recently, the dual n-back task was developed. This involves the presentation of two n-back tasks simultaneously, usually using different types of stimuli, such as visual and auditory.

(Raven, Raven, & Court, 2003). The findings suggested that cognitive training may indeed show general effects that extend beyond the task type used during training. The results were particularly exciting because both fluid intelligence (Rohde & Thompson, 2007) and memory ability (Pickering, 2006) are associated with scholastic success.

Jäeggi and colleagues (Jäeggi, Studer-Luethi, Buschkuehl, Su, Jonides, & Perrig, 2010) later found that performance on the n-back task is more strongly correlated with two measures of Gf than with measures of working memory. In a second experiment reported in their 2010 paper, two groups of students were trained for four weeks with either a single or a dual n-back intervention. A control group received no training. The researchers reported that improvements in Gf were more marked than improvements in working memory following practice at either n-back test compared to the outcome for the control group (see also Jäeggi et al., 2011, for a similar study that also demonstrated maintenance of Gf increases across a three-month follow-up period).

It is important to understand that fluid intelligence is only one component of general intelligence and improvements in fluid intelligence should not be mistaken for improvements in full-scale IQ (see Flynn, 1987). More specifically, fluid intelligence is associated strongly with working memory and attentional skills such as speed of information processing. Full-scale IQ, however, is measured across a broader ranger of skills than this. Moreover, in full-scale IQ testing, scores on tasks that measure working memory and speed of processing information (e.g., on the Weschler Intelligence Scale for Children [WISC]) can be ignored in calculating overall IQ if the clinician or psychometrician believes the test taker has attention deficits. Nevertheless, memory and attentional skills are important in an educational context, and it is likely that n-back procedure training works by improving these skills, thus enhancing the individual's ability to attend to and remember key aspects of problems, solutions to which the individual is already capable of providing.

Behavioral psychologists have also made occasional efforts to improve intelligent behavior skills (and therefore IQ scores), usually with special needs populations. The late O. Ivar Lovaas (1987) reported IQ gains up to 30 points (roughly two standard deviations) following a three-year applied behavior analysis (ABA) intervention for autism. Nearly half of the autistic children in that study were not noticeably intellectually different from normally functioning children after the three-year program (Reed, Osbourne, & Corness, 2005). However, even within behavior analysis, concerns were raised that such rises in IQ were unlikely to be reliable (Connor, 1998; Gresham & MacMillan, 1997; Reed et al., 2005). For instance, Magiati and Howlin (2001) criticized the study on the grounds of methodological flaws regarding subject selection, treatment condition assignment, differing treatment periods across the experimental and control groups, and the already high-functioning intellectual ability of the treatment group. They also noted that different IQ tests were often used at baseline and at follow-up. Nevertheless, in an independent replication of the Lovaas study, Sallows and Graupner (2005) recorded similar significant IQ rises among autistic children. In a further study, Smith, Eikeseth, Klevstrand, and Lovaas (1997) used an ABA treatment program to improve expressive speech and adaptive behavior among severely mentally retarded children with autistic features. They also measured IQs at follow-up. While behavioral problems diminished in both groups, children in the treatment condition displayed a higher mean IQ at follow-up and evinced more expressive speech than those in the comparison group.

The foregoing studies strongly suggest that IQ can be affected by broad intensive behavioral interventions. It is important to remember, however, that these studies did not specifically target general intelligence in their interventions but employed IQ measures as part of a larger range of dependent measures. However, in what follows we will outline a modern behavioral research program designed specifically to understand how the skills associated with high intelligence might be established in educational interventions.

A Relational Frame Approach to Nurturing Genius

Relational frame theory is an account that explains the human ability to derive stimulus relations. For example, most verbally able children will be able to understand that if any object, let's call it A, is bigger than a second object B, and if B is in turn bigger than C, that C *must be* smaller than A. This last conclusion was derived by the child, and this particular learned skill is known as derived relational responding (or arbitrarily applicable relational responding). Different researchers (e.g., Sidman, 1971; Sidman & Tailby, 1982) have described this ability using different terminology (such as *stimulus equivalence*), but RFT has identified three main features of derived relational responding, which it describes as *mutual entailment, combinatorial entailment*, and the *transformation of function* (Hayes, 1994).

Mutual entailment. Arbitrarily applicable relations are always bidirectional. If any stimulus (A) is related to (e.g., bigger than, before, etc.) another one (B), then a second relation between the two stimuli (i.e., from B to A) is automatically entailed. The type of relation entailed depends on the nature of the relation between the two stimuli. For instance, if A is opposite to B, then B is also opposite to A. In this case, the same relation as trained is entailed. However, if A is bigger than B, then B is smaller than A—a novel relation is entailed.

Combinatorial entailment. If a stimulus A is related to B, and B is related to C, then a relation between A and C is combinatorially entailed. Once again the nature of the combinatorially entailed relation depends on the nature of the trained relations. For example, if A is more than B and B is more than C, then A is more than C (i.e., the same relation as trained is derived). However, if A is opposite to B and B is opposite to C then a relation of coordination or sameness is combinatorially entailed between A and C (i.e., a relation different to that trained).

Transformation of function. If a stimulus A is related to another stimulus B, and a response function is established for A, then the functions of stimulus B will be transformed in accordance with the A-B relation (given appropriate contextual cues). For example, if A is in a combinatorially entailed relation with a stimulus C, and A elicits a fear response in context X, C will also elicit the same fear response in that context.

Perhaps the most important feature of RFT is its view that the ability to derive relations in accordance with relational frames is an acquired skill. In other words, RFT maintains that humans must learn the various ways in which stimuli can be related. This ability is most likely established during early development as the child navigates normal social interactions with caregivers. For example, suppose a mother wishes to teach a child to say the word "doll" when presented with a doll (doll first, word second). This would require multiple exemplars of the object-word relation, perhaps with the mother first holding up a doll, followed by speaking the word "doll" aloud and then asking the child to repeat the word.

Now suppose that the mother then reverses this relation across multiple other exemplars. Specifically, the mother first says the word "doll" and asks the child to point to the doll (word-object relation). Once this word-object relation has been reliably established the relation has become *bidirectional*. Importantly, however, the relation was not derived by the child; it was directly established in both directions *by the mother*. Across a sufficient number of such directly trained bidirectional relations established across numerous objects and words, a pattern of spontaneous bidirectional relational responding will eventually emerge for new objects and words (see Hayes, Fox, Gifford et al., 2001, pp. 26-27). For example, the mother might teach the child a novel object-name relation by pointing to a novel object (e.g., a cat), producing its name and prompting the child to repeat that name (e.g., "This is a cat. Can you say *cat?*"). This trains a relation from "object" to "name." If the mother subsequently asks "Where is the cat?" the child might spontaneously point out the animal, thus showing the derived or untrained "name-object" (i.e., reverse) relation. Derivation might also happen in the opposite direction so that being given a novel name (e.g., "chocolate") and taught to pick the correct object (e.g., a chocolate bar) results in the untrained response that given the object (e.g., seeing a similar chocolate bar on TV) a particular name is the correct one (e.g., the child says "chocolate" without prompting).

Behavioral research has long suggested that the ability to derive relations between stimuli in this way is likely a very important skill for language learning (e.g., Barnes, McCullagh, & Keenan, 1990; Devany, Hayes, & Nelson, 1986). This is because language is replete with word-sound associations that are entirely arbitrary (i.e., a child cannot figure out what the sound "dog" refers to in print because it is an arbitrary sound and its relation to the printed letters D-O-G must be taught). Where the ability to derive stimulus relations is very fluent, we should expect to see excellent vocabulary acquisition and rapid and improved ability to remember word meanings, because the ability to derive (and, if necessary, "re-derive") relationships supports these repertoires.

Relational frame theory researchers maintain, for both theoretical and empirical reasons, that the ability to derive relations must be learned (i.e., it is not an innate ability). RFT explains how this emergence occurs and attempts to identify the most important types of relations (e.g., more, less, before, after, opposite, different), or relational frames, involved in intellectual, behavioral, and emotional development. It may sound radical, but RFT researchers attempt to understand the full array of cognitive skills (e.g., language, deductive reasoning, problem solving) in terms of a relatively small range of relational frames. From an RFT perspective, much of what is measured in standard IQ tests can be understood in terms of relational frames. It is both a conceptual and empirical matter to work out precisely which relations or combinations of relations are involved in which types of intellectual skills. Nevertheless, the idea that we may have already identified a basic behavioral unit (i.e., relational responding) of intelligence is exciting to say the least. The most obvious implication of this is that by enhancing those fundamental relational framing skills, we may be able to move the entire intellectual skills repertoire in one single intervention.

Importantly, the ability to derive relations between new words and objects will remain under *contextual control* so that the relevant relationship between any two items is always specified by a cue, such as the word "Same." That is, in speech we will always use (in one way or another) one of the relational frame labels to specify for a child which relation we are talking about when we refer to two objects, or a word-object relation (e.g., "show me something *bigger than* your doll").

Through ongoing exposure to and interactions with the socioverbal community, relational framing becomes increasingly fluent, and the relations involved become more and more abstracted so that the ability to frame events relationally becomes increasingly unhinged from any particular words and objects. It might be helpful for the reader to think of mathematical relationships (e.g., $3 + 5$ is the same as 8) as examples of fully abstracted relations that are arbitrarily applicable to any set of items (e.g., sheep, apples, widgets). In simple terms, the child has now learned the very rules of derived relational responding and can even state them. It is at this point that we can ask a child, for example, to imagine x number of items that is more than y number of items. The relations and the rules of derived relational responding are not violated by the use of the algebraic terms x and y, but in this case there are no particular stimuli specified at all.

So fundamental is derived relational responding ability to a whole host of cognitive tasks that RFT theorists have suggested that it may underlie intelligence itself (see Barnes-Holmes, Barnes-Holmes, & Roche, 2001; Barnes-Holmes, Barnes-Holmes, Roche et al., 2001; Cassidy, Roche, & O'Hora, 2010). Several published studies have supported this idea. For instance, one study found that relational responding ability predicts performance on several IQ measures. Specifically, O'Hora, Pelaez, and Barnes-Holmes (2005) assessed people's ability to show complex rule following conceptualized in terms of patterns of derived coordinate (sameness) combined with temporal (before/after) relational responding. They found that 31 participants who successfully completed the derived relational protocol involved performed significantly better on the *Vocabulary* and *Arithmetic* subtests of the WAIS-III than the 44 subjects who had failed the task. (Task completion did not predict differences in the *Digit-symbol coding* subtest score). Moreover, correlations were observed between performance in *before/after responding* and the Vocabulary ($r = .342$, $p = .002$) and Arithmetic ($r = .231$, $p = .003$) subtests of the WAIS-III. In a follow-up study, O'Hora, Pelaez, Barnes-Holmes, Rae et al. (2008) found further correlations between performance in *before/after* relational ability and Full Scale ($r = 0.437$, $p < .0005$), Verbal ($r = 0.302$, $p = .006$), and Performance ($r = 0.419$, $p < .0005$) IQ. The strongest correlations were observed for the Verbal Comprehension ($r = .40$) and Perceptual Organization ($r = .41$) factors of the WAIS-III IQ test. In that study, significant moderate correlations were also observed between relational responding and scores on the Verbal Comprehension ($r = 0.403$, $p < .0005$) and Perceptual Organization indices ($r = 0.409$, $p < .0005$). Correlations with Working Memory ($r = 0.052$) or Processing Speed indices ($r = 0.203$) were not significant.

O'Toole and Barnes-Holmes (2009) employed a complex relational task known as the Implicit Relational Assessment Procedure (IRAP; Barnes-Holmes, Hayden, Barnes-Holmes, & Stewart, 2008) to test before/after and same/different relational responding fluency. They found that fluency at this task correlated with IQ as measured by the Kaufman Brief Intelligence Test (Kaufman, 1990). Specifically, correlations of $r = .38$ and $r = .35$ were found for before/after and same/different responding fluencies, respectively. Finally Gore, Barnes-Holmes, and Murphy (2010) found significant correlations between performance on a test for deictic relations (i.e., perspective-taking relations involving "I" and "You," and "Here" and "There" relations) and Full Scale (r ≐ .43), Verbal (r = .45) and Performance IQ (r = .45; p. 12) as measured by the Wechsler Abbreviated Scale of Intelligence (WASI; Weschler, 1999).

Some Relational Frames and Their Role in Intelligent Behavior

In this section, we illustrate a very basic RFT account of intelligence by outlining the roles of specific and common forms of derived relational responding. However, we will deal here with only the most common relations. More complex relations, such as deictic relations and relations among relations, also play an important role in higher level cognitive functioning (see Cassidy et al., 2010).

Frames of Coordination. A frame of coordination is essentially a relation of sameness. We think of this as the simplest relational frame, largely because it appears to emerge first in the behavioral repertoire and also because all of the relations derived in accordance with this frame are of the same kind as those trained. For example, if A is the same as B, and B is the same as C, this implies a relation between C and A that is also one of sameness. Laboratory findings also indicate that the derivation of *Same* relations requires less response time than deriving other relations (see O'Hora, Roche, Barnes-Holmes, & Smeets, 2002; Steele & Hayes, 1991). This confirms for us that understanding Sameness is probably the most fundamental and earliest type of relational ability to emerge. This is not surprising because words are usually taught to stand for (i.e., are the same as) things, or for other words, when they are first encountered by children. For example, a parent will likely teach a child that "this" (pointing to a doll) *is* a "doll," before they teach a child that "this" (pointing to an apple) is something *different to* a doll. Frames of coordination, therefore, are absolutely foundational in early language training.

A well-honed ability to respond to and derive frames of coordination is crucial for the acquisition of a broad and well-organized vocabulary. Most IQ tests examine vocabulary in some form and to some extent or other. Vocabulary is a fundamental and basic prerequisite to normal language development, the extent of which is both predicted by and predicts general intelligence.

Frames of Opposition. One important gauge of a child's understanding of opposition relations is that he or she can choose not just stimuli that are opposite to a range of objects or words but also that are the same as or in other relations with those stimuli. More specifically, we cannot conclude with confidence that a child understands what "opposite" means, just because he or she always chooses the opposite of any stimulus presented (e.g., choosing the word "hot" from an array of words when we present the word "cold"). This is because the child may make the same choices regardless of what instructions we provide to identify the relation of interest. For example, he or she may also choose the opposite stimulus to our sample stimulus when instructed to choose one that is the *same as* the sample. In order to fully establish that the word "opposite" has some properties as a cue for a specific type of relational responding, we need to contrast the effects of its use with those of other relational terms, such as "same." IQ tests often ensure that such contrasting control is exerted by same and opposite cues or words, even within the same test item. For example, the Heim AH4 intelligence test (Heim, Watts, & Simmonds, 1968/1975) presents the following task: "Near means the opposite of 1) close, 2) road, 3) speed, 4) far, 5) distance." A person for whom the words "same" and "opposite" provide little control over responding (i.e., in simple terms, he or she does not understand them well) will likely be drawn to respond to this test item by always producing a default coordination response (i.e., ignoring the relational cue "opposite"). In this case he or she may respond to *close* as the opposite of *near*. However, if he or she can reliably respond to opposite in preference to same relations in the presence of the 'opposite' cue and can do so across a variety of exemplars, this strongly suggests that both coordination and opposition responding repertoires are likely well established. This is indicative of a well-formed vocabulary because not only are the words meaningful, they are specifically meaningful *in relation to one another.*

Frames of Comparison. These relations are defined by Cassidy et al. (2010, p. 44) as being required when responding "to a novel stimulus in terms of its directional displacement from a known stimulus (e.g., more than/less than, half of, above, below)." Such frames appear to be particularly relevant to the types of mathematical skills assessed in standard IQ tests. The *Arithmetic* subtest of the WISC-IIIUK for example, poses several questions on subtraction that require the application of relational comparisons between numbers (e.g., which is bigger than which). Consider the numbers 1-5, for instance. For a child to be able to answer any question regarding the subtraction of any number in the range 1-5 from any other number in this range requires that the sequence of numbers from one to five be very well established and elaborated across countless exemplars in the past. The task of truly counting from one to five in the relational sense (as opposed to "parroting" the number sequence, as very young children and many animals can do) is more complex than the reader may have previously considered. Figure 1 provides just a few examples of the numerous relations of comparison that obtain between the numbers 1, 2, 3, 4, and 5. There are 15 possible two-digit subtraction problems that can be generated using just five digits that lead to nonnegative solutions (there are many more such problems if we are to include negative solutions). If a child cannot answer at least these positive solution questions correctly, we can fairly say that the relational frames of comparison have not yet been fully established and elaborated for this child across this number range.

Clearly, it is inefficient to teach the interrelations between the five numbers by rote. It is far more efficient to teach the framing skill itself so that the same relational responses can be applied to the numbers 1-5 and the numbers 100-105, 1,000-1,005, 1,000,000-1,000,005, and so on. This can be achieved using multiple exemplar training (MET) using a wide variety of objects (e.g., coins, cups, playing cards, etc.) as we teach children to subtract using this number range. It might escape some caregivers, but the broader the range of stimulus objects used, the more effective will be the generalization of the framing responses established. It may even be necessary to train the generalization of the subtracting responses to the numbers 100-105 and to 1,000-1,005 and so on until it eventually generalizes to any sequence with the same relational characteristics.

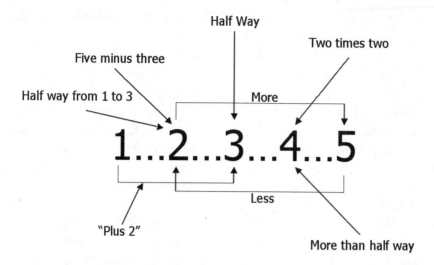

Figure 1: Examples of just some of the derived relational frames of comparison entailed by the number sequence 1-5, when each number in the range is sequentially trained as being directionally displaced by one unit from the previous number.

Of course, children do learn arithmetic tables by rote, and this is of use in establishing a basic ability to deal with numbers in everyday life. However, a truly relational response could be arrived at using generalized relational responding alone, as employed by, for example, highly trained mathematicians when dealing with numbers in ranges not dealt with in school-based rote learning or in unusual tasks (e.g., working out square or cubed roots of large numbers or mentally counting through the prime numbers ad infinitum).

While the use of multiple exemplar training no doubt lays the ground work for relational abilities in the first instance with small numbers, the skill is arbitrarily applicable (though applied only in appropriate contexts) to any set of numbers at higher ranges (e.g., we can imagine the directional displacement of 100 and 200 in the same way once a sufficiently large number of interrelations amongst numbers in the 1-10 range have been established).[3]

Once relational skills involving numbers have become sufficiently generalized across stimulus sets, it should even be possible for the child to identify a question (i.e., the context of division) from its answer (i.e., "the numbers are 36 and 4 and the answer is 9. What is the question?"). This latter skill is a high-order skill related to executive function that we associate with high-level problem solving and is referred to as *pragmatic verbal analysis*. An outline of pragmatic verbal analysis is beyond the scope of this paper, but the reader is referred to Hayes, Gifford, Townsend, and Barnes-Holmes (2001).

More complex mathematical problems may involve control by multiple contextual cues simultaneously or in sequence. For instance, a child may be asked how many of 6 sweets he will have finally when he gives half away and then is subsequently given three times more than what he had left. Such a problem involves the application of division and multiplication in sequence and represents a considerable challenge even to many normally functioning adults.

Temporal Relational Frames. Responding to an event in terms of its temporal displacement from other events represents an example of responding in accordance with temporal relations, such as before/after. We normally understand these relations as types of comparison relations, but this is a matter of conceptual convenience rather than an empirical matter. Several common IQ subtests measure the fluency of before/after responding. For example, in the WISC, the *Information* subtest examines the before/after relations that obtain between the months of the year and days of the week (e.g., "Which month comes next after April?"). When one looks across subtests and considers test items carefully, it is apparent that before/after responding is also being examined in other contexts. For instance, a naturalistic test for before/after relational responding can be found in the *Picture Arrangement* subtest of the WISC. In the third edition (UK) of this test, a child is asked to

---

3   The reader should note that establishing fluency from 1-10 is required for full numerical competence because in the modern Western world we use a numerical system to the base of 10. If we decided to switch to a number base system of 5, we would need only to establish full relational fluency with the numbers 1-5 to allow counting to infinity and the effective dealing with mathematical problems in precisely the same way as we do presently.

arrange sequentially a number of cards with images on them so that they tell a meaningful story. The idea is that all of the images (e.g., money, a wallet, a vending machine, a chocolate bar) are effectively randomly presented from the child's point of view, and unless the child has previously been shown how to perform this task with that precise stimulus set, he or she is likely to be producing relational frames of before and after using this stimulus set for the first time (i.e., the frame is arbitrarily applicable).

Hierarchical Relational Frames. Hierarchical relational responding might be roughly thought of as responding to things in terms of higher or lower order relationships to each other. The most common example might be assigning class membership and categorization. So for example, a rose is a type of flower. In this case, a rose is responded to in terms of its lower order relationship to flowers. The mutually entailed relation in this case is not the same as that established; in this example, a flower is not a type of rose. This type of relational responding has been studied extensively by Piagetian researchers, who refer to its unfolding in the developmental process as the emergence of the *operation of classifications.* Interestingly, the latter pattern typically emerges relatively late in child development (between 7 and 8 years), indicating the relative complexity of hierarchy, how many relational repertoires involving more basic relations must likely be first established, and how much training it takes to become reasonably fluent in it.

Hierarchical relations are crucial to understanding the organization of language itself (classes of words), and the fully abstracted form is commonplace in mathematics (e.g., x is a member of the set of y). They are also applied in describing attributes of objects and are therefore crucial in controlling complex transformations of functions. For example, the WISC asks the question, "What is the main material used to make glass?" Of course to answer this correctly the child will have to respond to glass as made of sand and not to sand as made of glass. More interestingly, however, once the relation is applied, the psychological response to glass is altered such that it now evokes some of the same responses normally produced by sand. A child may, for example, now continue to be reminded of sand or beaches whenever she sees glass, or she may imagine that the inside of a pane of glass may have a gritty texture, and so on. Later on she will learn that the sand itself is transformed utterly in the glass-making process, and so this will in turn involve the application of further frames of hierarchy (among others). For instance, sand is made of stone, which melts at high temperatures, and so forth. Each application of another frame of hierarchy, involving further specific attributes (i.e., response functions specified in that context), such as transparency, makes the psychological functions produced by glass and sand more numerous and richly interacting, and requires further and further degrees of refined contextual control so that the appropriate features of either stimulus are responded to in the appropriate context (for example, glass is responded to as transparent, but sand and stone are not).

Summary

Clearly, there are many more types of relational frames that we might analyze in the current chapter (e.g., deictic or "perspective" relations, analogical relations, etc.). However, the foregoing was intended only to illustrate the types of interpretive analyses possible given the nomenclature and concepts developed by RFT. They are all provisional and open to correction by empirical analysis. The important point to take away, however, is that by conceiving intellectual ability as measured by IQ tests and other forms of educational assessment as relational framing ability, at least to some extent, the possibility of improving this ability immediately presents itself, at least if relational skills can themselves be taught and enhanced.

Improving Relational Skills

The strategy of teaching relational skills by training multiple examples of the very skill we are trying to establish is known as *multiple exemplar training* (MET). Relational frame multiple exemplar training involving feedback and response correction (e.g., showing the child the correct answer to relational questions) continues indefinitely across a potentially infinite range of stimuli until regular testing without prompts or feedback demonstrates that the child can provide the correct response to the same problem but with novel stimuli on every occasion. For example, we might teach a child that given any statement of the form A is opposite to B, which is opposite to C (where A, B, and C are randomly selected stimuli that bear no consistent physical relationship to each other across statements), it follows that A is the same as C, C is the same as A, B is opposite to A, and C is opposite to B. Problems of this kind cannot be solved by looking at the forms of the stimuli because these are randomly selected and unrelated to each other. Rather, only the relations between the stimuli presented in the question can be used as a basis for the answer. The task is abstract and entirely relational (as in algebra). Of course, in some cases, one may need to establish the basic skill set using nonarbitrarily selected stimuli. For instance, we might begin to teach the frame of comparison by showing a child that if a large ball A is larger than a small ball B, then B must be smaller than A. In this case, however, exemplars will still be required to generalize this form of nonarbitrary relational responding to sets of stimuli where the non-arbitrary relationships no longer provide a guide to correct responding (e.g., coins of the same size but different in value; see Vitale, Barnes-Holmes, Barnes-Holmes, & Campbell, 2008).

We already have a healthy literature base illustrating that MET interventions can be successfully employed to enhance repertoires of derived relational responding. For example, Barnes-Holmes, Barnes-Holmes, and Roche (2001) employed exemplar training to produce generalization of a relational skill in accordance with mutual entailment for a sample of young children. More specifically, children were trained across four experiments (using various methods including MET) to reverse action-object relations (i.e., see object, perform an action). This effect was replicated by Barnes-Holmes, Barnes-Holmes, Roche, and Smeets (2001) and extended by Gomez, Lopez, Martin, Barnes-Holmes, and Barnes-Holmes (2007). A similar finding was reported by Luciano, Becerra and Valverde (2007).

Generalization of more complex derived relational responding involving Same and Opposite has also been demonstrated empirically with child populations using a MET procedure. In one study (Barnes-Holmes, Barnes-Holmes, & Smeets, 2004) children were trained to relate stimuli in accordance with relations of opposition and then to derive novel *same* and *opposite* relations across several sets involving three stimuli rather than just two. Specifically, the derived relational feature tested for was what we defined earlier as combinatorial entailment. That is, if any two stimuli are opposite to a third, they must be the same as each other. This is a concept that might not be properly established even in many fully developed adults. Yet in the Barnes-Holmes et al., (2004) study, cited above, children were trained to near perfect levels of fluency in deriving such combinatorially derived relations with novel stimuli across multiple test trials.

In another study, relational frame repertoires of *More than* and *Less than* relational responding were established for a group of young children, who previously were unable to demonstrate such relational response repertoires (Barnes-Holmes, Barnes-Holmes, Smeets, Strand, & Friman, 2004; see also Berens & Hayes, 2007, and Vitale et al., 2008, for further demonstrations of the use of MET to establish generalized relational frames of comparison).

The foregoing clearly illustrates that the use of MET to establish improved fluency in relational framing skills is a relatively successful enterprise. The central question here, however, is whether such improvements are accompanied by rises in general or specific intellectual abilities. This was the focus of one recent study that examined the effect of a large relational frame training battery across two experiments, with both normally developing and educationally challenged children. In Experiment 1 of a study by Cassidy, Roche, and Hayes (2011), four children were exposed to multiple exemplar training in stimulus equivalence (effectively a simple frame of coordination) and later a battery of MET for *Same, Opposite,* and *More than/Less than* relational responding across several regular sessions and across several months. Computer software administered blocks of training for stimulus equivalence and later for the four relations. Tests, without feedback, for equivalence and relational frames using novel stimuli required a 100% correct level of responding in order to be completed successfully. If an error was made on a test block, training was readministered using the stimulus set previously employed on the failed test. In effect, children were being trained to form relations (using trial-by-trial feedback) with the very stimuli that had appeared in a test in which they had failed to derive relations without feedback. Following retraining, further training was administered with a further novel stimulus set, followed by a further test with another novel stimulus set. This training-testing-retraining-retesting cycle continued until the child could produce 100% correct derived relational responding on a test without feedback and with a novel stimulus set. Each of the five derived relational skills was established this way in sequence.

Baseline IQ scores were calculated using the Wechsler Intelligence Scale for Children (WISC-IIIUK), which was re-administered following both the stimulus equivalence (Time 2) and the relational frame (Time 3) training batteries. Administrations of the test were separated by at least three months to preclude the possibility of test-retest effects, which account for rises of less than one standard deviation. The four experimental participants were matched against a no-treatment control group. The treatment group showed significant improvements in full-scale IQ following stimulus equivalence training but an asymptotic rise in IQ following the relational frame training battery. Table 1 shows participants' Full Scale IQs at times 1, 2, and 3 as well as their composite Verbal and Performance IQs at these measurement points. The table shows that mean Full Scale, Verbal, and Performance IQ scores rose from baseline to postrelational frame training by unprecedented factors, well in excess of one standard deviation. This is particularly impressive when one considers that IQ tests are carefully designed to preclude such a possibility by chance or transient environmental circumstances alone.

Table 1

		Control			Experimental		
		Mean	SD	Range	Mean	SD	Range
Full Scale IQ	Baseline	106.50	3.32	104-111	105.50	10.66	96-119
	SE Training	107.25	4.79	101-111	110.25	5.74	105-118
	Relational Training	104.25	3.86	99-108	132.75	4.03	128-137
Verbal IQ	Baseline	108.25	4.86	101-111	109.25	8.88	101-120
	SE Training	107.50	6.66	98-113	107.75	9.03	100-120
	Relational Training	108.50	8.85	99-117	127.00	12.99	111-139
Performance IQ	Baseline	102.75	6.13	94-107	100.25	11.24	91-115
	SE Training	105.00	7.07	96-113	111.50	3.32	107-115
	Relational Training	98.75	8.58	88-109	132.75	2.99	130-137

Means, standard deviations, and IQ ranges for control and experimental participants at baseline, following stimulus equivalence (SE) and relational frame training in Experiment 1 of Cassidy et al. (2011).

In Experiment 2, a further eight children, this time with educational difficulties and below-normal IQs, were exposed to a slightly modified multiple exemplar-based relational frame training intervention. There was no comparison group employed, because by this stage in our research we felt that it was unethical to deny what appeared to be a viable treatment to children with learning deficits. Time and monetary resources also precluded a full multiple baseline design being employed, and so a simple A-B (baseline measurement of IQ followed by a relational training intervention) was used. In this study, full-scale IQ as measured by the WISC-IVUK, rose by at least one standard deviation for seven of the eight children. This change was also significant at the group level (see Table 2). To put these IQ rises in context, the relational frame training intervention succeeded in raising the IQs of almost all of the educationally challenged children to such an extent that seven of eight of them changed IQ band (e.g., from below average to average or above average).

More recently, all eight children were revisited for follow-up IQ testing, almost four years since the completion of the relational training intervention (see Table 2). In all cases IQ rises were maintained well across this very large follow-up period. Only scores on one of the four IQ domains (processing speed) decreased across the follow-up period. The other three IQ domain scores continued to rise (at the group level across this extended follow-up period). Full-scale IQ dropped slightly since the postintervention assessment (i.e., due to the drop in processing speed scores) but was still considerably higher than at baseline.

Interestingly, processing speed is a measure of the ability to focus on a visual task, work quickly, and follow through in its completion under strict time constraints. This measure is highly subject to the effects of transitory, as well as more sustained motivational and attentional problems. Indeed, full-scale IQ scores can be calculated without this index (and/or the working memory index), where the clinician feels that attentional problems may detract from a representative index of general cognitive ability in contexts in which the latter is of primary concern. Thus, what the follow-up data reported in Table 2 suggest is that in terms of cognitive ability, scores on core IQ domains continued to rise over time postintervention, but in those domains not targeted directly by the intervention, deterioration was observed. It may be of relevance that all of the children were currently out of the school setting for a one-year period to attain workplace experience and undergo personal development when follow-up testing took place. It may well be, therefore, that attentional skills were deteriorating during this period in the absence of the usual scholastic contingencies. Nevertheless, skills in those IQ domains representing pure relational ability continued to grow and develop across time since the intervention. This is not at all surprising from a relational frame theory perspective. We would fully expect a relational training intervention to enhance repertoires that would make learning more sensitive to instruction and experience on an ongoing basis. The effect of a relational frame training intervention, therefore, should be accumulative as well as immediate. The fact that the improved full-scale IQs reported in Experiment 2 of Cassidy et al. (2011) have maintained well across time strongly suggests that the relational training intervention successfully targeted skills sets that were of enduring importance in the ongoing intellectual and educational activities of the children.

Table 2

	Baseline			PostIntervention			Four-Year Follow-Up		
	Mean	SD	Range	Mean	SD	Range	Mean	SD	Range
Full Scale IQ	82.9	8.3	70-92	95.9	10.6	76-111	102.57	12.19	91-126
Verbal Comprehension	82.3	7.3	73-93	92.4	9.2	83-110	100.86	6.91	90-112
Perceptual Reasoning	82.1	10.3	65-96	94.5	6.7	84-106	103.14	16.12	83-123
Working Memory	94.9	16.6	59-116	97.5	12.3	77-116	88.14	14.78	65-103
Processing Speed	91.0	9.8	83-109	107.0	15.6	78-121	98.86	10.33	86-114

Means, standard deviations, and ranges in full-scale IQ in all four IQ domains at baseline and postintervention as reported in Experiment 2 of Cassidy et al. (2011). Previously unpublished four-year follow-up IQ scores in all four IQ domains are also provided in the rightmost columns of the table for the seven of the eight children that were available.

Given the considerable impact the relational training interventions had in the two experiments outlined above, it would appear that a relational frame approach to intellectual deficit treatment has the potential to not only help children and families in need but to change lives in a real and measurable way. Of course, the samples used in both experiments were small, and there were other methodological imperfections, such as the use of en masse training instead of a multiple baseline design or a blind randomized control trial technique. Nevertheless, the IQ data moved dramatically in the right direction, and there is little ambiguity in the findings.

Relational Training Exercises for Teachers, Parents, and Clinicians[4]

So far we have outlined a relational frame analysis of intelligence and suggested that intelligence may be considered to comprise a well-developed repertoire of relational skills. We have also shown that these skills can be enhanced and that improving relational skills may lead directly to improved intelligence levels. However, up to this point the methods for enhancing relational skills that we have considered have been entirely laboratory based and have involved computer-controlled task presentation. Of course, this use of such research methods is part and parcel of good scientific practice, but many of these laboratory techniques can be employed at home more casually using printed materials or simply by using spoken words. In this section, we will suggest some easily employed exercises that parents, teachers, and clinicians can use with any children, casually, in any context and for either short or extended periods of time. These exercises are suitable for children roughly in the 8-14 years age bracket. For each of the following exercises, nonarbitrarily related stimuli can be employed in the place of the types of arbitrary ones suggested here in the event that the child is having difficulty providing correct answers to the questions (e.g., due to developmental stage or age). Providing exemplars using nonarbitrary stimuli will serve as a good

---

4   For online relational frame training software visit RaiseYourIQ.com

foundation for improved fluency on the exercises as we have outlined them in Table 3. For instance, in the case of the relational frame of comparison, names for objects that are of actual different sizes to each other (e.g., penny, football, house) can be used in the place of the arbitrarily related stimuli (i.e., coins of different value) to illustrate the number of relations that can be derived from just a few statements, and the fact that relations other than those used in the statements may also be derived (e.g., A more than B, and B more than C entails C less than A).

It is essential that correct answers are met with praise and positive feedback, and that correct answers are provided for the child whenever there is an error. A child should be moved through these levels and relational frames at a pace that allows him or her to succeed and not so quickly that the effort becomes punishing. Practice these exercises often in casual conversation, in different contexts, and with various stimuli as the opportunity arises. You should provide as many such exercises as possible, moving from easier to more difficult questions (i.e., levels) as the child's fluency improves (across several weeks) and working roughly from the more basic relations to the more complex relations, such as in the order presented here (i.e., 1-6). Remember, you need to provide your own stimuli, such as colors, stimulus names, and words as suggested for each exercise, and to vary them across each and every delivery of the exercise so that the child is continuously being exposed to the same types of questions but with different stimuli used in each case.

There are many different variations on these exercises that the reader can make, and there are numerous other levels of complexity that can be invented ad hoc. There are even other relations that can be worked on, but the relational range presented in Table 3 is enough for most children to begin with. Please be aware that many children will find the higher levels of questioning very difficult, and many may be unable to reach 100% accuracy on the hierarchical and deictic relations exercises. However, if the exercises are worked through slowly and systematically, moving forward only when fluency has been reached at a given level of complexity and for a given relational frame, then the child will eventually finish the entire exercise set. This will likely take several months of regular practice.

In Table 3 we have included different ways of presenting the various questions within the exercises—sometimes as detailed questions regarding relationships between words and objects, and sometimes as true/false questions (known as relational evaluations in RFT). You should feel free to mix and match the styles and methods to suit yourself and the child.

Table 3. Sample Relational Training Exercises for Parents, Teachers, and Clinicians

1. Relational Frame of Coordination (Sameness)	2. Relational Frame of Comparison (More than /Less than)
Stimuli: Spoken words from different languages but with shared meaning.	Stimuli: Objects with various levels of arbitrary values (e.g., monetary, aesthetic, etc.).[5]
Level 1. "Manzana" is the Spanish word for apple. What is an apple in Spanish?	Level 1. If a dime is worth more than a nickel, is a nickel worth more or less than a dime?
Level 2. "Madra" is the Irish word for the French word "Chien." "Chien" is the French word for the English word "dog." What is a "dog" in Irish?	Level 2. If a dime is worth more than a nickel, and a nickel is worth more than a penny, is a dime worth more or less than a penny?
Level 3. "Coche" is the Spanish word for the English word "car." "Car" is the English word for the Swedish word "bil." "Bil" is the Swedish word for the Italian word "auto." What is an auto in Spanish?	Level 3. Imagine that I have four objects; A, B, C, and D. If A is larger than B, and B is larger than C, and C is larger than D, is D less than or more than A?

5   Note that in this particular example, coins of a larger size (e.g., a nickel) are worth less than coins of a smaller physical size (e.g., a dime), and so the monetary value of the stimuli is not ascertainable from the formal size of the coins (i.e., their nonarbitrary features). To create a potentially infinite variety of "coins" for use in these exercises, simply make them out of pieces of colored paper cut into circles.

Level 4. "Car" is the English word for the Swedish word "bil." "Car" is also the English word for the Italian word "auto." "Coche" is the Spanish word for the Italian word "auto." What is a coche in Swedish?	Level 4. Imagine that I have four objects; A, B, C, and D. If B is larger than C, and A is larger than B, and D is larger than C, is D less than or more than A?
3. Relational Frame of Opposite	**4. Temporal Relational Frames (Before/After)**
Stimuli: Pairs of words with opposite meanings or designations	Stimuli: Any temporally related events
Level 1. I have two dogs, Aaron and Bart. If Aaron is really big and is opposite to Bart, then what is Bart?	Level 1. If Tuesday comes before Thursday, does Thursday come before or after Tuesday?
Level 2. If Jack (who is very tall) is opposite to Paul, and Paul is opposite to Charlie, then what is Charlie like?	Level 2. If Tuesday comes before Thursday, and Thursday comes before Friday, does Friday come before or after Tuesday?
Level 3. If A is opposite to B, and B is opposite to C, and C is opposite to D, are A and D the same or opposite? What about A and C? If A is really big, then what is D?	Level 3. Imagine that we give each day of the week a color label. If blue day comes before red day, and red day comes before purple day, does purple day come before or after blue day?
Level 4. If A is opposite to B, and D is opposite to C, and B is opposite to C, are A and D the same or opposite? What about C and A? If D is hot, then what is A?	Level 4. Imagine that we give each day of the week a color label. If blue day comes before red day, and red day comes before purple day, and yellow day comes after purple day, does yellow day come before or after blue day?

5. Relational Frame of Hierarchy	6. Deictic Relational Frames (to enhance perspective taking)
Stimuli: Category labels and names of category members	Stimuli: The words *I*, *you*, *here*, *there*, *now* and *then*
Level 1. If a broad bean is a type of bean, is a bean a type of broad bean?	Level 1. If I am here and you are there, where are you and where am I?
Level 2. If an Alsatian is a type of dog, and a dog is a type of mammal, is an Alsatian a type of mammal? Is a mammal a type of Alsatian?	Level 2. If I am here and you are there, and if I were you and you were me, where would you be? Where would I be?
Level 3. If an object A is a type of object B and an object B is a type of object C, then is an object A a type of object C?	Level 3. If yesterday I felt sad and today I feel happy, and if now were then and then were now, how did I feel then?
Level 4. If a broad bean is a type of pulse and a pea is a type of pulse, is a broad bean a type of pea? (This is a tricky question. We cannot know the answer to this.)	Level 4. If I feel sad and you feel happy, and if I were you and you were me, and if sad were happy and happy were sad, how would you feel? How would I feel?

Conclusion

The current chapter examined a behavior-analytic and RFT conceptualization of intelligence and illustrated how it might help us to better understand in practical terms precisely which skill sets IQ tests measure. In doing so, we have been able to point the way toward intervention formats that may prove capable of helping to raise intelligence levels. This is a feat that was previously considered impossible by psychologists. Of course, our analysis is somewhat speculative and far from complete. It is presented here only as a starting point from which other researchers can embark on exciting investigations and analyses of their own. This is only the beginning of a potential revolution in behavioral and educational psychology. No doubt, as it comes in, the data will shape the analysis. In the meantime, we have a starting point from which to move forward, alongside our colleagues in the positive psychology movement, to address the challenge of improving the human condition rather than merely maintaining it.

There are many challenges ahead in honing the relational training interventions outlined here. A whole host of variables influence the functioning of such interventions, including biological variables, such as diet, sleep, and motivation, and social variables, such as family structure, the quality of the schooling system, and levels of social skills. For instance, it has been argued that a child's level of self-discipline is twice as good a predictor of his or her school grades as IQ (Duckworth & Seligman, 2005). Thus, there are several dependent measures that also need to be taken in future research to fully assess the impact of relational training interventions, including standardized scholastic measures, school grades, and reports, as well as scores on specific tests of aptitude across various domains. However, the outlook is good. The confluence of various RFT research strands regarding the relationship between relational responding fluency and measured intelligence is promising indeed. This research has at least given us a direction in which to head to make improvements in the lives of others. The more recent findings of Cassidy et al. (2011) are even more promising and suggest that, maybe for the first time in the history of psychology, we have in our grasp the roughly hewn semblance of a technology with which we can literally *nurture genius*.

References

Ball, K., Berch, D. B., Helmers, K. F., Jobe, J. B., Leveck, M. D., Marsiske, M., Morris, J. N., Rebok, G. W., Smith, D. M., Tennstedt, S. L., Unverzagt, F. W., & Willis, S. L. (2002). Effects of cognitive training interventions with older adults: A randomized controlled trial. *Journal of the American Medical Association, 288*, 2271-2281.

Barnes, D., McCullagh, P., & Keenan, M. (1990). Equivalence class formation in non-hearing impaired children and hearing impaired children. *Analysis of Verbal Behavior, 8*, 1-11.

Barnes-Holmes, D., Hayden, E., Barnes-Holmes, Y., & Stewart, I. (2008). The Implicit Relational Assessment Procedure (IRAP) as a response-time and event-related-potentials methodology for testing natural verbal relations. *The Psychological Record, 58*, 497-516.

Barnes-Holmes, Y., Barnes-Holmes, D., & Roche, B. (2001). Exemplar training and a derived transformation of function in accordance with symmetry. *The Psychological Record, 51*, 287-308.

Barnes-Holmes, Y., Barnes-Holmes, D., Roche, B., Healy, O., Lyddy, F., Cullinan, V., & Hayes, S. C. (2001). Psychological development. In S. C. Hayes, D. Barnes-Holmes, & B. Roche (Eds.), *Relational frame theory: A post-Skinnerian account of human language and cognition* (p. 161). New York: Plenum.

Barnes-Holmes, Y., Barnes-Holmes, D., Roche, B., & Smeets, P. (2001). Exemplar training and a derived transformation of function in accordance with symmetry II. *The Psychological Record, 51*, 589-603.

Barnes-Holmes, Y., Barnes-Holmes, D., & Smeets, P. (2004). Establishing relational responding in accordance with opposite as generalized operant behavior in young children. *International Journal of Psychology and Psychological Therapy, 4*, 559-586.

Barnes-Holmes, Y., Barnes-Holmes, D., Smeets, P., Strand, P., & Friman, P. (2004). Establishing relational responding in accordance with more-than and less-than as generalized operant behavior in young children. *International Journal of Psychology and Psychological Therapy, 4*, 531-558.

Basso, M. R., Schefft, B. K., Ris, M. D., & Dember, W. N. (1996). Mood and global-local visual processing. *Journal of the International Neuropsychological Society, 2*, 249-255.

Belleville, S., Gilbert, B., Fontaine, F., Gagnon, L., Menard, E., & Gauthier, S. (2006). Improvement of episodic memory in persons with mild cognitive impairment and healthy older adults: Evidence from a cognitive intervention program. *Dementia and Geriatric Cognitive Disorders, 22*, 486-99.

Berens, N. M., & Hayes, S. C. (2007). Arbitrarily applicable comparative relations: Experimental evidence for a relational operant. *Journal of Applied Behavior Analysis, 40*, 45-71.

Cassidy, S., Roche, B., & Hayes, S. C. (2011). A relational frame training intervention to raise intelligence quotients: A pilot study. *The Psychological Record, 61*, 173-198.

Cassidy, S., Roche, B., & O'Hora, D. (2010). Relational frame theory and human intelligence. *European Journal of Behavior Analysis, 11*, 37-51.

Cattell, R. B. (1963). Theory of fluid and crystallized intelligence: A critical experiment. *Journal of Educational Psychology, 54*, 1-22.

Ceci, S. J. (1991). How much does schooling influence general intelligence and its cognitive components? A reassessment of the evidence. *Developmental Psychology, 27*, 703-722.

Chabris, C. F. (1999). Prelude or requiem for the "Mozart effect"? *Nature, 400*, 827-828.

Connor, M. (1998). A review of behavioural early intervention programmes for children with autism. *Educational Psychology in Practice, 14*, 109-117.

de la Fuente-Fernandez, R. (2006). Impact of neuroprotection on incidence of Alzheimer's disease. *PLoS ONE, 1*, e52.

Deary, I. J., Strand, S., Smith, P., & Fernandes, C. (2007). Intelligence and educational achievement. *Intelligence, 35*, 13-21.

Devany, J. M., Hayes, S. C., & Nelson, R. O. (1986). Equivalence class formation in language-able and language-disabled children. *Journal of the Experimental Analysis of Behavior, 46*, 243-257.

Dickins, D., Singh, K., Roberts, N., Burns, P., Downes, J., Jimmieson, P., & Bentall, R. (2000). An fMRI study of stimulus equivalence. *NeuroReport, 12*, 1-7.

Duckworth, A. L., & Seligman, M. E. P. (2005). Self-discipline outdoes IQ in predicting academic performance of adolescents. *Psychological Science, 16*, 939-944.

Duckworth, A. L., Steen, T. A., & Seligman, M. E. P. (2005). Positive psychology in clinical practice. *Annual Review of Clinical Psychology, 1*, 629-651.

Estrada, C. A., Isen, A. M., & Young, M. J. (1994). Positive affect improves creative problem solving and influences reported source of practice satisfaction in physicians. *Motivation and Emotion, 18*, 285-299.

Flynn, J. R. (1987). Massive IQ gains in 14 nations: What IQ tests really measure. *Psychological Bulletin, 101*, 171-191.

Fredrickson, B. L. (1998). What good are positive emotions? *Review of General Psychiatry, 2*, 300-319.

Frey, M. C., & Detterman, D. K. (2004). Scholastic Assessment or g? The relationship between the Scholastic Assessment Test and general cognitive ability. *Psychological Science 15*, 373-378.

Gomez, S., Lopez, F., Martin, C. B., Barnes-Holmes, Y., & Barnes-Holmes, D. (2007). Exemplar training and a derived transformation of function in accordance with symmetry and equivalence. *The Psychological Record, 57*, 273-294.

Gore, N. J., Barnes-Holmes, Y., & Murphy, G. (2010). The relationship between intellectual functioning and relational perspective-taking. *International Journal of Psychology and Psychological Therapy, 10*, 1-17.

Gresham, F. M., & MacMillan, D. L. (1997). Autistic recovery? An analysis and critique of the empirical evidence on the Early Intervention Project. *Behavioral Disorders, 22*, 185-201.

Hayes, S. C. (1994). Relational frame theory: A functional approach to verbal events. In S. C. Hayes, L. J. Hayes, M. Sato, & K. Ono (Eds.), *Behavior analysis of language and cognition* (pp. 9-30). Reno, NV: Context Press.

Hayes, S. C., Barnes-Holmes, D., & Roche, B. (Eds.). (2001). *Relational frame theory: A post-Skinnerian account of human language and cognition.* New York: Plenum Press.

Hayes, S. C., Fox, E., Gifford, E. V., Wilson, K. G., Barnes-Holmes, D., & Healy, O. (2001). Derived relational responding as learned behavior. In S. C. Hayes, D.

Barnes-Holmes, & B. Roche (Eds.), *Relational frame theory: A post-Skinnerian account of human language and cognition* (pp. 26-27). New York: Plenum.

Hayes, S. C., Gifford, E. V., Townsend, R. C., & Barnes-Holmes, D. (2001). Thinking, problem-solving and pragmatic verbal analysis. In S. C. Hayes, D. Barnes-Holmes, & B. Roche (Eds.), *Relational frame theory: A post-Skinnerian account of human language and cognition* (pp. 87-101). New York: Plenum.

Heim, A. W., Watts, K. P., & Simmonds, V. (1968/1975). AH4 Question Book. UK: NFER-Nelson Publishing Company Ltd.

Isen, A. M., Daubman, K. A., & Nowiki, G. P. (1987). Positive affect facilitates creative problem solving. *Journal of Personality and Social Psychology, 52*, 1122-1131.

Jäeggi, S. M., Buschkuehl, M., Jonides, J., & Perrig, W. J. (2008). Improving fluid intelligence with training on working memory. *Proceedings of the National Academy of Sciences (USA), 10*, 14931-14936.

Jäeggi, S. M., Buschkuehl, M., Jonides, J., & Shah, P. (2011). Short- and long-term benefits of cognitive training. *Proceedings of the National Academy of Science, 108*, 10081-10086.

Jäeggi, S. M., Studer-Luethi, B., Buschkuehl, M., Su, Y., Jonides, J., & Perrig, W. J. (2010). The relationship between n-back performance and matrix reasoning: Implications for training and transfer. *Intelligence, 38*, 625-635.

Kaufman, A. S. (1990). *Assessing adolescent and adult intelligence* (1st ed.). Boston: Allyn and Bacon.

Lohman, D. F. (1989). Human intelligence: An introduction to advances in theory and research. *Review of Educational Research, 59*, 333-373.

Lorant-Royer, S., Spiess, V., Goncalvez, J., & Lieury, A. (2008). Programmes d'entraînement cérébral et performances cognitives: Efficacité, motivation… ou marketing? De la Gym-Cerveau au programme du Dr Kawashima. *Bulletin de Psychologie, 61*, 531-549.

Lovaas, O. (1987). Behavioral treatment and normal educational and intellectual functioning in young autistic children. *Journal of Consulting Clinical Psychology, 55*, 3-9.

Luciano, C., Becerra, I. G., & Valverde, M. R. (2007). The role of multiple-exemplar training and naming in establishing derived equivalence in an infant. *Journal of the Experimental Analysis of Behavior, 87*, 349-365.

Magiati, I., & Howlin, P. A. (2001). Monitoring the progress of preschool children with autism enrolled in early intervention programmes: Problems in cognitive assessment. *Autism, 5*, 399-406.

McKelvie, P., & Low, J. (2002). Listening to Mozart does not improve children's spatial ability: Final curtains for the Mozart effect. *British Journal of Developmental Psychology, 20*, 241-258.

Newman, J., Rosenbach, J. H., Burns, K. L., Latimer, B. C., Matocha, H. R., & Vogt, E. R. (1995). An experimental test of "The Mozart Effect": Does listening to his music improve spatial ability? *Perceptual and Motor Skills, 81*, 1379-1387.

O'Hora, D., Pelaez, M., & Barnes-Holmes, D. (2005). Derived relational responding and performance on verbal sub-tests of the WAIS-III. *The Psychological Record, 55,* 155-175.

O'Hora, D., Pelaez, M., Barnes-Holmes, D., Rae, G., Robinson, K., & Chaudary, T. (2008). Temporal relations and intelligence: Correlating relational performance with performance on the WAIS-III. *The Psychological Record, 58,* 569-584.

O'Hora, D., Roche, B., Barnes-Holmes, D., & Smeets, P. M. (2002). Response latencies to multiple derived stimulus relations: Testing two predictions of relational frame theory. *The Psychological Record, 52,* 51-76.

O'Toole, C., & Barnes-Holmes, D. (2009). Three chronometric indices of relational responding as predictors of performance on a brief intelligence test: The importance of relational flexibility. *The Psychological Record, 59,* 119-132.

Pickering, S. (Ed.). (2006). *Working memory and education.* Oxford: Elsevier.

Ramsden, S., Richardson, F. M., Josse, G., Thomas, M. S. C., Ellis, C., Shakeshaft, C., Seghier M. L., & Price, C. J. (2011). Verbal and non-verbal intelligence changes in the teenage brain. *Nature, 479,* 113-116.

Rauscher, F. H., Shaw, G. L., & Ky, K. N. (1993). Music and spatial task performance. *Nature, 365,* 611.

Raven, J., Raven, J. C., & Court, J. H. (2003). *Manual for Raven's Progressive Matrices and Vocabulary Scales.* San Antonio, TX: Harcourt Assessment.

Reed, P., Osborne, L., & Corness, M. (2005). The effectiveness of early intervention programmes for autistic spectrum disorders. *A Report for the South East Regional Special Educational Needs Partnership.* Research Partners: Bexley, Brighton & Hove, East Sussex, Kent, Midway, Surrey, West Sussex.

Rohde, T. E., & Thompson, L. A. (2007). Predicting academic achievement with cognitive ability. *Intelligence 35,* 83-92.

Sallows, G. O., & Graupner, T. D. (2005). *Replicating Lovaas' treatment and findings: Preliminary results.* PEACH. Putting Research into Practice Conference, London.

Schmidt, F. L., & Hunter, J. E. (1998). The validity and utility of selection methods in personnel psychology: Practical and theoretical implications of 85 years of research findings. *Psychological Bulletin, 124,* 262-274.

Seligman, M. E. P., & Csikszentmihalyi, M. (2000). Positive psychology: An introduction. *American Psychologist, 55,* 5-14.

Seligman, M. E. P., Ernst, R. M., Gilham, J., Reivich, K., & Linkins, M. (2009). Positive education: Positive psychology and classroom interventions. *Oxford Review of Education, 35,* 293-311.

Sidman, M. (1971). Reading and auditory-visual equivalences. *Journal of Speech and Hearing Research, 14,* 5-13.

Sidman, M., & Tailby, W. (1982). Conditional discrimination versus matching to sample: An expansion of the testing paradigm. *Journal of the Experimental Analysis of Behavior, 37,* 5-22.

Smith, G. E., Housen, P., Yaffe, K., Ruff, R., Kennison, R. F., Mahncke, H. W., & Zelinski, E. M. (2009). A cognitive training program based on principles of brain plasticity: Results from the Improvement in Memory with Plasticity-based Adaptive Cognitive Training (IMPACT) study. *Journal of the American Geriatrics Society, 57,* 594-603.

Smith, T., Eikeseth, S., Klevstrand, M., & Lovaas, O. (1997). Intensive behavioral treatment for preschoolers with severe mental retardation and pervasive developmental disorder. *American Journal on Mental Retardation, 102,* 238-249.

Spector, A., Thorgrimsen, L., Woods, B., Royan, L., Davies, S., Butterworth, M., & Orrell, M. (2003). Efficacy of an evidence-based cognitive stimulation therapy programme for people with dementia: Randomised controlled trial. *British Journal of Psychiatry, 183,* 248-254.

Steele, D. L., & Hayes, S. C. (1991). Stimulus equivalence and arbitrarily applicable relational responding. *Journal of the Experimental Analysis of Behavior, 56,* 519-555.

Steele, K. M., Bass, K. E., & Crook, M. D. (1999). The mystery of the Mozart effect: Failure to replicate. *Psychological Science, 10,* 366-369.

Sternberg, R. J. (2003). Driven to despair: Why we need to redefine the concept and measurement of intelligence. In L. G. Aspinwall & U. M. Staudinger (Eds.), *A psychology of human strengths: Fundamental questions and future directions for a positive psychology* (pp. 319-329). Washington, DC: American Psychological Association.

Vitale, A., Barnes-Holmes, Y., Barnes-Holmes, D., & Campbell, C. (2008). Facilitating responding in accordance with the relational frame of comparison: Systematic empirical analyses. *The Psychological Record, 58,* 365-390.

Wechsler, D. (1944). *The measurement of adult intelligence.* (3rd ed.). Baltimore, MD: Williams & Wilkins.

Wechsler, D. (1999). *The Wechsler Abbreviated Scale of Intelligence.* San Antonio: The Psychological Corporation.

Willis, S. L., Tennstedt, S. L., Marsiske, M., Ball, K., Elias, J., Koepke, K. M., Morris, J. N., Rebok, G. W., Unverzagt, F. W., Stoddard, A. M., & Wright, E. (2006). Long-term effects of cognitive training on everyday functional outcomes in older adults. *Journal of the American Medical Association, 296,* 2805-2814.

Wilson, R. S., Mendes de Leon, C. F., Barnes, L. L., Schneider, J. A., Bienias, J. L., Evans, D. A., & Bennett, D. A. (2002). Participation in cognitively stimulating activities and risk of incident Alzheimer disease. *Journal of the American Medical Association, 287,* 742-748.

CHAPTER 13

The Genuine Conversation

Steven C. Hayes

University of Nevada

Wh   hat you hold in your hands is the beginning of a conversation. This book opens a dialogue between two traditions, positive psychology and the acceptance and mindfulness traditions, particularly as represented by contextual behavioral science (CBS) and its subcomponents of ACT and RFT, but spreading into related approaches such as MBCT or DBT.

A conversation or dialogue involves an exchange of thoughts, opinions, and feelings between two or more persons, and they can be of two kinds: rote or genuine. A rote conversation is a kind of oral turn taking, in which the familiar and well-practiced statements or ideas of one party serve primarily as an occasion for the familiar and well-practiced statements of the other. A genuine conversation involves perspective taking, sharing, and the risk of change. It means being willing to see the world through the eyes of another, to share one's own views, and to allow similarities, distinctions, and innovations to emerge in an honest way that can alter the previously held views of both parties.

In social interchanges, rote conversations leave each party largely unchanged, while genuine conversations offer the opportunity for growth and transformation. Political conversations are almost always rote, as any observer of modern political discourse has undoubtedly noted. There is a reason for that: the participants are more interested in being right (and being viewed as such by others) than in learning. Conflicted social conversations (e.g., the well-worn battles between spouses) are usually rote and for much the same reason. Genuine conversations are different.

They are not about being right or ending up on top; they are not about power and politics; they are not about who thought of it first or last; they are about seeing what can be gained through mutual understanding.

Most books that are meant to be conversations are structured in a relatively rote way for structural reasons: books are linear, it is easier for authors to state again what they have stated before, and the ideas of others have to be considered by authors with different views, which is difficult. But with the right posture of authors, and indeed of readers, even the linear dictates of the written page can yield a genuine conversation. Instead of authors arriving ready to defend their views, and readers arriving ready to be proven right in their existing beliefs, authors can do their best to consider other points of view, and readers can bring an open posture to the experience of reading the sequential monodies in the volume, integrating them into a larger conversation.

Even before the exchange of ideas begins, a real conversation is made more likely if these processes are embraced psychologically in the interests of the positive potential of dialogue. People who are interested in positive psychology, or in acceptance, mindfulness, and values, seem particularly likely to have the psychological tools needed to enter such a genuine conversation as writers and readers. Both of these areas address issues such as values, relationship, empathy, compassion, and perspective taking that are central to any genuine social interchange.

I was allowed the opportunity in this brief closing chapter to consider the other chapters and to reflect on what this project may mean going forward. It is my sense that the editors and authors of this book have created a genuine serial conversation, and if the reader has approached these pages with openness to possibilities, there is much to be gained by the experience. Most of the chapters made serious attempts to consider the interconnections between these different ideas and traditions, and they have done so in a transparent way that readers can build upon. It does, however, require openness on the part of readers to make sure that the potential of a genuine conversation is realized.

In this chapter I would like to explore a few of the areas of overlap and connection that I saw, looking broadly across the chapters. Rather then get into details I will try to bring these areas down to the ground by speaking more generally, focusing on what practitioners and researchers might do going forward. This book is meant to help guide teachers, therapists, coaches, and health professionals among others. What does it say for now, and for the future?

What ACT Has to Teach Positive Psychology: Not Positive Form, Positive Function

In the earliest days of positive psychology (e.g., Seligman & Csiksentmihalyi, 2000), it was easy to see this tradition primarily as one that had turned away from the almost obsessive focus in applied psychology on disorder and dysfunction toward positive human traits and virtues. Instead of considering how we might treat anxiety and depression, we would study, say, flourishing or meaning. Rather than dealing primarily with the abnormal, we would deal with the positive potential of the normal.

The founders of positive psychology invited this characterization by seemingly presenting certain traits as *inherently* "positive":

> The field of positive psychology at the subjective level is about valued subjective experiences: well-being, contentment, and satisfaction (in the past); hope and optimism (for the future); and flow and happiness (in the present). At the individual level, it is about positive individual traits: the capacity for love and vocation, courage, interpersonal skill, aesthetic sensibility, perseverance, forgiveness, originality, future mindedness, spirituality, high talent, and wisdom. At the group level, it is about the civic virtues and the institutions that move individuals toward better citizenship: responsibility, nurturance, altruism, civility, moderation, tolerance, and work ethic. (Seligman & Csiksentmihalyi, 2000, p. 5)

Despite the above quote, positive psychology was never completely bound to a mere list of so-called positive traits, even in what Steger, Sheline, Merriman, and Kashdan (Chapter 11 of the present volume) rightfully label "Positive Psychology 1.0." There was always acknowledgement of the importance of so-called negative emotions, for example, but formally positive features were emphasized, even over-emphasized in an effort to put better balance into the field (Duckworth, Steen, & Seligman, 2005).

In the same way that health and flourishing is not merely a bipolar opposite of disorder and dysfunction, however, positive experiences are not the bipolar opposite of negative ones. As Ciarrochi, Kashdan, and Harris (Chapter 1 of the present volume) point out, there have at times been excesses in the thinking of some wings of positive psychology that are put right by finding the contextual boundary conditions for all of these experiences and actions. There are healthy ways to relate to emotions, positive and negative, and these depend on context; there are healthy ways to act, and sometimes these are not merely "the more virtue the better"—it depends on context. In every area, meaning, purpose, and context matter (Steger et al., Chapter 11).

The list where this has been shown to be true is impressive. A recent article by McNulty and Fincham (2012) documents this fact in some detail. For example, although forgiveness predicts relationship adjustment overall (e.g., Toussaint, Williams, Musick, & Everson, 2001), in some contexts forgiveness can be pathological. Women with high levels of forgiveness who are the victims of domestic violence are more likely to return to an abusive spouse (Gordon, Burton, & Porter, 2004) and once there will experience continuing or increasing levels of psychological and physical aggression, not the declining rates experienced by less forgiving partners (McNulty, 2010). There are contextual limits to altruism, which can at times be pathological (Oakley, Knafo, Madhavan, & Wilson, 2011; Vilardaga & Hayes, 2011). McNulty and Fincham (2012) document the same kind of contextual limits on other so-called positive traits such as optimism, benevolence, or kindness. In each case these traits correlate with well-being and good relationships overall, but in some contexts they predict problems. Optimists tend to keep gambling after financial loses (Gibson & Sanbonmatsu, 2004); benevolent people with severe relationship problems experience declining satisfaction because their problems did not improve as much as less benevolent people (McNulty, O'Mara, & Karney, 2008); wives' unkind behaviors during problem-solving discussions (e.g., rejection, criticism) predicted more stable relationship satisfaction over four years among both spouses (Karney & Bradbury, 1997). It is hard to avoid a conclusion: virtually any "positive" trait one can name can function negatively in some contexts and the vast majority of so-called negative traits can function positively in some contexts (Biswas-Diener, Kashdan, & Minhas, 2011). Malouf, Youman, Harty, Schaefer, and Tangney (Chapter 10 of this volume) provide an excellent example, and one with profound lessons for the field: negative emotions such as guilt have a positive social role to play. The acceptance and mindfulness wing has helped show that experimentally (e.g., Luoma, Kohlenberg, Hayes, & Fletcher, 2012).

The literature of this kind is now becoming voluminous, and it is simply no longer tenable to support the view that psychological experiences and traits can be meaningfully sorted into "positive" and "negative" piles based on their form. If it was ever held firmly as an intellectual belief, science has shown it to be false. If we are interested in the *function* of experiences, traits, or actions, we have to be concerned with their *impact in given contexts*. In other words, it is not merely a matter of positive versus negative forms; it is a matter of contextually bound positive versus negative functions.

In this area, the acceptance and mindfulness traditions can add something useful to positive psychology as it transitions into "Positive Psychology 2.0" (Wong, 2011). Contextual behavioral scientists and practitioners are well suited to this task because their focus on context affords a more dynamic and less judgmental approach to human experience. ACT and CBS more generally help show that in many contexts *there are functionally positive ways to relate to so-called negative events.*

The psychological flexibility model that undergirds ACT suggests that felt emotions—"positive" and "negative"—are generally worth noticing and experiencing as they are. In some context that process of experiencing with open curiosity may be extensive. For example, when a difficult emotion has long been avoided or denied, it may be helpful to dive into it consciously, to watch it rise and fall, or to watch what one's body does when it occurs. It may be worth noting what memories rise up in association with the emotion or what urges co-occur with it. At other times that process of noticing and experiencing may be very brief. For example, when noticing the re-occurrence of a frequently felt and well-explored emotion (e.g., the rise of anxiety before giving a talk), noticing may entail little more than tipping one's hat to this "old friend" and then directing attention to the purpose of the task at hand (e.g., the values and actions involved in giving a talk). It is even possible that there are some contexts in which noticing itself is not helpful. For example, it appears that emergency care workers or children with life-threatening illnesses may do better (at least over moderate time frames) if they are focused on the task challenges at hand rather than attending much to emotion at all (Mitmansgruber, Beck, & Schüßler, 2008; Phipps, 2007). It is not clear how long such a coping approach can be used without harm, but it is another demonstration of the contextual nature of all psychological adjustments.

It is not possible to be conditional in how difficult emotions are dealt with unless other aspects of the psychological flexibility model are present. For this process to be conscious and chosen, there has to be a degree of defusion from the automatic thoughts that emerge in connection with emotion. Fused thoughts mean that emotions seemingly *demand* attention; they literally *dictate* it. Mindfulness skills help the person hear the dictator's voice as merely one of many ideas or perspectives rather than viewing a world structured by that dictation without being aware of the process of the mind creating that structure.

Similarly, learning flexible attention to the present moment fosters attention as a *choice*. Acceptance does not mean wallowing. It is a bit of a misunderstanding to say, as Parks and Biswas-Diener do in Chapter 7 of this volume, that "an acceptance-based approach makes no attempt to change a client's experience." Acceptance-based approaches change client's experience in two fundamental ways. First, an emotion struggled with is no longer *functionally* the same when it is openly embraced in the moment. It may still be called by the same name, but it is not the same experience. Ironically, that functional change quickly alters even the form of the emotion. Second, being present with what is present in an open and curious way allows other responses to emerge. The repertoire narrowing impact of avoidance and fusion eases, and attention can more easily flow toward chosen purposes as afforded by the external and internal situation. That is a huge change in the client's experience as well, and it allows what positive psychology is learning to be applied in a healthy way. Chosen purpose is the exact domain in which "positive" experiences reside (Steger et al., Chapter 11). A deep connection with meaning and purpose is inherently positive and has been the focus of positive psychology from the beginning.

Said in another way, one thing ACT and the psychological flexibility model has to offer positive psychology is a more certain way to be positive *in a functional sense*. When a negative emotion is noted as it is, with openness and curiosity, without judgment, the function of the emotion can be determined more voluntarily by the greater flexibility this posture affords, which becomes behaviorally important in the ability then to make an attentional turn toward values-based action without it being an unhealthy act of suppression or avoidance. That one-two punch seems important over the long run because so-called negative emotions contain the seeds of positive values. Sadness over a betrayal contains the seeds of love and loyalty as a value—without access to pain in a deep sense love is impossible (see Walser, Chapter 3 in this volume). Anxiety over a social failure contains the seeds of social contribution as a value—without knowing where you hurt and fear, it is harder to know where your caring resides. Like bread crumbs, pain can help us find the way: even trauma can encourage our growth (Park & Helgeson, 2006). The psychological flexibility model helps show how it is possible for negative emotions to lose their negativity in a functional sense, even when they are present. We can experience them, learn from them, and yet not be dominated by them. Instead, they can become an ally in the creation of a values-based life.

This matters for positive psychology because that exact process is the process that is needed for positive emotions to be held in a healthy way. There is a growing body of evidence that experiential avoidance and psychological inflexibility not only increase the harmful impact of negative emotions, they undermine the ability to experience positive emotions (Kashdan & Breen, 2008; Kashdan & Steger, 2006). Such findings present a flashing yellow warning sign to the commonsense idea that "a positive intervention aims to *replace* negative experiences with positive ones" (Parks & Biswas-Diener, Chapter 7 in this volume, emphasis in original). It matters *how* negative events become positive. The desire to replace negative events is understandable, but it is only a small step from that posture to avoidance and suppression—precisely the posture that tends to build negativity and ironically undermines positive emotional experience. From an ACT perspective, positivity linked to a replacement agenda is needlessly dangerous. Positivity linked to open choice is far safer, but that agenda cannot be mounted without knowing how to move into a psychological space in which open choice is possible when difficult experiences have occurred.

One way to think about this that makes the general message easy to remember is to think of positive and negative as also meaning additive and subtractive. Just as psychology has been too focused on the negative, it has been too focused on the subtractive approach to experience. Efforts in experiential subtraction are rarely functionally positive regardless of their putative purpose. Acceptance and mindfulness methods teach people how to live more additively, and in that sense "positively," in which present events are present, regardless of form, and the key question is what to add next. Ironically, negative emotions can be a great arena in which to learn these "additive" psychological skills such as mindfulness, curiosity, and noticing without judgment, but these same skills apply equally to positive emotions. In some contexts it is helpful to appreciate and savor positive emotions; in others it is more a matter of tipping one's hat to them and moving on to the next challenge or opportunity. As Jack Kornfield said in the title of his book, "After the ecstasy, the laundry" (2001).

What Positive Psychology Has to Teach ACT: Building Positive Change

As McCracken rightly points out in Chapter 6, committed action is the least well worked out part of the psychological flexibility model. There was a reason for that. ACT was built within behavior analysis 30 years ago. The technologies of behavior change were relatively well developed for that time, and they were taken as a given. The goal was to bring emotional and cognitive openness, conscious present moment awareness, and chosen values to the process of behavior change. The concept of "commitment" was added (namely that behavior change was deliberately linked to a self-amplifying process of building values-based action), but the hard work was elsewhere.

Now the times are different. The entire field of psychology has created hard-won gains in the areas that were almost untouched 30 years ago: acceptance, mindfulness, attentional flexibility, and so on. These processes are not a panacea, but they are worthwhile and their evidentiary basis is now so strong that it seems highly unlikely that 30 years from now students of applied psychology will not deal reasonably extensively with such matters. What is less well developed is how to bring values work into behavior change.

In its very name, ACT is committed to that area and has made good progress in understanding values, but positive psychology has provided many useful leads about how to build out a positive agenda of change. Let me give some concrete examples.

The broaden-and-build approach of Fredrickson and colleagues (e.g., Fredrickson, 2004) described by Garland and Fredrickson in Chapter 2 in this volume, rightly guides the attention of practitioners toward opportunities for growth that can fill a kind of content vacuum in an ACT approach.

An example of that vacuum that ACT clinicians know how to fill will help explain what I mean by a vacuum. In ACT exposure work with anxiety disorders (say, a person with panic disorder and agoraphobia), the goal of exposure is not the reduction of anxiety per se but response flexibility. During exposure (say, being in a shopping mall) the clinician works first on present moment awareness, acceptance, and defusion, but when there is a sense of openness the clinician inserts new response functions (e.g., What would you most like to buy here? Who is wearing the most interesting clothes?). What is inserted is not well specified—it is left up to the creativity of the therapist and the spontaneous comments of the client.

In this case it is generally not difficult to do so, but my point is to note the content vacuum that can occur. If you expand out the issue from this specific example, you will see how broadly applicable this point is and how positive psychology might support and enhance the psychological flexibility model by providing useful content leads. Suppose an ACT practitioner helps a depressed client be more skilled in coming into the present moment and doing so with increased emotional and cognitive flexibility through acceptance, defusion, and mindfulness work. What might be inserted into the next moment of work? The usual answer is that values will be a guide, which is an excellent idea, but inside that functional structure it can help to consider proximal steps. Actions focused on positive emotions such as gratitude, compassion, love, or appreciation of beauty could be extremely helpful—not because the emotions replace other emotions but because they mark actions of importance. The exercises and methods of positive psychology fit comfortably into many such moments in the acceptance and mindfulness work. In the right moment a gratitude journal, or exercises in forgiveness, or a focus on the appreciation of beauty, or consciously practicing compassion can take advantage of the more psychologically flexible moments that acceptance and mindfulness work often produces.

Even cognitive reappraisal has a role here, once it is stripped of any subtractive agenda that can undermine its functional positivity. If handled deftly, Garland and Fredrickson's concepts of "mindful reappraisal" and "positive reappraisal" can fit within the functional contextual perspective. ACT clinicians have always believed in reappraisal in the sense of cognitive flexibility (e.g., the "pick an identity" exercise, Hayes, Strosahl, & Wilson, 1999, pp. 196; the rewrite your story exercise, Hayes, Strosahl, & Wilson, 2011, pp. 227-228; among many others); their concern has been to avoid the natural pull toward suppression by implying that there is a "correct" or "true" way to think and that doing so can subtract or eliminate more difficult thoughts. This issue can best be understood as a matter of variation and selection. Cognitive reappraisal, meaning healthy variation, can be linked to values-based selection based on workability. That kind of "mindful reappraisal" can indeed be encouraged inside an ACT approach.

There is another way that this same idea enhances an ACT approach: prevention. The impact of ACT for those in distress is quite consistent across the literature, but the same cannot be said for prevention. You cannot use creative hopelessness and other classic ACT methods to reach those who are doing well. What can you use?

Positive interventions can fit very well here, and if put toward a psychological flexibility agenda there is no reason ACT practitioners should resist doing so. This is essentially what has already been happening if you look at successful ACT prevention trials. For example, Fledderus, Bohlmeijer, Pieterse, and Schreurs (2011) created an ACT prevention intervention and cast it in terms of "positive mental health." Successful ACT programs that are not based on the hook of personal psychological pain often include group processes that create what Biswas-Diener calls a "microculture" that is supportive of growth (Chapter 9 in this volume).

Building Out Contextual Behavioral Approaches

ACT is a positive research program, but RFT (relational frame theory) is more important than ACT, and CBS (contextual behavioral science) is more important than RFT. There are three dominant features that a contextual behavioral approach brings to the table that hold our hope for progress as part of this genuine conversation between positive psychology and the acceptance and mindfulness traditions: a contextual approach, the pragmatic embrace of middle-level terms and analytic-abstractive theory, and an interest in a bottom-up account.

Positive psychology has sometimes been based on elemental realist assumptions (see Ciarrochi et al., Chapter 1 of this volume), which have made it more difficult to understand the kind of studies that show the contextual limits of positive psychological traits (McNulty & Fincham, 2012; Sheldon, Kashdan, & Steger, 2011). While assumptions can only be owned, not truly evaluated, it is worthwhile noting how easy it is to understand contextual limits when all concepts are viewed as being contextually embedded and to be evaluated relative to purpose (Hayes, Hayes, Reese, & Sarbin, 1993). There is no guarantee that a particular set of assumptions will work equally well in all contexts. It does seem that in the world of applied psychology there is ample evidence that elemental realist assumptions have notable limits (Biglan & Hayes, 1996), in part because these assumptions contain ontological assurances that do not demand that concepts be vetted against their utility in creating systematic change (Hayes et al., 2011). It is relatively easier in that case to be right but not useful—which such a comfortably unhelpful end· point is impossible if "right" means "useful in this context."

Practitioners need models that simplify the world, but it is hard to create such models in extremely high precision/high scope language alone. Contextualistic assumptions allow theories to be useful as a given level because truth is a matter of contextually situated workability. A baseball coach describing hitting to a player does not necessarily need to know the mathematical formula that describes the parabolic path of a struck baseball, just as scientists interested in characterizing the path of a ball in flight do not necessarily need to know how relativity applies to gravity. But in a scientific system there should be consilience across all of these difference levels.

A bottom-up approach that seeks such consilience seems to be particularly useful when linked to contextualism. Almost everyone agrees that applied psychology needs to be concerned with basic principles, but when linked to a functional contextual perspective, basic principles can become high precision/high scope verbal guides to successful intervention efforts in basic and component research (Levin, Hildebrandt, Lillis, & Hayes, in press), without demanding that practitioners understand the details of basic accounts. This volume contains good examples of that very process, such as in Roche, Cassidy, and Stewart's program for "nurturing genius" (Chapter 12 in this volume) or Stewart and McHugh's approach to perspective taking (Chapter 5 in this volume). Instead of hypothetico-deductive theories, these researchers are building up theories that abstract the pragmatically key features such as perspective taking or intellectual behavior.

It is also possible to use such principles to understand other approaches. Foody, Barnes-Holmes, and Barnes-Holmes (Chapter 8 in this volume) do that with a set of issues in positive interventions. In the brief time I have remaining I would like to give such a broad overview to the issue of compassion and self-compassion (see Neff and Tirch in Chapter 4 of this volume). I am drawing here on the work of Yadavaia, and his dissertation, which was a randomized controlled trial examining the impact of ACT on self-compassion (Yadavaia, 2012).

Neff (2003b) defines self-compassion in terms of three components that emerge primarily from a Buddhist perspective: self-kindness, common humanity, and mindfulness:

> Self-compassion ... involves being touched by and open to
> one's own suffering, not avoiding or disconnecting from it,
> generating the desire to alleviate one's suffering and to heal
> oneself with kindness. Self-compassion also involves offering
> nonjudgmental understanding to one's pain, inadequacies and
> failures, so that one's experience is seen as part of the larger
> human experience. (p. 87)

Each of these are thought to be dimensional and to describe relatively healthy ways of relating to the self. Most work on self-compassion defined in this way has been done using the "self-compassion scale"

(SCS—Neff, 2003a) and as Neff and Tirch document, the benefits are considerable.

From the point of view of the psychological flexibility model that underlies ACT, self-acceptance and self-kindness overlap rather clearly. Being touched by, open to, not avoiding, and not disconnecting from experience as part of a kind effort to heal or be whole (the etymology of "heal" is "make whole") would be a fairly good definition of acceptance in ACT. Self-kindness represents an attitude of benevolence and is characterized by the absence of self-criticism and harsh self-judgment. These latter features harken to an ACT posture of defusion and the choice to embrace one's own experience.

The same could be said of mindfulness. Neff's approach to mindfulness (e.g., being nonjudgmental and in the moment) is shared not just with ACT but with most of the mindfulness-based approaches. In that context is it not surprising that Neff and Tirch report that the SCS correlates .65 with the Acceptance and Action Questionnaire (Hayes et al., 2004; Bond et al., 2011), which is the most popular measure of ACT processes—and in our laboratory we have found a similar relationship between these two measures.

My point is not that self-compassion offers nothing new. Such a claim would be inconsistent with a contextual approach to language. Different ways of speaking offer new opportunities. For example, I have found that speaking of "self-kindness" with clients is a very useful way to communicate the kind of posture of acceptance ACT is trying to foster.

The reason I am making the connection in this context is that the work on RFT analyses of acceptance or mindfulness (as an example) should thus be directly relevant to the work on self-compassion. So far as I am aware, self-compassion theory is not based on an experimental laboratory science, and CBS brings something broadly useful to the table as a result.

This can be seen most directly in the last attribute: the sense of common humanity. Neff discusses this attribute as involving a sense of connectedness with humanity at large and the sense that one's experiences, including those that are painful, are shared as part of the human condition.

Here the work on deictic relational frames, as described by Stewart and McHugh (Chapter 5 in this volume), provides a way forward. A concept like "common humanity" began as a middle-level theoretical term, but if it can be linked to basic analyses, it is possible to have both the benefits of ready understanding and the possible progressivity of experimental behavioral science. Being able to bring perspective-taking skills to one's own experience and that of others, embeds them in a sense of shared experience in a more precise way that the term "common humanity" alone can do. Thus, it could be that a genuine conversation could help build out contextual behavioral approaches with new data, intervention ideas, and connections for the betterment of all.

Genuine Engagement

In the beginning of their chapter, Parks and Biswas-Diener (Chapter 7) tell the story of being asked in workshop what the difference is between a positive intervention and ACT. They say "Obscured within this polite statement are the questions they *really* want to ask: Is there anything new about positive interventions?" Parks and Biswas-Diener go on to try to show how positive interventions are distinctive and new.

I like to think that the questioners were not really asking "what is the difference" in some "prove yourself" way. A more interesting way to view the exchange is to suppose that the questioner is seeing or sensing a deep relationship and asking whether these two fit together: Can they be usefully integrated? Are they fellow travelers?

This book provides an answer to these three questions: "it depends" and "probably so" and "we shall see."

If positive interventions are really committed to replacing negative emotions, and to a "more is better" philosophy applied to any content that is topographically "positive," then the two do not fit other than for some useful borrowing. But if *that* is the agenda, then it appears to me from the outside that the research literature within positive psychology itself is rapidly trimming back this perspective. The pruning shears of science can be harsh, but they are necessary. I think that pruning is already happening, as several chapters show. That agenda, in my opinion, does not comport well with what is known about human psychology, and as positive psychology has matured there is a growing realization that positive functions and positive forms (and negative functions and negative forms) are just not the same thing. That moment of realization provides an opening, and the acceptance and mindfulness traditions, and especially ACT, RFT, and CBS, are stepping forward ready to engage fully with "Positive Psychology 2.0."

That leaves the questions of whether they can be usefully integrated, gradually becoming mutually supportive fellow travelers. Is it possible for this genuine conversation to blossom into a kind of genuine engagement: an ongoing relationship that is based on common interests, shared perspectives, and mutual respect?

In my own view, I hope so. I think we have much to gain from each other. As for what the future holds, I do not know; but let's start with where we are. Hope and optimism are here, now, in the present: they have filled these pages. Readers reaching these last two sentences of the volume will be the ones to decide whether they can be realized going forward. We shall see, but it is worth taking the time to savor and appreciate this moment: a genuine conversation is an excellent place to start.

References

Biglan, A., & Hayes, S. C. (1996). Should the behavioral sciences become more pragmatic? The case for functional contextualism in research on human behavior. *Applied and Preventive Psychology: Current Scientific Perspectives, 5*, 47-57. doi: 10.1016/S0962-1849(96)80026-6

Biswas-Diener, R., Kashdan, T. B., & Minhas, G. (2011). A dynamic approach to psychological strength development and intervention. *Journal of Positive Psychology, 6*, 106-118.

Bond, F. W., Hayes, S. C., Baer, R. A., Carpenter, K. M., Guenole, N., Orcutt, H. K., Waltz, T., & Zettle, R. D. (2011). Preliminary psychometric properties of the Acceptance and Action Questionnaire—II: A revised measure of psychological inflexibility and experiential avoidance. *Behavior Therapy, 42*, 676–688.

Duckworth, A. L., Steen, T. A., & Seligman, M. E. P. (2005). Positive psychology in clinical practice. *Annual Review of Clinical Psychology, 1*, 629-651. doi: 10.1146/annurev.clinpsy.1.102803.144154

Fredrickson, B. L. (2004). The broaden-and-build theory of positive emotions. *Philosophical Transactions of the Royal Society B, 359*, 1367-1378.

Gibson, B., & Sanbonmatsu, D. M. (2004). Optimism, pessimism and gambling: The downside of optimism. *Personality and Social Psychology Bulletin, 30*, 149-160. doi: 10.1177/0146167203259929

Hayes, S. C., Hayes, L. J., Reese, H. W., & Sarbin, T. R. (Eds.). (1993). *Varieties of scientific contextualism.* Oakland, CA: Context Press/New Harbinger.

Hayes, S. C., Strosahl, K., & Wilson, K. G. (1999). *Acceptance and Commitment Therapy: An experiential approach to behavior change.* New York: Guilford Press.

Hayes, S. C., Strosahl, K., & Wilson, K. G. (2011). *Acceptance and Commitment Therapy: The process and practice of mindful change* (2nd ed.). New York: Guilford Press.

Hayes, S. C., Strosahl, K. D., Wilson, K. G., Bissett, R. T., Pistorello, J., Toarmino, D., Polusny, M. A., Dykstra, T. A., Batten, S. V., Bergan, J., Stewart, S. H., Zvolensky, M. J., Eifert, G. H., Bond, F. W., Forsyth, J. P., Karekla, M., & McCurry, S. M. (2004). Measuring experiential avoidance: A preliminary test of a working model. *The Psychological Record, 54,* 553-578.

Karney, B. R., & Bradbury, T. N. (1997). Neuroticism, marital interaction, and the trajectory of marital satisfaction. *Journal of Personality and Social Psychology, 72,* 1075-1092. doi: 10.1037/0022-3514.72.5.1075

Kashdan, T. B., & Breen, W. E. (2008). Social anxiety and positive emotions: A prospective examination of a self-regulatory model with tendencies to suppress or express emotions as a moderating variable. *Behavior Therapy, 39,* 1-12.

Kashdan, T. B., & Steger, M. F. (2006). Expanding the topography of social anxiety: An experience sampling assessment of positive emotions and events, and emotion suppression. *Psychological Science, 17,* 120-128.

Kornfield, J. (2001). *After the ecstasy, the laundry: How the heart grows wise on the spiritual path.* New York: Bantam.

Levin, M. E., Hildebrandt, M. J., Lillis, J., & Hayes, S. C. (in press). The impact of treatment components suggested by the psychological flexibility model: A meta-analysis of laboratory-based component studies. *Behavior Therapy.*

Luoma, J. B., Kohlenberg, B. S., Hayes, S. C., & Fletcher, L. (2012). Slow and steady wins the race: A randomized clinical trial of Acceptance and Commitment Therapy targeting shame in substance use disorders. *Journal of Consulting and Clinical Psychology, 80,* 43-53. doi:10.1037/a0026070

McNulty, J. K. (2010). Forgiveness increases the likelihood of subsequent partner transgressions in marriage. *Journal of Family Psychology, 24,* 787-790.

McNulty, J. K., & Fincham, F. D. (2012). Beyond positive psychology? Toward a contextual view of psychological processes and well-being. *American Psychologist, 67,* 101-110. doi:10.1037/a0024572

McNulty, J. K., O'Mara, E. M., & Karney, B. R. (2008). Benevolent cognitions as a strategy of relationship maintenance: "Don't sweat the small stuff" but it's not all small stuff. *Journal of Personality and Social Psychology, 94,* 631-646. doi: 10.1037/0022-3514.94.4.631

Mitmansgruber, H., Beck, T. N., & Schüßler, G. (2008). "Mindful helpers": Experiential avoidance, meta-emotions, and emotion regulation in paramedics. *Journal of Research in Personality, 42,* 1358-1363.

Neff, K. D. (2003a). The development and validation of a scale to measure self-compassion. *Self and Identity, 2,* 223-250.

Neff, K. D. (2003b). Self-compassion: An alternative conceptualization of a healthy attitude toward oneself. *Self and Identity, 2,* 85-101.

Oakley, B., Knafo, A., Madhavan, G., & Wilson, D. S. (Eds.). (2011). *Pathological altruism*. New York: Oxford University Press.

Park, C. L., & Helgeson, V. S. (2006). Introduction to the special section: Growth following highly stressful life events—Current status and future directions. *Journal of Consulting and Clinical Psychology, 74*, 791-796.

Phipps, S. (2007). Adaptive style in children with cancer: Implications for a positive psychology approach. *Journal of Pediatric Psychology, 32*, 1055-1066. doi:10.1093/jpepsy/jsm060

Seligman, M. E., & Csikszentmihalyi, M. (2000). Positive psychology: An introduction. *American Psychologist, 55*, 5-14.

Sheldon, K., Kashdan, T. B., & Steger, M. F. (2011). *Designing positive psychology: Taking stock and moving forward*. New York: Oxford University Press.

Toussaint, L. L., Williams, D. R., Musick, M. A., & Everson, S. A. (2001). Forgiveness and health: Age differences in a U.S. probability sample. *Journal of Adult Development, 8*, 249-257. doi:10.1023/A:1011394629736

Vilardaga, R., & Hayes, S.C. (2011). A contextual behavioral approach to pathological altruism. In B. Oakley, A. Knafo, G. Madhavan, & D. S. Wilson (Eds.), *Pathological altruism* (pp. 31-48). New York: Oxford University Press.

Wong, P. T. P. (2011). Positive psychology 2.0: Towards a balanced interactive model of the good life. *Canadian Psychology/Psychologie Canadienne, 52*, 69-81.

Yadavaia, J. (2012). Using Acceptance and Commitment Therapy to decrease high-prevalence psychopathology by targeting self-compassion: A randomized controlled trial. Unpublished doctoral dissertation, University of Nevada, Reno.

Todd B. Kashdan, PhD, is an associate professor of psychology and senior scientist at the Center for Consciousness and Transformation at George Mason University. Kashdan has published over one hundred peer-reviewed articles on meaning and purpose in life, happiness, mind-fulness, how to deal with stress and anxiety, and social relationships. He is the author of several books, including *Curious? Discover the Missing Ingredient to a Fulfilling Life*, and a TEDx speaker. His work has been featured in the *New York Times* and the *Washington Post*, and on CNN, National Public Radio, and other media outlets. Kashdan received the 2013 American Psychological Association (APA) Distinguished Scientific Award for Early Career Contribution to Psychology.

Joseph Ciarrochi, PhD, is a professor at University of Western Sydney. He has published over eighty scientific articles in the area of well-being, and a number of books, including *Get Out of Your Mind and Into Your Life for Teens* and *Emotional Intelligence in Everyday Life*. His work on emotional intelligence is among the most highly cited in the area of emotional intelligence. He is currently investigating mindfulness, accep-tance, values, and other core processes that promote well-being and effectiveness.

Index

230–232; values clarification
process in, 222–223
Review of General Psychology, 4
RFT. *See* relational frame theory
rituals/traditions, 203–205
Roche, Bryan, 267
role induction, 205–206
rote conversations, 303

S

savoring: definition of, 74;
interventions based on, 154–155;
positive reappraisal and, 50–52
Schaefer, Karen, 215
schizophrenia, 114
scholastic success, 269, 272
self: ACT approach to, 171–178;
positive psychology and, 167–
168; RFT approach to, 168–171
self-as-content, 94, 121–122,
172–175
self-as-context, 11, 95, 122–123,
176–178
self-as-process, 122, 175–176
self-compassion, 15, 78–101; ACT
and, 78–79, 93–96, 99–101,
314–315; clinical interventions
and, 90–93; common humanity
and, 80–81, 315–316; elements
or components of, 79–82, 314;
evolutionary basis of, 96–98;
family functioning and, 89–90;
interpersonal relationships and,
20, 88–89; interventions based
on, 167; mindfulness and, 81–82,
91–92, 98, 315; motivation and,
85–86; self-esteem vs., 87–88;
self-kindness and, 79–80, 315;

techniques for practicing, 83, 86;
well-being and, 82–84. *See also*
compassion
Self-Compassion Scale (SCS), 82,
314–315
self-concept, 22, 248
self-control, 15, 117–118
self-criticism, 85
self-determination theory, 161
self-discipline, 297
self-esteem, 87–88
self-kindness, 79–80, 315
self-other transcendence, 116,
121–125
self-reflection, 41
self-transcendence, 261
set-shifting process, 47
seven foundations of well-being,
7–15; behavioral control, 9, 14;
cognitive skill, 9, 14–15;
experiential acceptance, 9,
13–14; functional beliefs, 7, 10;
linking to character strengths,
15–16; list of chapters discussing,
23–25; mindfulness and
awareness, 8, 10–11; perspective
taking, 8, 11–12; values, 8, 12–13
shame, 218–219, 237
shared experiences, 207–208
sharpening perceptions, 154
Sheline, Kelly, 240
social anhedonia, 114
social change, 198
social connections, 151–153
social intelligence, 117
Socratic questioning, 54
solutions focus approach, 206

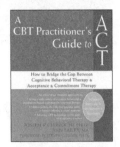
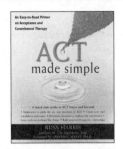
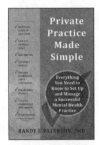
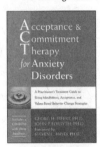
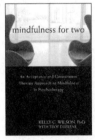
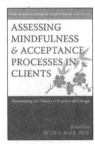